REINVENTING PUBLIC HEALTH

More Praise for *Reinventing Public Health*

Reinventing Public Health is a triumph in reconceptualization of public health with a bold public policy orientation to improve U.S. population health and to reduce health disparities. Its translation of research into practical actionable policies across an extraordinary range of social domains merits attention and acclaim.

The book is highly well organized, with a consistent theme carried from front to back through every chapter. Each chapter has been crafted with great care, making for smooth reading and clarity. All chapters are interesting and present either original and fresh ideas or syntheses that are worthy of attention.

Most importantly, the book is an original, evocative formulation of the proper role of a new public health grounded in social and societal factors and public policies. The book contributes powerful ideas for public policy formulation, teaching, research, and for providing young students with a fresh vision of the potential of public health as a field for them.

Tour de force is a tired phrase by now, but the book does overflow with new and fresh ideas. The book points out the initiatives taken by several other nations, and rightly so, because they have actually and deliberately adopted policies to redress inequities in social advantage. But none of those nations has presented such fresh formulations so completely and persuasively as this book does.

Reinventing Public Health is the most comprehensive science-based synthesis of public policies to improve population health and to reduce health disparities ever advanced. It provides a fresh understanding of the dynamic processes of health production. It should spark a great awakening in public health for which we all have been searching.

Alvin R. Tarlov, M.D.
Executive director, Texas Program for Society and Health (retired 2005)
James A. Baker III Institute for Public Policy
Rice University

REINVENTING PUBLIC HEALTH

Policies and Practices for a Healthy Nation

Lu Ann Aday
Editor

Foreword by Kenneth I. Shine

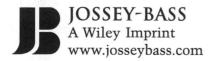

JOSSEY-BASS
A Wiley Imprint
www.josseybass.com

Library of Congress Cataloging-in-Publication Data

Reinventing public health : policies and practices for a healthy nation
    / Lu Ann Aday, editor ; foreword by Kenneth I. Shine. -- 1st ed.
        p. ; cm.
    Includes bibliographical references and index.
    ISBN 0-7879-7561-3 (alk. paper)
    1. Public health--Social aspects. 2. Social medicine. 3. Health
—Social aspects. I. Aday, Lu Ann.
    [DNLM: 1. Public Health. 2. Socioeconomic Factors. 3. Health
Policy. 4. Health Services Accessibility—economics. 5. Health
Status Indicators.   WA 30 R375 2005]
    RA418.R425 2005
    362.1—dc22   2005021187

Printed in the United States of America
FIRST EDITION
HB Printing   10 9 8 7 6 5 4 3 2 1

CONTENTS

Figures, Tables, and Exhibits   vii

Foreword   xi

Preface   xv

Acknowledgments   xix

The Editor   xxiii

The Contributors   xxv

1   Analytic Framework   1
    Lu Ann Aday

2   Fundamental Determinants of Population Health   35
    Kathryn M. Cardarelli, Janet S. de Moor, M. David Low, Barbara J. Low

3   Sustainable Development   65
    Sondip K. Mathur, Carl S. Hacker, Lu Ann Aday

4   Human Development   106
    Barbara J. Low, M. David Low, Kathryn M. Cardarelli, Janet S. de Moor

5 Economic Development   183

Luisa Franzini, J. Michael Swint, Yuki Murakami, Rafia S. Rasu

6 Community Development and Public Health   237

Cynthia Warrick, Dan Culica, Beth E. Quill, William D. Spears, Rachel Westheimer Vojvodic

7 Toward a Healthy (Re)Public   285

Lu Ann Aday, Beth E. Quill, Hardy D. Loe Jr., Charles E. Begley

Name Index   333

Subject Index   000

FIGURES, TABLES, AND EXHIBITS

Figures

1.1 Comparisons of Disciplinary, Multidisciplinary, Interdisciplinary, and Transdisciplinary Research Paradigms 20

1.2 Ecosocial Transdisciplinary Paradigm 21

1.3 Racial Segregation as a Fundamental Determinant of Racial Disparities in Health 24

1.4 Pathways for Evaluating Policies 27

2.1 Conceptual Framework of Fundamental Determinants of Population Health 40

3.1 Epidemiology of the Marketplace 70

3.2 General Model of Ecosystem Function: The Natural Cycle 76

3.3 The Ecological Determinants of Population Health 79

3.4 Closed Model of Economic System: The Economic Cycle 84

3.5 Current Policies That Affect Ecological Determinants 89

3.6 Framework for Corporate Social Responsibility for Population Health 91

4.1 Principal Components of the Life-Course Health Development Framework and Their Influence on Health Outcomes 110

4.2 Average Reading, Math, and General Knowledge Standardized Test Scores Within Income-to-Needs Groups, 1998 115

4.3   Readiness to Learn at School by Family Income: National
       Longitudinal Study of Canadian Youth, 2000   117
4.4   Adult Mortality Related to Socioeconomic Conditions During
       Childhood   129
4.5   Fourth-Grade Standardized National Assessment of Educational
       Progress Math Scores by Percent of U.S. Students Eligible for
       National Free or Reduced-Cost Lunch Program, 2000, by State and
       District of Columbia   151
5.1   Relationships Between Economic Policies and Population Health   190
5.2   Life Expectancy and Gross Domestic Product (GDP) per Capita, 2000   200
5.3   Evaluation of Economic Policies   219
6.1   Healthy People in Healthy Communities: A Systematic Approach
       to Health Improvement   240
6.2   Community Development Model for a Healthy (Re)Public   253
7.1   Framework for Designing and Evaluating the Impact of Population
       Health–Centered Policy   324

Tables

1.1   Framework for Moving Toward a Healthy (Re)Public   5
1.2   Comparisons of Political Philosophies and Implications
       for Public Health   11
1.3   Differing Perspectives on Population Health and Health Disparities   22
1.4   Criteria for Evaluating Policies   28
3.1a   Examples of Atmospheric Changes and Potential Health Impacts   80
3.1b   Examples of Aquatic System Changes and Potential Health Impacts   81
3.1c   Examples of Terrestrial Ecosystem Changes and Potential
       Health Impacts   82
5.1   Time Line: Concurrent Policy Development in Nine European
       Countries   207
6.1   The Domains of Social Capital and Appropriate Neighborhood
       Policies to Support Them   245
6.2   Models of Community Development   260
6.3   Typology of Selected Community Development Policies   267
6.4   Evaluation of Selected Community Development Policies Based
       on Effectiveness, Efficiency, and Equity Criteria   268
7.1   Selected Policies Affecting Population Health and Health Disparities   287
7.2   Major Issues of Policy Effectiveness, Efficiency, and Equity   288
7.3   Dimensions and Criteria for a Healthy (Re)Public   294

7.4 Specific Policies Addressing Population Health Determinants in the United Kingdom   298

7.5 Categories of Policy Questions and Related Research for a Population Health–Centered Policy   304

7.6 Building Blocks for an Intersectoral Public Health System   305

7.7 Models for Collaborative Decision Making   310

7.8 Population Health–Centered Public Health Practice   314

Exhibits

5.1 Approaches for Addressing Socioeconomic Inequalities in Health   208

7.1 Blueprint for the Design of an Intersectoral Local Public Health Agency   308

7.2. A Model Public Health University for the 21st Century   321

FOREWORD

Throughout the world the concept of sustainability has recently received considerable attention. Sustainability has emphasized the use of renewable fuels and other natural resources to sustain the planet. Sustainability engenders considerable discussion because of its complexity and because of the implications it has for economic, social, organizational, and political aspects of society. Although human health is sometimes included in these discussions, the importance of sustainability of the human population has not yet been articulated as elegantly as by the authors of this book. They have highlighted the intersections between research and policy that must occur if one is to optimize the impact of education, housing, urban development, economics, community, and corporate responsibility on the health of a population.

A prominent recent example of this intersection has been the impact that tobacco taxes and no-smoking areas have had on the decrease of cigarette smoking in the United States. At the same time, economic policies facilitating the importation of increasing amounts of tobacco into developing countries emphasize the negative impact that such policies can have on health. When China was accepted into the World Trade Organization, member nations paid little attention to the behavior of privatized state industries that sought competitiveness by dropping health benefits for their workers.

The compelling evidence for the relationships between education and health status emphasizes the complexities of these interactions. Children with poorly managed chronic illnesses, such as asthma, do not learn well. Schools that do not help young people develop healthy lifestyles have profound impacts such as the growing epidemic of childhood obesity or teenage pregnancy. At the same time, the increased reliance of the United States on a knowledge-driven economy, and strong evidence that individual and family income are linked to levels of educational accomplishment as well as health status, should make the nexus between education and health among the nation's highest priorities.

There are still many unknown factors. With the possible exceptions of Costa Rica and the Indian state of Kerala, it is clear that socioeconomic stratification has a profound impact on health status, irrespective of average income in countries around the world. The United States is a conspicuous and unhealthy example. The authors have wisely emphasized the requirements for research and better evidence as we examine the role of socioeconomic stratification on population health.

The intersection between the various factors that the authors identified—including environmental influences, housing, economic development, corporate responsibility and equity—poses important challenges for the relationship of policy to advocacy and politics. Evidence is essential if public health is to affect policy. Such evidence requires both analysis and interventions, which will fulfill a kind of Koch's postulates for public health, not dissimilar to their application to infectious diseases, that is, following rigorous procedures for understanding in this case the social causes or determinants of population health, much as German bacteriologist Robert Koch did in demonstrating how a certain bacterium causes a particular disease. Although it is appropriate to advance policy based on logical inferences from the data, these must be carefully reasoned and supported by objective science, as difficult as this may be in these complicated arenas. Short of these data, sustainability quickly becomes very ideologically driven on all sides.

There is understandable frustration in public health for the incredible imbalance between the resources employed in health care delivery versus those designated to enhance the health of the population. When an individual becomes ill, he or she and family members understandably want the very best in care to cope with illness. Moreover, the economic incentives for all of those involved in the health care system are aligned to offer more and better of the same. However, the increasing rate of health care spending in the United States is not a phenomenon that we can sustain over the long term. Moreover, the present rationing of health care, which is an inevitable consequence of unrelenting health care costs, comes through limitations of access for significant portions of the population.

Rather than rationing care, a public policy that improves the health of the population is ultimately a more promising approach to the control of costs. There is increasing evidence that illness can be compressed into a significantly shorter period of an individual's life as the population ages. Although health care spending is highest in the last year of life, if for no other reason than that this is the time when the final illness is diagnosed, evaluated, and treated, there is also reason to believe that spending in the last year of life is lower as people age. Population health could contribute to a growing healthy population living without chronic illness and experiencing only a very brief and, hopefully, less expensive illness at a more advanced age.

A partnership between medicine and public health is critically important in obtaining these objectives. The education of physicians in population health will become increasingly necessary and will benefit from better data, the electronic health record, and the preventative strategies that arise out of population health. Moreover, medicine and public health can be important partners in moving policy in many of the areas that this book identifies.

Recent evaluations of community preparedness for terrorist attacks have highlighted the fragmentation of the public health care system, police, fire, media, intelligence agencies, and communication with racial and ethnic groups that characterize national and local responses. Some progress has been made in the face of recent natural and man-made infectious disease threats, but it remains to be seen how well these partnerships will fully develop and, even more importantly, how sustainable they will be.

It has been shown in understanding medical errors and chronic disease management that systems of care are essential for success. In a similar manner, the authors have outlined the importance of systems in the organization of community and national efforts to maintain a healthy population. They have made a series of sensible and well-supported recommendations to accomplish these goals.

Population health can have no greater importance than in dealing with health disparities. The knowledge economy will become increasingly dependent on a healthy and well-educated workforce. Underrepresented minorities not only are becoming an increasing proportion of the overall population but represent a disproportionate number of youth, on whose shoulders the older population must rest over the next several decades. Those in our society who do not understand issues of equity and distributive justice must understand this inevitability. The authors have created a convincing set of arguments, for the most pragmatic reader, of the wisdom of their approach and of their recommendations.

As immediate past president of the Institute of Medicine, I am very proud of contributions by the Institute's Reports on Public Health. They have been wise and compelling. In this volume the authors have extended those visions conceptually and practically into ideas that are essential to the health and well-being of the republic as well as its citizens. The challenge will be to communicate these ideas and the evidence that support them to policymakers in an objective and convincing manner based on logic and reason. It will be a challenging task. This book provides empirically grounded and thoughtfully designed guidance for undertaking the challenge.

August 2005   Kenneth I. Shine, M.D.
                       Executive Vice Chancellor for Health Affairs
                       University of Texas System
                       Immediate Past President of the Institute of Medicine

PREFACE

Research from a variety of disciplines in recent decades has amply documented the role of fundamental nonmedical versus medical determinants of population health and health disparities. These include environmental, social, and economic factors, such as environmental risks, education, occupation, employment, income, and social support and related community empowerment, which health care services or policy does not typically or directly address.

The research in this area has, however, not been effectively translated into a broad health policy agenda for addressing these fundamental determinants of population health and health disparities at the national, state, and local levels in many countries, and in the United States in particular. Further, public health, health care, and health services research professionals are often not aware of the research, practice, and policy in fields of study and practice that may affect these determinants, such as sustainable, human, economic, and/or community development programs and policies. And professionals in these arenas of development practice and policy often do not take into account the implications of their work for the health and health risks of individuals and populations that their efforts target.

The book introduces a framework for identifying, arraying, and evaluating the evidence regarding the fundamental social, economic, and ecological determinants of population health and health disparities; explores the role of related development policies in influencing these fundamental determinants; and suggests alternative models of more health-centered policy and program design incorporating a consideration of the fundamental determinants of health. The vision for reinventing public health is grounded in the concept of a healthy republic—in which public decision making takes into account the impacts of policies related to fundamental determinants on the health of the populations that these policies target.

The central thesis of the book is that to effectively improve population health and reduce health disparities, policymaking in a *variety* of domains must take into account policies that address the fundamental social, economic, and ecological determinants of health.

The book project emanated from the Rural Economic and Community Health (REACH) project. The original aim of the REACH project was to support collaborative policy-oriented research, community service, and teaching activities between three sets of partners: academic partners (the University of Texas School of Public Health and the Texas Tech University Health Sciences Center), state and regional partners (the Texas Department of Health and others), and an inaugural community partner (Morton, Cochran County, TX). The project was directed toward understanding and addressing the impact of rural community and economic development on the health and well-being of rural residents and communities. Support for the REACH project was provided through an interagency agreement between the University of Texas School of Public Health and the Texas Tech University Health Sciences Center, under contract with the Rural Health Unit, Office of Rural Community Affairs (Texas State Office of Rural Health Policy). REACH collaborators contributed a series of papers to a special issue of the *Texas Journal of Rural Health* (vol. 20, no. 4, 2002) that focused on rural development and health, based on REACH project activities.

Though the REACH project initially focused on the linkages between development and health in rural communities, it expanded to encompass a look at these issues more broadly in both rural and urban settings, and in the United States as well as internationally. The expanded goal of REACH was to provide a collaborative forum for developing the conceptual, methodological, and empirical foundations for integrating community, economic, and sustainable development, and public health and health care research and policy, in improving population health and reducing health disparities. This book resulted from these collaborations.

The book will be an important resource for students and professionals who want to understand the implications of the growing body of research on the fundamental determinants of health for the design of more health-centered programs and policies in a variety of policy arenas. The book critically evaluates the knowledge base for guiding the formulation of such policies and identifies what we still need to know and do to address persistent health disparities.

Further, the book will acquaint students with the literature in this area and provide them a framework to use in identifying groups most at risk as well as both the specific and common determinants of health and well-being. It will provide health and public health professionals guidance for translating the growing body of research on the fundamental determinants of population health into operational programs and policies. It offers a new set of tools and insights for development specialists to identify and evaluate the health consequences of their policies and actions. Finally, it can serve as a reference source for policymakers who need a quick review of the issues and corresponding guidance regarding how best to innovate effective policy options for addressing them.

Houston, Texas   Lu Ann Aday
August 2005

ACKNOWLEDGMENTS

The authors gratefully acknowledge the thoughtful and constructive comments provided by the anonymous Jossey-Bass and Wiley reviewers.

We want to extend a particular thank-you to the following individuals who graciously reviewed earlier drafts of selected chapters of the book:

Chapters 1 and 7

Edward Baker, M.D., M.P.H., M.Sc., University of North Carolina School of Public Health

Bernard J. Turnock, M.D., M.P.H., University of Illinois at Chicago School of Public Health

Chapter 2

Barbara Krimgold, Center for the Advancement of Health–Washington, DC

Chapter 3

Thomas R. Saving, Ph.D., Private Enterprise Research Center, Texas A&M University

Chapter 4

> Elizabeth Baumler, Ph.D., Center for Health Promotion and Prevention, University of Texas School of Public Health (UTSPH)–Houston
>
> Phuong Huynh, Ph.D., International Program in Health Policy, The Commonwealth Fund, New York
>
> Susan Tortolero, Ph.D., Center for Health Promotion and Prevention, UTSPH–Houston

Chapter 5

> M. David Low, M.D., Ph.D., UTSPH–Houston
>
> John Lynch, Ph.D., M.P.H., University of Michigan School of Public Health

Chapter 6

> Ellen Cushman, Ph.D., Michigan State University
>
> James E. Rohrer, Ph.D., Texas Tech University Health Sciences Center
>
> Richard Warnecke, Ph.D., University of Illinois at Chicago

Special thanks go to Anne D. Wiltshire, B.D.S., M.P.H., who helped to compile and edit the extensive set of references for the book. Her hard work, patience, and attention to detail were immensely valuable to all of us who worked on the book.

We also gratefully acknowledge the contributions of Manish Aggarwal, M.B.B.S.; Yu-Chia Chang, M.P.H.; Paula Cronin, B.A.; Dritana Marko, M.D.; and Nykiconia Preacely, M.P.H., to locating and compiling sources for the manuscript, as well as the helpful administrative support provided by Regina Fisher, Chantel Johnson, and Elizabeth S. Brown.

We want to especially recognize colleagues at the Texas Tech University Health Sciences Center—Patti J. Patterson, M.D.; James E. Rohrer, Ph.D.; and James B. Speer Jr., Ph.D.—as well as community leaders in Morton, Cochran County, Texas, who supported the collaborations under the auspices of the Rural Economic and Community Health project, from which the book emanated.

The editor also gratefully acknowledges the editorial assistance of Katherine V. Wilcox in ensuring that the text read clearly to someone other than the editor!

We are grateful for the flexible environment at the University of Texas School of Public Health, which supported the rewarding task of writing the book as a routine component of faculty roles and responsibilities.

The work on the book was truly a stimulating and collaborative project. It expanded our individual and collective understanding of the role that fundamental social, economic, and environmental determinants play in influencing the health of the public and generated new ways of thinking regarding how best to address them. Our hope is that those who read it will be similarly rewarded.

L.A.A.

THE EDITOR

Lu Ann Aday, Ph.D., earned her B.S., with high honors, in agricultural economics at Texas Tech University and her M.S. and Ph.D. degrees in sociology at Purdue University. She is the Lorne Bain Distinguished Professor in Public Health and Medicine at the University of Texas School of Public Health. Her principal research interests are equity of access to health and health care for vulnerable populations. You may contact her at the University of Texas School of Public Health–Houston, 1200 Herman Pressler Street, Room E-321 (RAS), Houston, TX 77030; tel.: (713) 500-9177; e-mail: lu.a.aday@uth.tmc.edu

THE CONTRIBUTORS

Charles E. Begley, Ph.D., received his B.S. in business administration from Northern Arizona University and his M. A. and Ph.D. in economics from the University of Texas at Austin. Begley is professor of management, policy, and community health at the University of Texas School of Public Health, where he teaches health economics and policy. His research emphasizes the economic aspects of health policies and programs at the national, state, and local levels. You may contact him at the University of Texas School of Public Health–Houston, 1200 Herman Pressler Street, Room E-317 (RAS), Houston, TX 77030; tel.: (713) 500-9179; e-mail: charles.e.begley@uth.tmc.edu

Kathryn M. Cardarelli, Ph.D., received her B.A. in biology from the University of Texas at Austin, her M.P.H. from the University of North Texas School of Public Health, and her Ph.D. in epidemiology from the University of Texas School of Public Health. She is an assistant professor of epidemiology at the University of North Texas School of Public Health. Her primary research interests are the social influences on health and the interface of epidemiology and health policy. You may contact her at the University of North Texas School of Public Health, 3500 Camp Bowie Boulevard, Fort Worth, TX 76107; tel.: (817) 735-5192; e-mail: kcardare@hsc.unt.edu

Dan Culica, M.D., Ph.D., received his M.D. in medicine from the University of Bucharest, Romania, and his M.A. in health services management from the University of Manchester, England. He became a specialist doctor in surgery and public health in Romania and received his Ph.D. in health policy and management from the University of Iowa. He is an assistant professor in management, policy, and community health at the University of Texas School of Public Health, and his teaching and research interests are in public health management, community health planning, and outcomes of care. You may contact him at the University of Texas School of Public Health–Dallas, 5323 Harry Hines Boulevard, Room V8.300, Dallas, TX 75390; tel.: (214) 648-1070; e-mail: dan.v.culica@uth.tmc.edu

Janet S. de Moor, M.P.H., Ph.D., is a postdoctoral fellow at Harvard University School of Public Health. She has a B.S. from Penn State University and an M.P.H. and Ph.D. from the University of Texas School of Public Health. Her research interests are social disparities in cancer prevention with an emphasis on tertiary prevention and the pathways through which patients' economic and psychosocial resources shape cancer-related outcomes. You may contact her at the Center for Community Based Research, Dana Farber Cancer Institute, 44 Binney Street, Smith 342, Boston, MA 02115; tel.: (617) 632-6120; e-mail: janet_demoor@dfci.harvard.edu

Luisa Franzini, Ph.D., received her B.Sc., M.Sc., and Ph.D. in economics and econometrics from the London School of Economics and is an associate professor of health policy at the University of Texas School of Public Health. After several years of working as a theoretical econometrician, she is currently engaged in the fields of health economics, cost analysis, and social determinants of health. You may contact her at the University of Texas School of Public Health–Houston, 1200 Herman Pressler Street, Room E-919 (RAS), Houston, TX 77030; tel.: (713) 500-9487; e-mail: luisa.franzini@uth.tmc.edu

Carl S. Hacker, Ph.D., J.D., is an ecologist and an attorney. He received a B.S. in biology from the College of William and Mary, a Ph.D. in biology from Rice University, and a J.D. from the University of Houston Law Center. His research and teaching at the University of Texas School of Public Health consider the effect of urban environments on ecosystems and the relationship between law and the public's health. You may contact him at the University of Texas School of Public Health–Houston, 1200 Herman Pressler Street, Room W-312 (RAS), Houston, TX 77030; tel.: (713) 500-9185; e-mail: carl.s.hacker@uth.tmc.edu

Hardy D. Loe Jr., M.D., M.P.H., received his M.D. degree from the University of Texas Medical Branch at Galveston and his M.P.H. from the University of

California at Berkeley. He is past associate dean and associate professor of community health at the University of Texas School of Public Health. His public health practice and research interests include public health practice, community decision making, health planning, and community health information systems. You may contact him at 1844 Kipling Street, Houston, TX 77098; tel.: (713) 524-2682; e-mail: hardyloe@yahoo.com

Barbara J. Low, M.P.H., Dr.P.H., received her graduate degrees in health education and health promotion at the University of Texas School of Public Health and completed her postdoctoral training at the university's Center for Health Promotion and Prevention Research. Her research focuses on the determinants of child and adolescent health-risk behavior, particularly violence, risky sexual behavior, and dropping out of school, and on the associations between these behaviors and youth health status. You may contact her at the Center for Health Promotion and Prevention Research, UTSPH–Houston, 7000 Fannin Street, Suite 2664B, Houston, TX 77030; tel.: (250) 468-1825; e-mail: mdlow@shaw.ca

M. David Low, M.D., Ph.D., FRCP(C), is past Health Science Center president and professor emeritus of public health, University of Texas–Houston Health Science Center; a charter member of the Communitarian Council; cofounder of the National Medicine–Public Health Initiative; founder of the Texas Program in Society and Health; and the first holder of the Rockwell Chair in Society and Population Health at the University of Texas School of Public Health. You may contact him at 1621 Marina Way, Nanoose Bay, BC V9P 9B5 (Canada); tel.: (250) 468-1825; e-mail: David.Low@uth.tmc.edu

Sondip K. Mathur, Ph.D., received his B.A. with honors in economics from Delhi University, his M.A. in economics from Cleveland State University, and his Ph.D. in economics from Texas A&M University. He is an assistant professor at the Texas Southern University College of Pharmacy and Health Sciences. His principal research interests are institutional economics, managerial economics, public policy, health economics, and population health. You may contact him at Texas Southern University, College of Pharmacy and Health Sciences, 127 Gray Hall, 3100 Cleburne Street, Houston, TX 77004; tel.: (713) 313-1839; e-mail: mathursk@tsu.edu

Yuki Murakami, M.P.H., received her B.A. in economics from Aoyama Gakuin University in Japan and her M.P.H. at the University of Texas School of Public Health. She is currently attending the Harvard School of Public Health in Boston. Her interest is in economics and financing of health care sectors in developing countries and Japan. You may contact her at 19 Green Street #5, Brookline, MA 02446; tel.: (617) 566-5611; e-mail: ymurakam@hsph.harvard.edu

Beth E. Quill, M.P.H., received her R.N. from Massachusetts General Hospital, her B.A. in sociology from Emmanuel College, and her M.P.H. from the University of Pittsburgh in health administration. She has extensive administrative experience with federal, state, and local public health agencies and is currently an associate professor of management, policy, and community health and associate director of the Center for Transforming Public Health Systems at the University of Texas School of Public Health. Her primary research interests are public health practice and management, rural health, and vulnerable populations. You may contact her at the University of Texas School of Public Health–Houston, 1200 Herman Pressler Street, Room E-909 (RAS), Houston, TX 77030; tel.: (713) 500-9159; e-mail: beth.e.quill@uth.tmc.edu

Rafia S. Rasu, Ph.D., M. Pharm., M.B.A., received her Ph.D. in management, policy, and community health from the University of Texas School of Public Health. She is an assistant professor at the University of Missouri School of Pharmacy in Kansas City. Her primary research interests are the economic evaluation of public health programs, health care interventions, and outcomes research. You may contact her at University of Missouri-Kansas City, School of Pharmacy, 2411 Holmes M3-C19, Kansas City, MO 64108; tel.: (816) 235-5498; e-mail: rasur@umkc.edu

William D. Spears, Ph.D., received his B.A. and M.A. in sociology from Texas Tech University and his Ph.D. from the University of Texas School of Public Health. He is an assistant professor in management, policy, and community health at the School of Public Health. His major research interests are health information systems and community health and community assessment. You may contact him at the University of Texas School of Public Health–San Antonio, 7703 Floyd Curl Drive, San Antonio, TX 78284; tel.: (210) 567-5930; e-mail: william.d.spears @uth.tmc.edu

J. Michael Swint, Ph.D., received his B.A. in economics from California State University, Humboldt, and his M.A. and Ph.D. degrees in economics from Rice University. He is professor of economics at the University of Texas School of Public Health and the University of Texas Medical School–Houston. His principal research interests are economic evaluation of public health programs and policies and health care interventions. You may contact him at the University of Texas School of Public Health–Houston, 1200 Herman Pressler Street, Room E-933 (RAS), Houston, TX 77030; tel.: (713) 500-9158; e-mail: john.m.swint@uth.tmc.edu

Rachel Westheimer Vojvodic, M.P.H., received her B.S. in health professions and health care administration from Texas State University and her M.P.H. in health services organization from the University of Texas School of Public Health. Her interests regard how health system structure and policies translate into the delivery of services. You may contact her at the Center for Health Promotion and Prevention Research, UTSPH–Houston, 7000 Fannin Street, 25th Floor, Houston, TX 77030; tel.: (713) 500-9752; e-mail: rachel.w.vojvodic@uth.tmc.edu

Cynthia Warrick, Ph.D., received her B.S. in pharmacy from Howard University, her M.S. in public policy from the Georgia Institute of Technology, and her Ph.D. in environmental science and public policy from George Mason University. She is an associate professor of environmental health at the Florida A&M University Institute of Public Health. Her principal research interests are environmental justice and health disparities in minority populations. You may contact her at the Institute of Public Health, FAMU, Science Research Center, Suite 207B, Tallahassee, FL 32307; tel.: (850) 599-8145; e-mail: cynthia.warrick@famu.edu

CHAPTER ONE

ANALYTIC FRAMEWORK

Lu Ann Aday

Chapter Highlights

- The fundamental determinants of population health represent essential resources that serve to enhance the prospects of health and well-being at a variety of levels. These resources include natural capital (environmental resources), human capital (education), material capital (occupation, employment, and income), and social and cultural capital (social support and community empowerment).
- In a healthy republic, public decision making takes into account the impacts of policies related to fundamental determinants on the health of the populations that these policies target.
- Policy domains that directly influence the fundamental determinants of population health have not traditionally been fully integrated into public health policy and practice; this includes sustainable development, human development, economic development, and community development policy.
- The effectiveness, efficiency, and equity criteria can be used in identifying the actual or potential success of policies in each of these domains.

- **Effectiveness assesses the weight of the evidence regarding the impact of policies on the fundamental determinants of population health.**
- **Efficiency evaluates the mix and level of investments in alternative policies required to improve population health, given available resources.**
- **Equity addresses the fairness and effectiveness of policies in minimizing population health disparities.**

A growing body of research on the fundamental determinants of health has documented that people's lived experiences and the institutions that shape them (families, economies, and communities, for example) influence the overall health and well-being of individuals and populations. The fundamental determinants of health represent essential resources such as education, income and wealth, social support, and physical and environmental resources that serve to enhance the prospects of health and well-being. Wide disparities in health risks and outcomes across subgroups and communities are associated with variant levels of these resources (Link & Phelan, 1995).

Institutions such as families, schools, neighborhoods, and workplaces and the local, state, regional, national, and international economies that delimit the availability and distribution of goods, services, and wealth represent powerful influences on these fundamental determinants and subsequently on the health and well-being of the individuals and populations nested within such institutions. The operation and impact of major social institutions are shaped by decisions and policies within broader private and public spheres of decision making, including the actions of federal, state, and local governments; regional, national, and international markets; and civic organizations and communities.

The percentage of the gross domestic product devoted to health care has steadily increased while major health disparities between socioeconomic and racial and ethnic groups have steadily persisted in the United States and other countries (Aday, Begley, Lairson, & Balkrishnan, 2004). Nations such as Australia, Great Britain, Canada, and Sweden, among others, have sought to translate research on the fundamental determinants of population health and health disparities into a broad health policy agenda for improving health and reducing disparities (see Chapter Two). The United States has, however, not adopted this broad focus on population health–centered policy.

Public health, health care, and health services research professionals often do not consider other domains of policy or practice that may affect the fundamental determinants of population health, such as sustainable, human, economic, and/or community development programs and policies, in their decision making. And professionals in various arenas of development practice and policy often do not take into account the implications of their work for the health and health risks of individuals and populations that their efforts target.

This book examines the implications of research on the fundamental determinants of health on the formulation of more health-centered public policy. The central thesis of the book is that *to effectively improve population health and reduce health disparities, policymaking in a variety of policy domains must take into account the fundamental social, economic, and ecological determinants of health.*

The vision for reinventing public health is grounded in the concept of a healthy republic—in which public decision making takes into account the impacts of policies related to fundamental determinants on the health of the populations that these policies target. The health of what we call the (re)public is intended to reflect the inextricable linkage between the health of populations and policies related to the fundamental determinants of health. The word *public* refers to populations that are the focus of public policy decisions. The word *republic* refers essentially to a form of government in which power ultimately resides in a body of citizens entitled to vote and is exercised by elected officers and representatives responsible to citizens and governing according to law. A healthy republic produces healthy citizens. Healthy citizens contribute to building and sustaining a healthy republic. The final chapter of this book presents the blueprint for a healthy republic grounded in more population health–centered public health policies and practices.

The Canadian Institute for Advanced Research (CIAR, 2004), which has conducted much of the foundational research on population health and related social determinants, has created the Successful Societies Program. The program is essentially concerned with two questions: How do social relations condition collective levels of health, well-being, and human development? How might policies be designed to create successful societies? The vision of a successful society presented here is that of a healthy republic.

The book introduces a framework for identifying, arraying, and evaluating the evidence regarding the fundamental social, economic, and ecological determinants of population health and health disparities in the context of the vision of a healthy republic; it assesses the impact of policies in a variety of domains in influencing these fundamental determinants; and it suggests alternative models of more health-centered policy and program design incorporating a consideration of the fundamental determinants of health.

Chapter One summarizes the overall framework for the book and the specific topics that the respective chapters will address.

Framework for Moving Toward a Healthy (Re)Public

Table 1.1 summarizes the book's framework. It is grounded most essentially in fields of study and related policy domains directly or indirectly influencing the fundamental determinants of population health.

Fields of Study

Population health as a field of study refers to "the health outcomes of a group of individuals, including the distribution of such outcomes within the group. . . . The field of population health includes health outcomes, patterns of health determinants and interventions that link these two" (Kindig & Stoddart, 2003, p. 380). Chapter Two reviews the field of population health and related research on the fundamental determinants of health.

Public health is broadly "what we, as a society, do collectively to assure the conditions in which people can be healthy" (Institute of Medicine, Committee for the Study of the Future of Public Health, 1988, p. 1). Policy domains that directly influence the fundamental determinants of population health have, however, not traditionally been fully integrated into public health policy and practice.

The fundamental determinants of population health include natural capital (renewable and nonrenewable resources), human capital (levels of education and skills); material capital (the distribution of wealth and income); and social and cultural capital (quantity and quality of social ties and community values and empowerment). The fields of study underlying an understanding of the impact of these various determinants and related policies on population health are based on different units of analysis and related theories, summarized in Table 1.1. The chapters that follow will critically examine these determinants both independently and in an ecological context—that is, in terms of their primary contributions as well as the interactions among them, in predicting population health and health disparities.

Policy Domains

Recent Institute of Medicine reports (Committee on Assuring the Health of the Public in the 21st Century, 2003; Committee on Educating Public Health Professionals for the 21st Century, 2003) argue for more broadly grounding innovations in the design and implementation of public health policies and programs in an ecological model of population health, based on research on the multifactorial determinants of health. This book provides guidance regarding the specific

TABLE 1.1. FRAMEWORK FOR MOVING TOWARD A HEALTHY (RE)PUBLIC.

Policy Domains	Fundamental Determinants	Unit of Analysis	Underlying Theories	Policy Models and Examples
Chapters 2 and 7: Public health	Population health and health disparities	Population	• Ecosocial theory • Public health research • Health services research • Policy analysis	Population health–centered policy: public health system and policy development
Chapter 3: Sustainable development	Natural capital (renewable and nonrenewable resources): environmental resources and risks	Ecosystem, corporations	• Ecology • Managerial economics • Corporate social responsibility	Market: corporate models of internalizing incentives for optimizing profitability and sustainability
Chapter 4: Human development	Human capital (levels of education and skills): education	Individuals	• Human capital and development theory • Life-course epidemiology	Government: public policies grounded in the social determinants of health
Chapter 5: Economic development	Material capital (distribution of wealth and income): occupation, employment, and income	International, national, regional, state, and/or local economies	• Macroeconomic theory	Government: public policies grounded in the economic determinants of health
Chapter 6: Community development	Social capital (quantity and quality of social ties): social support Cultural capital (community values): community empowerment	Community	• Deliberative democracy • Social capital theory • Community development theory • Participatory action research	Community: sustainable participatory models of community decision making

Fields of Study

policy domains that stakeholders may draw on in implementing this broader public health policy agenda, including sustainable, human, economic, and community development policy.

Sustainable development refers to practices that simultaneously create economic vitality, environmental stewardship, and social equity for present and future generations. *Human development* policy is concerned with investments in people's skills and capabilities (such as early childhood or vocational education) that enable them to act in new ways (for example, to master a trade) or enhance their contributions to society (to enter the labor force). *Economic development* focuses on enhancing the efficiency of a national, regional, state, or local economy by investing in business in an area, which would in turn yield multiplier effects in terms of creating new jobs and increasing the wealth and income of target residents. *Community development* addresses the equity of social and economic arrangements in a given locality, grounded in assessments of the extent to which the affected parties fully and effectively participate in shaping the decisions that affect them.

Why does this book focus on development? *Development* fundamentally refers to growth or maximizing gains—either economic gains, growth in human productive potential, or growth in the assets and capacities within a community. Gains can, however, be uneven across communities and groups; that is, some areas or populations may benefit more than others, and growth in one sector, for example, the corporate economy, may have untoward consequences in others, for example, the environment (Mathur & Aday, 2002). Understanding the impact of the respective realms of development on the fundamental determinants of population health provides an essential blueprint for designing a new intersectoral policy approach to addressing these determinants.

Chapter Two looks at the field of population health and related conceptual and empirical research on understanding the fundamental determinants of population health. The chapters that follow review the following development strategies for addressing these determinants:

- Sustainable development (Chapter Three)
- Human development (Chapter Four)
- Economic development (Chapter Five)
- Community development (Chapter Six)

The outline for these chapters is as follows:
Introduction
Overview
Fields of study
Policy domains

Evidence regarding research on fundamental determinants
Current policies that address fundamental determinants
Strengths and limitations of current policies
Recommendations

Chapter Three introduces the concept of sustainable development. The sustainability perspective appears first in the book because it serves to present the following important concepts and perspectives:

- Sustainable development deals with the broadest and most comprehensive unit of analysis and impact—the earth's ecosystem.
- It acknowledges the essential interdependence and impact of decisions made in one sector (e.g., corporate policy) on others (e.g., environmental quality).
- Sustainable development by definition acknowledges the importance of balancing the development goal of *growth* or *maximizing gains* with the sustainability principle of *maintenance* or *minimizing losses* (for example, to both sustain rural natural environments and resources *and* develop rural economies and communities).
- Sustainable development policy argues for the centrality of environmental, efficiency, *and* equity criteria in evaluating the success of public decision making.
- The sustainability concept introduces a long-term rather than short-term perspective, in that the goal of sustainability is to ultimately maintain benefits and resources across generations.
- Sustainable development policy also argues that innovative approaches to improving the health of populations may call for the essential engagement of what might appear to be unconventional allies (e.g., the corporate business sector and local public health agency in a community).

In summary, Chapter Three sets the stage for the chapters that follow by introducing a broad, interdependent, innovative, and long-term perspective on the environmental underpinnings of population health.

Chapter Four turns analytic lenses on the microcosm of the essential human impacts of the fundamental determinants of population health—the development of productive potential throughout the life course. That chapter's review of the human development perspective offers the following insights:

- It illuminates the defining and desired end point of population health–centered policies and research: to improve the health and developmental opportunities for individuals throughout their lives.

- It grounds the future-oriented time horizon introduced through the sustainability perspective in an acknowledgement of how investments in the earliest stages of life can manifestly shape the future prospects for health and well-being throughout the life course.

- As does the sustainability chapter, Chapter Four documents the impact of nonhealth sectors (e.g., education) on individual and population health outcomes.

- It also convincingly points out the role of economic factors (e.g., poverty), as well as education, in accounting for positive human development and health at all stages of development and cumulatively over a lifetime.

In summary, the human development perspective introduced in Chapter Four grounds a look at what must be the ultimate goal of population health–centered policies and programs—*enhancing the human capacities and productive potential of individuals throughout their lives*—and acknowledges that policies that lie outside the conventional province of health policies (that is, education and economic policies) may offer the greatest prospects for achieving this goal.

Chapters Five and Six, on economic development and community development, respectively, present what some may view as competing policy contexts for maximizing the prospects for community and individual health and well-being. Economic development strategists may be at odds with community development goals when they ignore the consequences for economic growth–oriented policies or business strategies on the values, identities, autonomy, integrity, or health of the neighborhoods toward which the policies and strategies are directed. Community development strategies, on the other hand, may fail to acknowledge the powerful economic, political, and global forces that constrain the prospects of success of local community empowerment or issues-centered initiatives. Chapters Five and Six present different points of leverage in influencing population health–macroeconomic policy versus local community action. On the other hand, they also share important common ground in arguing that assuring the success of these policies and interventions will require the full participation of affected parties in formulating them.

Chapter Five points to the following specific remedy for addressing and improving population health: support economic policies that reduce poverty, increase labor market participation, improve the balance of trade benefits for developing countries relative to developed countries, as well as health policies that are explicitly intended to improve population health.

Chapter Six offers the following specific guidance to the field of public health in enhancing the prospects of successful community development: train public health practitioners in facilitating community development—particularly in the context of promoting deliberative democracy, local leadership, community values, and political action—to facilitate positive change in the communities through collective action.

Both chapters conclude that neither economic nor community development is likely to be successful unless those whom major policy decisions affect—at either the international, national, state, or local levels—are engaged in shaping them.

The final chapter, Chapter Seven, discusses the implications of the framework and related analyses for innovative public health system and policy development to improve population health and reduce health disparities.

Table 1.1 summarizes the principal policy models and related examples reviewed in Chapters Two through Seven, and the following section reviews the political and philosophical underpinning for them.

Policy Models and Examples

The discussion that follows reviews the changing political and economic landscape and related transformations that have taken place in the policies of nation-states, as well as the ways that these changes have affected the field of public health. This backdrop is intended to provide a context for understanding both the constraints and potential for the field of public health as the millennium unfolds.

The World Health Organization (WHO) has struggled to reevaluate the role of health in contributing to economic well-being, as well as the role of economic forces and factors in influencing health (Kickbusch, 2003; WHO, 1999, 2000; WHO, Commission on Macroeconomics and Health, Working Group 1, 2002). Canada has sought to balance the social-structural change and political action agenda emanating from the Ottawa Charter and related Health Promotion program focus with what some view as the more politically conservative research-oriented agenda of the Population Health Research Program of the Canadian Institute for Advanced Research (CIAR) (Coburn et al., 2003; Evans & Stoddart, 2003; Glouberman & Millar, 2003; Raphael & Bryant, 2002). In the United States, the Institute of Medicine (Committee on Assuring, 2003; Committee on Educating, 2003) has assumed leadership in charting new directions for the field that move beyond governmental public health and forge partnership with diverse sectors, including business and the media, among others, to create and activate an intersectoral public health system.

These reflections on new directions for the field are taking place in the context of immense political, economic, and cultural changes nationally and internationally.

Most notable among these changes is the dominance of economic forces in the globalization of markets and financial capital and corollary policies to devolve the role of centralized governments and welfare states in providing safety nets of publicly supported services.

Table 1.2 displays the conventional political continuum ranging from the politics of the left to those of the right. Though a diversity of political parties and beliefs can exist within countries, one can broadly contrast and compare nation-states according to the dominant political forces within them (Aday, 1997; Navarro, 2002; Navarro & Shi, 2001). The table highlights examples of selected categories of nation-states that may manifest the dominant political philosophies across the political spectrum. This is not to imply that diverse political philosophies do not exist within each of them as well, as is certainly the case in the United States. The author provides the template, however, to serve as a point of reference for more fully understanding the larger political and economic environment that public health faces and to which it must respond and adapt.

The politics of the left has conventionally seen a large role for government, ranging from more authoritarian communist regimes that have dominated nation-states such as the former Soviet Union countries, Cuba, and the People's Republic of China to the heavily tax-supported social welfare states of the Nordic countries, such as Norway and Sweden, to the liberal democratic politics in the United States that have had a strong human rights emphasis and corollary investments in major social welfare programs, such as Social Security, Medicare, and Medicaid.

The politics of the right—grounded at its most fundamental in the libertarian philosophy, which valorizes property rights and the operation of free market forces—eschews taxation or any other models of income and wealth distribution and argues for a greatly diminished and in some cases minimal or nonexistent role for government (Mulhall & Swift, 1996). The United States, dominated most notably by a very strong and successful capitalist economy, anchors probably one of the strongest expressions nationally and internationally of the central role of the market in political, economic, and social life.

Communitarian philosophy balances a look at the role of the community and related cultural and family values in shaping private and public lifeworlds (Mulhall & Swift, 1996). It seeks to find a place between the dominance of the market and government to express and enforce deeply held community or cultural beliefs and values. The central role of community in national and international politics can be found in the dominance of the religious right in the United States and other countries, as well as in large-scale social movements such as the civil rights and environmental justice movements, in assuring that deeply held cultural and/or community values make their way to the national political agenda.

TABLE 1.2. COMPARISONS OF POLITICAL PHILOSOPHIES AND IMPLICATIONS FOR PUBLIC HEALTH.

	Political Left	*Decision-Making Domains*			Political Right
	Government	Civil society	Community	Third Way	Market
Political and economic issues and trends	Devolution of government	Civil society	Deliberative democracy	Third Way	Globalization
Nation-states (examples)	Authoritarian communist (former Soviet Union nations, Cuba, People's Republic of China)	Social democratic (Denmark, Finland, Norway, Sweden)	Christian democratic (Belgium, France, Germany, Italy, Netherlands)	Liberal democratic (Australia, Canada, United Kingdom)	Neoliberal democratic (United States)
Public health	Governmental public health	Canadian Institute for Advanced Research (CIAR) Population Health Research program	Ottawa Charter ("New Public Health") Health Promotion program	Public-private partnerships	Privatized medical care

Intersectoral Public Health System

Against this long-standing backdrop of right- versus left-wing politics, monumental economic and social forces over the last half of the 20th century have dominated and have set some very important new trends into play at the beginning of the 21st century. One of the most notable and influential is the phenomenon of globalization. International trade has been a component of the human economy and experience from the earliest stages of history. Its expression in the global economy of the late 20th and early 21st centuries has, however, assumed a hegemony and velocity that is unprecedented in previous centuries and generations. The advent of information technologies (computers and the Internet in particular) has provided unprecedented opportunities for the rapid and widespread movement of financial capital and the interdependence of financial markets nationally and internationally. The resulting globalization of the economy has led to less rooted investments on the part of the international corporate economy in localized labor forces and material resources and capital. As a consequence the role of organized labor in influencing wages and benefits and corollary public support for social welfare spending has greatly declined in many countries (Hardt & Negri, 2000).

A neoliberal political philosophy has come to replace the liberal democratic politics that supported the rise of the social welfare state in the social democracies of Europe and within the United States through President Franklin D. Roosevelt's New Deal, for example. Neoliberalism places central importance on the role of the free market, reduced taxation, and the government's minimal role in interfering in the operation of free market forces. Its seeds are present in libertarian politics, but its dominance as a political value has become greater as global markets have assumed a larger role in influencing the economies and cultures of nation-states (Coburn, 2000).

With the collapse of the authoritarian communist states of the Soviet Union and Eastern Europe, the political far left also collapsed. Organized labor, which had been an important political force for maintaining a strong social welfare state in more moderate social democracies, has been weakened in many countries as the forces of globalization have led to the rapid disengagement of international businesses from local labor markets in the search for lower-priced wage workers and/or material resources and capital. The dominance of the neoliberal political philosophy and the related weakening of effective political advocacy of the political left show up in national, state, and local politics in calls for the devolution of government, structural readjustments to downsize and/or privatize government services, and reduced taxes especially on the wealth-holding classes.

During the 1980s President Ronald Reagan in the United States and Prime Minister Margaret Thatcher in Great Britain were strong and effective allies for a neoliberal, market-dominated political philosophy, which found expression in successful initiatives on the part of their administrations to downsize and/or to introduce market-oriented mechanisms for reducing or managing large-scale social programs, such as health and welfare services.

Many credit the neoliberal political philosophy with shifting economic policy from a strategy of demand stimulation to one of profit stimulation. The demand-stimulation strategy that characterized the economic policy of the New Deal programs under the Roosevelt administration of the 1930s and the Great Society Initiatives under Lyndon Johnson in the 1960s sought to stimulate the economy and produce greater social and economic opportunities for the poor, working, and middle class. The profit-stimulation approach, which has characterized the neoliberal political agenda of the late 20th and early 21st centuries, is designed to reduce the cost of production and thereby encourage private economic growth and investment. The term for the ideological framework characterizing this trend is *recapitalization,* which is reflected in tax cuts for corporations and those with the greatest wealth-holding assets, the contracting out (privatization) of public services to private providers, deregulation, reductions of public spending (especially for health and social services), and the enactment of international policies (such as the North American Free Trade Agreement and the General Agreement on Tariffs and Trade) that have greatly facilitated the mobility of global capital (Whiteis, 1998, 2000).

During the 1990s the financial flows from developed to developing countries shifted from largely public to private investments. Net loans and grants from the International Monetary Fund, for example, fell by more than half from 1990 to 2000, and net commercial lending (except for bonds) fell to almost nil. For example, during this period, financial flows from the public sector in developed countries to the public sector in developing countries dropped by 56% to around 9% of the total flows. On the other hand, funds flowing from the private sector in developed countries to the private sector in developing countries rose from 18% in 1980 to 38% in 1990 to 82% in 2000. Though there is some evidence that this growth has led to reduction in poverty overall in some countries, there is also strong evidence that income disparities have increased as a result of greater concentrations of wealth among a capital-holding minority in both developed and developing countries (Woodward, Drager, Beaglehole, & Lipson, 2004).

Interestingly, the administrations of President Bill Clinton in the United States and Prime Minister Tony Blair in Great Britain moved toward what some have characterized as a Third Way in politics (Giddens, 2000). Though there is no consensus regarding what exactly the Third Way represents in principle and philosophy, one may broadly characterize it as a centrist political strategy that attempts to balance the neoliberal and liberal democratic social welfare agendas. The Third Way sees a role for markets and the reduction of governmental responsibility and spending. It does not, however, argue, as would the strict neoliberal philosophy, that government should in effect get out of the business of taxing and redistributing income and wealth in order to provide public goods and services. Proponents of the Third Way argue that it offers a reasonable balance to the political excesses of either the political left or the right. Critics argue that in practice it is a fruit that has not fallen far from the tree of market-dominated neoliberalism (Bourdieu, 1998; Giddens, 2000).

The political battles between the giants of progovernment and promarket forces have not gone unnoticed by those concerned with the role of democratic political processes and the political voice of affected parties in mediating the excesses of either. These concerns have manifested themselves on two primary fronts for reinventing community: the call for the emergence and support of *civil society* and *deliberative democracy*, both of which this chapter discusses more fully.

The collapse of the communist-dominated socialist nation-states has also been accompanied in many cases by the collapse of social order, leading to large increases in violent crime, interethnic warfare, and political corruption. Many historical and political reasons might account for these costly human consequences of change. An important observation, however, is that a major legacy of the authoritarian and repressive regimes that dominated many of these countries was the suppression or elimination of mediating institutions, such as nongovernmental, fraternal, or religious organizations, that help to create a civil society and a basis for democratic and shared governance. On the other hand, the Western democratic nations, and especially the United States, have not been immune from the hegemony of the market and the media in standardizing and universalizing culture and values, nor from the dominance of neoliberal political values and weakening of progovernment sentiments that have led correspondingly to diminished public engagement in public affairs, voting, and an overall distrust of public officials and the government as a whole. Social critics call for the creation of a civil society (or public sphere) of involved and interested citizens to help mediate the excesses of either government or the market and to create a Third Way grounded in a more democratic political process (Habermas, 1996). This finds expression in the central role that private nongovernmental organizations play in either advocating for or providing needed programs and services, as well as the emergence of public-private partnerships to address identified needs that neither government nor the market is meeting.

A corresponding and important trend in reinventing community is the emergence of a call to deliberative democracy. Deliberative democracy is essentially concerned with (re)building civil society by assuring that all groups are involved in shaping the decisions that will affect them. Chapter Six more fully discusses the process and principles of deliberative democracy. Critics of modern and postmodern society argue that excessive reliance on either the government or the market has failed to develop effective mechanisms for addressing major social problems, such as growing wealth and income disparities, environmental degradation, and population health disparities; as a matter of fact, they claim, this reliance may have contributed directly to creating and/or exacerbating these and other problems (Habermas, 1996). Growing cultural diversity and related multiculturalism has led to significant challenges within nation-states as well as between nations regarding how to evolve peaceful and reasoned approaches to dealing with what may be very different political and cultural values in the service of developing new forms of shared governance. Those who call for the strengthening of civil society and deliberative democracy deem these to be ways to balance what may be the excesses of a communitarian philosophy that may support strongly held community values (e.g., racism or xenophobia) that may nonetheless not be supportive of diverse group interests and values.

Revolutionary changes in the scientific paradigms for understanding the operation of the physical world have widespread consequences for science and practice in the social, economic, and political spheres as well. The discussion that follows highlights trends that have had significant implications for public health research and practice. This provides a background and context for the review of the consequences of these trends in subsequent chapters.

Thomas Kuhn, in his book *The Structure of Scientific Revolutions* (1996), chronicles the challenges in the conduct of normal science that accompanied the succession of Copernican, Galilean, and Newtonian understandings of the universe. In the early part of the 20th century, Albert Einstein's theory of relativity and the accompanying growth of the field of quantum physics yielded revolutionary insights regarding the operation of the vast physical universe as well as the elementary and essential particles constituting it.

In contrast to the Galileian-Newtonian understanding of the world as structured by mechanistic and deterministic laws of nature, Einstein's work revealed a universe that behaves in ways that are often unpredictable and produces unexpected rather than fully predictable outcomes. Observations at the subatomic level document the interdependent and interactive, rather than independent and mechanistic, operation of the elemental transformations of matter into energy and of energy into matter.

The revolutionary impact of Einstein's work has reverberated throughout science and society. Mechanistic models of how the world is structured and operates have been challenged by more dynamic, process-oriented models of how physical and biological systems behave. *Complexity theory*, which posits a dynamic interactive view of reality, has challenged linear cause-effect traditional disciplinary approaches to theory development and testing ("Complex Systems," 1999). *Positivist science,* which assumes that there is an objective reality to be studied, captured, and understood and relies on the scientific method and related hypothesis testing, has been challenged by a postpositivist approach to knowledge that argues that one can never fully apprehend reality and that multiple methods, including capturing the stories and subjective lived experiences of study subjects, are required to fully understand human experience. *Postmodernism* argues that all experience is essentially subjective: there are no unassailable standards and conventions for judging ethics, politics, or art; such standards, if they do exist, reside uniquely in the eye and mind of the beholder (Denzin & Lincoln, 2000).

Critics of modern society have condemned the mechanistic, technical-rational approach to problem solving that has characterized the domination of the welfare state and the profit-oriented underpinnings of the market in shaping public policies and interventions. These critics have argued that not only have these mechanisms and means been unsuccessful in addressing major social problems, but they may in fact have led to the prospect of these problems worsening due to the diminishment of the mediating role of communities and related institutions and organizations that characterize a healthy civic life. *Critical theory,* for example, probes the deep structured inequalities in the distribution of economic and political power and the distinguishing role of race and gender in accounting for enduring social problems in modern societies; it also calls for reinvigorating democratic principles to mediate the excesses of governments and markets (Denzin & Lincoln, 2000; Habermas, 1996).

Approaches to bridging the subjectivity and uncertainty of human experience resulting from these pervasive scientific, political, and social influences include exploring the role of *communication* or *discourse* in helping to create common grounds of understanding for collective actions required to operate within human society. Jürgen Habermas's theory of communicative action (1996) and Paolo Freire's approach (1970) to empowering the disempowered through dialogue and associated social learning (see Chapter Six) represent approaches to building new forms of civil society and social equity through participatory discourse on the part of those whom public or corporate decision making affects. The offshoots of this type of discourse may arise in major social movements such as protests of the actions of the International Monetary Fund, World Bank, and World Trade Organization around globalization; neighborhoods organizing around issues of environmental justice; and/or coalitions developing to move toward a common political goal.

The advent of high-speed computers, the Internet, and related informational and communication technologies has greatly multiplied and accelerated the rate of connectivity that crosses traditional geographic or social boundaries. Electronic highways have increasingly become a way for individuals and organizations to connect across vast distances and for entities that have traditionally not communicated to do so.

The early part of the 21st century may be accurately characterized as an information age, one in which sharing of knowledge and information are key for promoting learning and generating innovation, as well as gaining access to conventional political and economic power.

Contemporary organization theory is challenging hierarchical bureaucracies and modern corporations to focus less on organizational structure and more on communication and information sharing, to maximize quality and/or profits. The *learning organization* is one in which there is a commitment to high-quality work that can result when teams work together to capitalize on the synergy of continuous group learning for optimal performance (Senge, 1994). Institutions have used approaches to creating a learning organization (or learning communities) to implement continuous quality improvement efforts within the corporate and health care sectors, for example. *Communities of practice,* or "groups of people informally bound together by shared expertise and passion for a joint enterprise" (Wenger & Snyder, 2000, p. 139), represent a specific model that some organizations use to develop members' capabilities and to build and exchange knowledge within and across organizations either electronically or through regular personal communication, such as e-mail discussion groups or listservs, for example. Members of communities of practice join them voluntarily; their passion, commitment, and identification with the group's expertise and interests hold the group together.

The discussion that follows illuminates the blueprint for reinventing public health, grounded in a realistic understanding of the political, social, and economic forces that shape the strategic environment in which the field of practice must operate as well as the growing body of knowledge regarding how best to define and address the health of the public.

Major Public Health Trends

Three public health revolutions have influenced the development and evolution of the field worldwide. The first public health revolution was essentially concerned with the role of public sanitation and the corollary use of medical police power, meaning the formulation and enforcement of public health laws and regulations to protect the health of individuals and the public. The second public health revolution, following on the Lalonde report in Canada in 1974, ignited public health investments in lifestyle and related behavioral change to reduce risky behaviors, such as smoking, alcohol consumption, and drug abuse, or to promote healthy practices, such as the use of screening or preventive services. The third public health revolution, credited with launching a new public health, acknowledged that macro social and economic forces are at play in exposing individuals and communities to risk and that a fuller engagement of affected parties and a broader policy agenda are required to successfully address or ameliorate these risks (Awofeso, 2004; Kickbusch, 2003; Szreter, 2003; Tesh, 1988).

As this chapter mentioned earlier, the neoliberal politics of the 1980s in the United States led to cutbacks in federal and state investments in health and social welfare programs, including public health. The call to reinvent government (Osborne & Gaebler, 1992) yielded a template for the Clinton administration to streamline, privatize, and contract out services that public agencies and entities had previously provided directly.

In the early 1990s the promise of significant health care reform was visible on the political horizon. The Clinton Health Care Plan sought to restructure the U.S. health care system by building on the growing consolidation of the system into large-scale, competing, managed care plans. Philip Lee, assistant secretary for health in the U.S. Department of Health and Human Services, saw that reform proposal as an opportunity to reinvent public health as well. Governmental public health had increasingly come to assume a role as a provider of the safety net for clinical care services for uninsured and particularly at-risk populations in many states and localities. Medicaid funding had also come to be a major source of revenue for supporting public health departments in many states and localities. As a result, however, governmental public health had begun to stray or had fewer resources to put into more population health rather than personal health care services and programs. The prospect of having more universal financing for health care services opened a window of opportunity for public health to more effectively serve its population health–oriented mission ("Lee Closes Meeting," 1993; Lee & Paxman, 1997).

These hopes were fundamentally dashed, however, with the failure of health care reform by the mid-1990s. The growing dominance of the for-profit managed care industry and the resulting competition for Medicaid enrollees who had traditionally been served by publicly supported agencies, including public health providers, have led to a significant diminishment of revenues for these safety-net providers. Governmental public health and the related public health infrastructure have undergone a significant period of reassessment and redesign in many states and localities.

A promising offshoot of these transformations, however, as well as of the mandate for change that the population health and related social determinants agenda have offered, is that there is an opportunity for governmental public health to assume leadership and a new vision for reinventing the field of public health in ways that strengthen its prospects for realizing its long-standing population health mission in new ways and with renewed promises of success.

Instructive guidance for reinventing public health to respond to the issues dominating the third public health revolution has been documented in various sources, including reports from the WHO (1999, 2000; Commission on Macroeconomics and Health, Working Group 1, 2002), the work of Canadian researchers (CIAR, 2004; Coburn et al., 2003; Evans & Stoddart, 2003; Glouberman & Millar, 2003), and Institute of Medicine reports (Committee for the Study, 1988; Committee on Assuring, 2003; Committee on Educating, 2003) on the future of the field.

Key elements of these calls for reform are as follows:

- Transdisciplinary (in contrast to a disciplinary, multidisciplinary, or interdisciplinary) research base
- Population health–centered
- Grounded in the fundamental social and economic determinants of health
- Participatory and inclusive
- Intersectoral in design

The Institute of Medicine report *The Future of the Public's Health in the 21st Century* (Committee on Assuring, 2003) calls for a transdisciplinary research paradigm for identifying and addressing public health problems in new ways.

Figure 1.1 provides an instructive contrast between disciplinary, multidisciplinary, interdisciplinary, and transdisciplinary research (Albrecht, Freeman, & Higginbotham, 1998). *Disciplinary research* turns itself on problem areas that permit theory development and hypothesis testing within a discipline. *Multidisciplinary research* acknowledges that research teams may need to represent more than one field of study, with appropriate division of labor or specialized expertise, to address a particular problem area. *Interdisciplinary research* more directly enforces team building in the service of addressing complex problems in which multicausal explanations might exist. A limited number of disciplines may be able to reach consensus regarding a common definition of problems or solutions. *Transdisciplinary research* moves to a different level of synthesis and integration through the formulation of a research framework for defining and addressing a problem, which integrates what may have previously been discrete or competing points of view for addressing the problem. The definition of the problem expands to include and integrate all relevant disciplinary insights. This book is inherently transdisciplinary in focus by drawing on a variety of disciplines and policy domains (summarized in Table 1.1) for identifying and addressing the determinants of population health.

FIGURE 1.1.   COMPARISONS OF DISCIPLINARY, MULTIDISCIPLINARY, INTERDISCIPLINARY, AND TRANSDISCIPLINARY RESEARCH PARADIGMS.

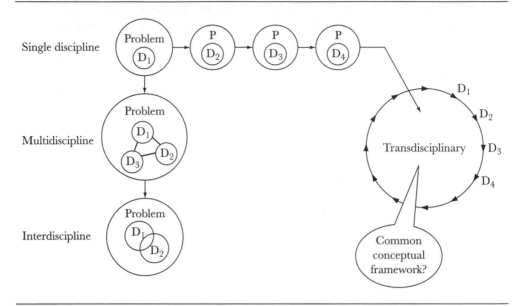

Note. D_1, D_2, D_3, and D_4 refer to different disciplines. P refers to different ways of viewing or defining the problem that may be emphasized by different disciplines. From "Complexity and Human Health: The Case for a Transdisciplinary Paradigm," by G. Albrecht, S. Freeman, and N. Higginbotham, 1998, *Culture Medicine and Psychiatry, 22*, p. 64, fig. 1. Used by permission of Springer Science and Business Media.

Improving the health of populations—and reducing health disparities—is the implicit and central policy agenda framing the book and the specific chapters that follow. Chapter Two more fully discusses issues related to the definition and measurement of population health. The following chapters are replete with discussion of the growing body of evidence regarding the importance of social, economic, and environmental factors in influencing the health of individuals and populations. The Institute of Medicine (Committee on Assuring, 2003) has suggested that an ecosocial paradigm guide the design of research and related development of an intersectoral public health system. Figure 1.2 and the related research and policy mandate are intended to highlight the central role of what some may view as more distal social, economic, and environmental factors that shape the risks and resources available to individuals, communities, and populations for preventing disease and producing and assuring good health.

There is a growing understanding, however, that different policy agendas may be informed and motivated by how researchers measure and model population

FIGURE 1.2.   ECOSOCIAL TRANSDISCIPLINARY PARADIGM.

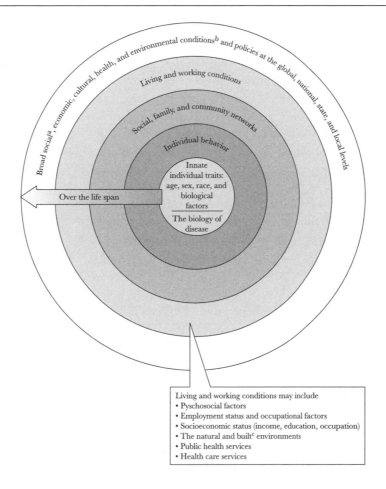

Living and working conditions may include
- Pyschosocial factors
- Employment status and occupational factors
- Socioeconomic status (income, education, occupation)
- The natural and built[c] environments
- Public health services
- Health care services

Note. From *The Future of the Public's Health in the 21st Century,* by the Institute of Medicine, Committee on Assuring the Health of the Public in the 21st Century (Washington, DC: National Academies Press, 2003), p. 52, fig. 2-2. Originally from *Policies and Strategies to Promote Social Equity in Health,* by G. Dahlgren and M. Whitehead (Stockholm, Sweden: Institute for Futures Studies, 1991), p. 11, fig. 1. Used by permission of the Institute for Futures Studies.

[a]Social conditions include but are not limited to economic equality, urbanization, mobility, cultural values, attitudes, and policies related to discrimination and intolerance on the basis of race, gender, and other differences.

[b]Other conditions at the national level might include major sociopolitical shifts, such as recession, war, and governmental collapse.

[c]The built environment includes transportation, water and sanitation, housing, and other dimensions of urban planning.

health and its determinants. Research on population health may be centrally intended to describe current levels or difference, measure change, explain what causes differing levels of health or illness, and/or evaluate the success of interventions in addressing it (McDowell, Spasoff, & Kristjansson, 2004).

Further, policy interventions may focus on *fundamental causes* or attempt to be *ameliorative* of the more immediate causes of illness (see Table 1.3). Fundamental causes refer to *distal* (macro) social-structural factors related to underlying material conditions or resources (such as income) and their distribution, whereas *intervening mechanisms* refer to more immediate *proximate* (micro) psychosocial-behavioral causes of illness (high-risk behaviors such as smoking or feelings of social isolation, for example) (Krieger, 2001; Link & Phelan, 1995; Tarlov, 2000). This book focuses on fundamental, distal social and economic determinants of population health in the service of guiding the formulation of a broad policy and action agenda for both improving population health and reducing health disparities.

Hilary Graham (2004a, 2004b) also importantly points out that frameworks for understanding the social determinants of *health disparities* would differ in important ways from those one might use to examine the social determinants of *population health*. The focus on the *health gap* between groups underlying health disparities and the focus on the *health gradient* in population health research (that is, better health tends to be associated with more material and social resources) may also lead to different political agendas and investments—focusing on the particularly socially disadvantaged versus growing the economy as a whole to improve everyone's health. The tensions between these competing points of view will be illuminated later in discussions of examples of the research and policy mandates

TABLE 1.3. DIFFERING PERSPECTIVES ON POPULATION HEALTH AND HEALTH DISPARITIES.

Dimensions	Perspectives	
	Fundamental Causes	*Ameliorative Interventions*
Focus	Social-structural	Psychosocial-behavioral
Predictors	Material conditions	Intervening mechanisms
Outcomes	Health disparities	Population health
Measurement	Health gap	Health gradient
Examples	Ottawa Charter ("New Public Health") Health Promotion program	Canadian Institute for Advanced Research (CIAR) Population Health program

emanating from these respective points of view, such as the Ottawa Charter Health Promotion and CIAR programs.

The framework for examining racial segregation as a fundamental determinant of population health (Schulz, Williams, Israel, & Lempert, 2002) (shown in Figure 1.3) illustrates the fundamental and sequential intermediate, proximate, and resulting health impacts of race-based residential segregation. Macrosocial factors such as historical racism, economic structures, and legal codes have resulted in concentrated patterns of race-based segregation in many U.S. localities, which has also exacerbated and subsequently been exacerbated by diminished employment and educational opportunities. The concentration of racially and socioeconomically disadvantaged populations in highly segregated communities has yielded a community infrastructure and social environment that has often led to land use and associated industrial practices that produce higher health risks in the community. Diminished social integration and support, the presence of social stressors such as violent crime and the illegal drug trade, and health-related high-risk behaviors and practices ultimately lead to the poorer health of residents in such areas. Perspectives such as those provided by the field of social determinants research and related applications, as in the framework from Schulz and associates (2002), underline the essential importance of a broader policy agenda to fundamentally and ultimately improve the health of populations and communities.

Critics of conventional (particularly governmental) public health practice have argued that it has paid insufficient attention to engaging affected populations in identifying and addressing community problems, focused on community deficits and ignored community assets, and dominated decision making regarding the design of programs and allocation of resources to address identified needs. As a consequence, programs have either been ineffective or failed to be sustained beyond the life of external funding or investments by outside entities or agencies in supporting them. Chapter Six reviews the importance of community development and associated participation and empowerment in addressing the weaknesses of previous public health interventions and in building successful new models for public health intervention and practice. The call to strengthen civil society and apply the principles of deliberative democracy in building institutions to support it mentioned earlier in a broader political context is echoing resoundingly in the field of public health as elaborated in Chapter Six.

And finally, public health as a field is being summoned to consider the design of an intersectoral public health system to more effectively address the fundamental determinants of population health that scholars are increasingly identifying and documenting. Since the inception of the field of public health, the health of populations has been a defining focus, in contrast to the focus on the health of individuals in the field of clinical medicine. Public health has, however, largely been

FIGURE 1.3. RACIAL SEGREGATION AS A FUNDAMENTAL DETERMINANT OF RACIAL DISPARITIES IN HEALTH.

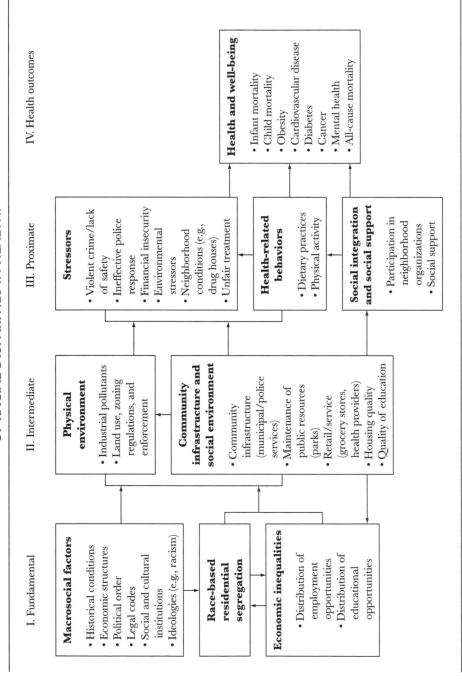

I. Fundamental   II. Intermediate   III. Proximate   IV. Health outcomes

Macrosocial factors
- Historical conditions
- Economic structures
- Political order
- Legal codes
- Social and cultural institutions
- Ideologies (e.g., racism)

Race-based residential segregation

Economic inequalities
- Distribution of employment opportunities
- Distribution of educational opportunities

Physical environment
- Industrial pollutants
- Land use, zoning regulations, and enforcement

Community infrastructure and social environment
- Community infrastructure (municipal/police services)
- Maintenance of public resources (parks)
- Retail/service (grocery stores, health providers)
- Housing quality
- Quality of education

Stressors
- Violent crime/lack of safety
- Ineffective police response
- Financial insecurity
- Environmental stressors
- Neighborhood conditions (e.g., drug houses)
- Unfair treatment

Health-related behaviors
- Dietary practices
- Physical activity

Social integration and social support
- Participation in neighborhood organizations
- Social support

Health and well-being
- Infant mortality
- Child mortality
- Obesity
- Cardiovascular disease
- Diabetes
- Cancer
- Mental health
- All-cause mortality

Note. From "Racial and Spatial Relations as Fundamental Determinants of Health in Detroit," by A. J. Schulz, D. R. Williams, B. A. Israel, and L. B. Lempert, 2002, *Milbank Quarterly, 80,* p. 682, fig. 1. Used by permission of Blackwell Publishing.

delimited—as was the case in a 1988 report by the Institute of Medicine—by governmentally supported public health departments and agencies at the national, state, county, and local levels. The broadened vision of public health as a field directed to improving population health reflected in the more recent Institute of Medicine reports (Committee on Assuring, 2003; Committee on Educating, 2003) signals the importance of the full partnership and leadership of conventional public health practice with other policy and practice arenas (e.g., medicine, business, media) in creating an intersectoral public health system. This book provides a more expansive and explicit policy blueprint for forging such a system.

Table 1.2 highlights the key elements in developing such a system and its corollary grounding in contributing to a healthy republic *and* healthy public.

As indicated earlier, public investments in federal, state, county, and city government public health departments have provided for the defining core of public health as a field of practice. Only 3% to 4% of federal health care expenditures are related to public health or related health promotion, prevention, or protection services (National Center for Health Statistics, 2003). Thus, governmental public health represents an important but relatively small public investment in population health.

In contrast, particularly in the United States, the medical care delivery system represents the lion's share of public and private expenditures for what is largely a private, increasingly market- and corporate-dominated purveyor of clinical services. The twin forces of competition and profitability have challenged the managed care industry to develop more of a population health perspective in calibrating enrollee risk profiles and related premium and fee structures. Other challenges have come from outside the industry, from public health and other population health advocates, to develop socially responsible managed care that provides more fundamental investments on the part of managed care in disease prevention and health promotion efforts in the service of both lower health care costs and improved population health (Schlesinger et al., 1998; Showstack, Lurie, Leatherman, Fisher, & Inui, 1996).

A Third Way that is increasingly at play in the public health and health care arena is the growth of public-private partnerships (Linder, Quill, & Aday, 2001). With the devolution and increasing privatization of what had been publicly funded and delivered services, governmental agencies, including health departments at all levels, have been forced into a position of reducing core staff and/or contracting out services. At its best, the growth of public-private partnerships has facilitated a combining of resources across agencies and/or with nongovernmental or business groups that recognize how to serve their mutual interests by investing in a public health problem that is creating major drains on both public and private resources (e.g., alcohol and drug addiction). Maintaining the power balance in such collaborations when resources and values may differ greatly has been and continues to be the challenge in forging and maintaining such partnerships.

The WHO has assumed leadership for addressing persistent population health problems and health disparities. In the 1970s it created its initiative of Health for All, forged through the 1978 Alma Alta Declaration, which focused on developing and providing primary care; in the mid-1980s it created the Health Promotion initiative, grounded in the 1986 Ottawa Charter (Kickbusch, 2003). The Ottawa Charter in particular argued for the greater activist involvement of affected communities in identifying assets and addressing identified needs. The WHO Healthy Cities and Healthy Communities initiatives represent prominent examples of the more holistic and social change orientation to public health action, working to engage communities and a variety of health and nonhealth sectors within the community to address fundamental health and health care needs (Awofeso, 2004).

Controversy has surfaced within Canada and other countries that the emergence of *population health* as a defined research and policy focus, most notably credited to the work of Robert Evans and his collaborators at the CIAR, has led to a more conservative and less participatory community change and political action agenda (Coburn et al., 2003; Evans & Stoddart, 2003; Glouberman & Millar, 2003; Raphael & Bryant, 2002). This debate is grounded in the variant perspectives on fundamental causes versus intervening mechanisms discussed earlier (Table 1.3). Chapter Two will review the issue more fully.

The CIAR policy agenda calls for a multisectoral focus on population health policy that engages the finance as well as other government ministries in considering the impact of their policies on the fundamental determinants of population health (e.g., the distribution of income and wealth) and corollary health disparities. The population health approach may then be viewed as concerned with creating new intersectoral policies and related institutions to address the fundamental determinants of population health. Critics argue that in doing so, population health fails to give sufficient weight to the underlying differences in the distribution of political and economic power shaping such policies and the need for more fundamental social and political change for policies to be successful in improving population health.

As summarized in Table 1.2, this book acknowledges that powerful economic and political values, forces, and trends fundamentally shape both the past and the future of public health and that the field must attend in actions and design to those values, forces, and trends. Creating a healthy republic in the service of a healthy public compels the design of an intersectoral public health system in the light of these changes. The blueprint for the design of such a system will emerge in the chapters that follow, and the final chapter of the book more fully describes its specific architecture.

As conveyed in Table 1.2, the design of such a system must acknowledge and balance the competing values and priorities of politics of the right and left; the roles of government, community, and market as agents of change and impact; the powerful political, economic, and social forces that shape nations, states, and provinces as well as the localities and institutions (including public health) within them; and effective public-private partnerships between and among governmental public health, privatized medical care, intersectoral population health–centered policies, and community-centered health and development initiatives.

The book purposely steps outside the boundaries that have conventionally defined the field of public health. In particular, the book draws on the domains of sustainable, human, economic, and community development policies and programs and critically reviews the evidence regarding the fundamental determinants of population health in the context of those determinants that the respective domains most importantly influence.

Policy Criteria

Figure 1.4 and Table 1.4 highlight the fact that policies in a variety of domains may directly or indirectly affect population health and related disparities. The chapters that follow assemble and evaluate existing evidence regarding the impact of *fundamental determinants* on *population health and health disparities* (pathway A). Such evidence provides the essential foundation for exploring the impacts of policies in a given domain on relevant determinants. *Current policies* in a given area, such as human development and educational policy, may affect *population health and health disparities* in one of two ways, either indirectly (pathway B) through influencing the *fundamental determinants* of population health (school achievement, level of education, and related

FIGURE 1.4.   PATHWAYS FOR EVALUATING POLICIES.

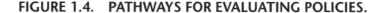

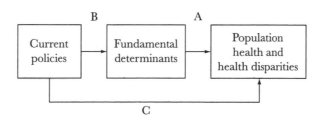

Note. The policy evaluation questions addressed by the relationships implied in causal pathways A, B, and C are presented in Table 1.4.

TABLE 1.4.   CRITERIA FOR EVALUATING POLICIES.

	Criteria[a]		
	Effectiveness	**Efficiency**	**Equity**
Definitions	Fundamental determinants of population health and health disparities	Mix and level of investments to maximize population health, given available resources	Fairness and effectiveness of policies for minimizing population health disparities
Indicators	Independent and direct effects	Technical (production) efficiency Allocative efficiency Dynamic efficiency	Intergenerational justice Distributive justice Deliberative justice Social justice
Evaluation[b]	**A.** Does research on the fundamental determinants addressed in a given domain document the independent and direct effect of these determinants on population health and health disparities?	**A.** What mix of inputs within and across domains seems to be most efficient in producing health improvements?	**A.** What equity criteria principally underlie research on fundamental determinants in a given domain?
	B and/or C. Do current policies serve to improve population health and reduce health disparities?	**B and/or C.** Do current policies invest in the most efficient mix of inputs to produce health improvements?	**B and/or C.** Do current policies satisfactorily address some or all of the equity criteria?

[a]See *Evaluating the Healthcare System: Effectiveness, Efficiency, and Equity,* by L. A. Aday, C. E. Begley, D. R. Lairson, and R. Balkrishnan (3rd ed.; Chicago: Health Administration Press, 2004).

[b]A, B, and C correspond to the pathways shown in Figure 1.4.

skills of individuals and groups) or *directly* (pathway C) through programs that explicitly target the health needs of selected populations (child nutrition, health education, and school health services, for example).

Table 1.4 highlights the major questions that this book will pose within a specific domain and across domains to assess major policies in the respective areas. A central hypothesis of the book is this:

The prospects for improving the health of individuals and communities are enhanced by policies that address the fundamental determinants of health.

This book's authors will use the criteria of effectiveness, efficiency, and equity in identifying and presenting available evidence regarding this hypothesis.

The *effectiveness* criterion will assess the weight of the evidence of the potential and actual impact of selected determinants on population health and health disparities. The *efficiency* criterion will guide an examination of the mix and level of investments (e.g., public education and/or economic development) that maximizes population health, given available resources. The *equity* criterion examines the extent to which one may judge policies to be fair, based on the application of explicit criteria of justice within and across policy domains (Aday et al., 2004; Handler, Issel, & Turnock, 2001).

The essential questions and related criteria to evaluate the effectiveness, efficiency and equity of current policies are summarized in Table 1.4.

The central question for determining effectiveness is this: Does research on the fundamental determinants addressed in a given domain document the independent and direct effect of these determinants on population health and health disparities? One would evaluate policies with respect to existing evidence regarding the extent to which the policies directly or indirectly improve population health and reduce health disparities.

The central question for determining efficiency is this: What mix of inputs within and across domains seems to be most efficient in producing health improvements? One can evaluate efficiency with respect to whether current policies invest in the most efficient mix of inputs to produce health improvements, taking into account the following efficiency dimensions:

- Technical (production) efficiency: whether the least possible resources are used to produce the intermediate outcomes (i.e., the fundamental determinants of population health such as education or income) [pathway B in Figure 1.4]
- Allocative efficiency: whether the mix of intermediate outcomes (i.e., fundamental determinants of population health) maximizes final outcome (population health improvement), given resource constraints [pathway A in Figure 1.4]
- Dynamic efficiency: whether inputs are used so as to maximize value over the long run, taking into consideration the need to entice technological and organizational changes needed to achieve that value (population health in this case) [pathways B and/or C in Figure 1.4]

Solid empirical evidence is not available at present to fully evaluate existing policies in terms of this array of efficiency criteria. Thus, the efficiency assessments of the policies in the chapters that follow will focus on qualitative assessments of whether greater or lesser investments of resources in a given domain, relative to others, may be warranted, based on available evidence regarding their documented impact on population health and health disparities.

The equity criterion poses the following two questions: (a) What equity criteria principally underlie research on fundamental determinants in a given domain? and (b) Do current policies satisfactorily address some or all of the equity criteria? One may apply the following criteria of justice in assessing the equity of existing policies:

- Intergenerational justice: maintenance of resources and benefits across generations
- Distributive justice: fair distribution of benefits and burdens across individuals and communities
- Deliberative justice: full and effective participation of affected parties in decision making
- Social justice: minimization of health disparities between groups

The equity analyses will identify the principal equity criteria that either explicitly or implicitly underlie a given policy domain, as well as the trade-offs in equity resulting from emphasizing a given criterion of fairness to the exclusion of others.

Conclusion

Public health and health services research in recent decades has amply documented the role of fundamental nonmedical versus medical determinants of population health and health disparities (see Chapter Two). These include environmental, social, and economic factors, such as environmental risks, education, occupation, employment, and income; social support; and related community empowerment, which health care services or policy do not typically or directly address.

Immense political, economic, and cultural changes nationally and internationally compel new directions for public heath and population health–centered policy. The dominance of economic forces in the globalization of markets and financial capital and corollary policies to devolve the role of centralized governments and welfare states in providing safety nets of publicly supported services have had major consequences for the health of nations and communities.

In order to successfully achieve its mission of improving the health of populations and reducing health disparities, the field of public health must expand to encompass broader domains of policy and practice that affect the fundamental determinants of population health. This book critically reviews the evidence regarding the impact of sustainable, human, economic, and community development on the fundamental determinants of population health and provides a blueprint for the redesign of the field of public health policy and practice to more fully encompass these domains. The blueprint is grounded in the vision of a healthy (re)public, in which public decision making takes into account the impacts of policies related to fundamental determinants on the health of the populations that these policies target.

This book is intended to be a resource to students and professionals in a variety of policy arenas in gaining an understanding of the implications of the growing body of research on the fundamental determinants of health for the design of more health-centered programs and policies.

This book extends and applies the growing body of evidence on the fundamental determinants of population health in designing more health-centered public policy based on the following:

- Enlarging the domains of policy to consider sustainable, human, economic, and community development policy, in addition to public health policy and practice
- Lodging the examination of these issues in the context of sustainability principles that take into account the balance of environmental, efficiency, and equity criteria in maintaining benefits and resources across generations
- Applying explicit criteria of effectiveness, efficiency, and equity in evaluating available evidence on the fundamental determinants of population health and health disparities
- Expanding training and practice in public health to encompass development research, policy, and practice and advancing the insights and understanding of development specialists regarding the impact of their activities on the health and health risks of the populations that their initiatives target

In summary, this book provides an integrative framework for guiding the development of more health-centered public policy and identifies what still needs to be known and done to improve population health and ameliorate health disparities. It presents a vision and a challenge (a) to the field of public health to design more effective means for addressing its long-standing commitment to promoting and protecting the health of the public and (b) to domains of intervention and influence that have traditionally been outside the purview of public health to revisit ways to enhance their successes by joining with public health in initiatives to improve population health and reduce health disparities.

References

Aday, L. A. (1997). Vulnerable populations: A community-oriented perspective. *Family and Community Health, 19*(4), 1–18.

Aday, L. A., Begley, C. E., Lairson, D. R., & Balkrishnan, R. (2004). *Evaluating the healthcare system: Effectiveness, efficiency, and equity* (3rd ed.). Chicago: Health Administration Press.

Albrecht, G., Freeman, S., & Higginbotham, N. (1998). Complexity and human health: The case for a transdisciplinary paradigm. *Culture, Medicine and Psychiatry, 22,* 55–92.

Awofeso, N. (2004). What's new about the "new public health"? *American Journal of Public Health, 94,* 705–709.

Bourdieu, P. (1998). *Acts of resistance: Against the tyranny of the market* (R. Nice, Trans.). New York: New Press.

Canadian Institute for Advanced Research. (2004, April 19). *Successful societies program.* Retrieved September 17, 2004, from http://www.ciar.ca/web/prdocs.nsf/0/6fe56f1 eb2f6bcfa85256cc600603ff8?

Coburn, D. (2000). Income inequality, social cohesion and the health status of populations: The role of neo-liberalism. *Social Science and Medicine, 51,* 135–146.

Coburn, D., Denny, K., Mykhalovskiy, E., McDonough, P., Robertson, A., & Love, R. (2003). Population health in Canada: A brief critique. *American Journal of Public Health, 93,* 392–396.

Complex systems. (1999, April 2). *Science, 284,* 79–109.

Dahlgren, G., & Whitehead, M. (1991). *Policies and strategies to promote social equity in health.* Stockholm, Sweden: Institute for Futures Studies.

Denzin, N. K., & Lincoln, Y. S. (Eds.). (2000). *Handbook of qualitative research* (2nd ed.). Thousand Oaks, CA: Sage.

Evans, R. G., & Stoddart, G. L. (2003). Consuming research, producing policy? *American Journal of Public Health, 93,* 371–379.

Freire, P. (1970). *Pedagogy of the oppressed* (M. B. Ramos, Trans.). New York: Continuum.

Giddens, A. (2000). *The Third Way and its critics.* Malden, MA: Blackwell.

Glouberman, S., & Millar, J. (2003). Evolution of the determinants of health, health policy, and health information systems in Canada. *American Journal of Public Health, 93,* 388–392.

Graham, H. (2004a). Social determinants and their unequal distribution: Clarifying policy understandings. *Milbank Quarterly, 82,* 101–124.

Graham, H. (2004b). Tackling inequalities in health in England: Remedying health disadvantages, narrowing health gaps or reducing health gradients? *Journal of Social Policy, 33,* 115–131.

Habermas, J. (1996). *Between facts and norms: Contributions to a discourse theory of law and democracy* (W. Rehg, Trans.). Cambridge, MA: MIT Press.

Handler, A., Issel, M., & Turnock, B. (2001). A conceptual framework to measure performance of the public health system. *American Journal of Public Health, 91,* 1235–1239.

Hardt, M., & Negri, A. (2000). *Empire.* Cambridge, MA: Harvard University Press.

Institute of Medicine, Committee for the Study of the Future of Public Health. (1988). *The future of public health.* Washington, DC: National Academies Press.

Institute of Medicine, Committee on Assuring the Health of the Public in the 21st Century. (2003). *The future of the public's health in the 21st century.* Washington, DC: National Academies Press.

Institute of Medicine, Committee on Educating Public Health Professionals for the 21st Century. (2003). *Who will keep the public healthy? Educating public health professionals for the 21st century.* Washington, DC: National Academies Press.

Kickbusch, I. (2003). The contribution of the World Health Organization to a new public health and health promotion. *American Journal of Public Health, 93,* 383–388.

Kindig, D., & Stoddart, G. (2003). What is population health? *American Journal of Public Health, 93,* 380–383.

Krieger, N. (2001). A glossary for social epidemiology. *Journal of Epidemiology and Community Health, 55,* 693–700.

Kuhn, T. S. (1996). *The structure of scientific revolutions* (3rd ed.). Chicago: University of Chicago Press.

Lalonde, M. (1974). *A new perspective on the health of Canadians: A working document.* Ottawa, Ontario, Canada: Department of National Health and Welfare.

Lee closes meeting with White House plan to reinvent public health. (1993). *The Nation's Health, 12,* 24.

Lee, P., & Paxman, D. (1997). Reinventing public health. *Annual Review of Public Health, 18,* 1–35.

Linder, L. H., Quill, B. E., & Aday, L. A. (2001). Academic partnerships in public health practice. In L. F. Novick & G. P. Mays (Eds.), *Public health administration: Principles for population-based management* (pp. 521–538). Gaithersburg, MD: Aspen.

Link, B. G., & Phelan, J. (1995). Social conditions as fundamental causes of disease. *Journal of Health and Social Behavior* [Special issue], 80–94.

Mathur, S. K., & Aday, L. A. (2002). Decision-making for rural community sustainability: The role of social capital in mediating the limitations of market and planning models. *Texas Journal of Rural Health, 20*(4), 52–61.

McDowell, I., Spasoff, R. A., & Kristjansson, B. (2004). On the classification of population health measurements. *American Journal of Public Health, 94,* 388–393.

Mulhall, S., & Swift, A. (1996). *Liberals and communitarians* (2nd ed.). Cambridge, MA: Blackwell.

National Center for Health Statistics. (2003). *Health, United States, 2003, with chartbook on trends in the health of Americans* (DHHS Publication No. PHS 2003–1232). Hyattsville, MD: Public Health Service.

Navarro, V. (Ed.). (2002). *The political economy of social inequalities: Consequences for health and quality of life.* Amityville, NY: Baywood.

Navarro, V., & Shi, L. Y. (2001). The political context of social inequalities and health. *Social Science and Medicine, 52,* 481–491.

Osborne, D., & Gaebler, T. (1992). *Reinventing government: How the entrepreneurial spirit is transforming the public sector.* Reading, MA: Addison-Wesley.

Raphael, D., & Bryant, T. (2002). The limitations of population health as a model for a new public health. *Health Promotion International, 17,* 189–199.

Schlesinger, M., Gray, B., Carrino, G., Duncan, M., Gusmano, M., Antonelli, V., et al. (1998). A broader vision for managed care, part 2: A typology of community benefits. *Health Affairs, 17*(5), 26–49.

Schulz, A. J., Williams, D. R., Israel, B. A., & Lempert, L. B. (2002). Racial and spatial relations as fundamental determinants of health in Detroit. *Milbank Quarterly, 80,* 677–707.

Senge, P. M. (1994). *The fifth discipline: The art and practice of the learning organization.* New York: Currency Doubleday.

Showstack, J., Lurie, N., Leatherman, S., Fisher, E., & Inui, T. (1996). Health of the public: The private-sector challenge. *Journal of the American Medical Association, 276,* 1071–1074.

Szreter, S. (2003). The population health approach in historical perspective. *American Journal of Public Health, 93,* 421–431.

Tarlov, A. R. (2000). Public policy frameworks for improving population health. In A. R. Tarlov & R. F. St. Peter (Eds.), *The society and population health reader: Vol. 2. A state and community perspective* (pp. 310–322). New York: New Press.

Tesh, S. N. (1988). *Hidden arguments: Political ideology and disease prevention policy.* New Brunswick, NJ: Rutgers University Press.

Wenger, E. C., & Snyder, W. M. (2000). Communities of practice: The organizational frontier. *Harvard Business Review, 78,* 139–145.

Whiteis, D. G. (1998). Third world medicine in first world cities: Capital accumulation, uneven development and public health. *Social Science and Medicine, 47,* 795–808.

Whiteis, D. G. (2000). Poverty, policy, and pathogenesis: Economic justice and public health in the U.S. *Critical Public Health, 10,* 257–271.

Woodward, D., Drager, N., Beaglehole, R., & Lipson, D. (2004). Globalization, global public goods, and health. In N. Drager & D. Vieira (Eds.), *Trade in health services: Global, regional, and country perspectives* (pp. 3–12). Washington, DC: Pan American Health Organization.

World Health Organization. (1999). *The world health report 1999: Making a difference.* Geneva: Author.

World Health Organization. (2000). *The world health report 2000: Health systems: Improving performance.* Geneva: Author.

World Health Organization, Commission on Macroeconomics and Health, Working Group 1. (2002). *Health, economic growth, and poverty reduction: The report of Working Group 1 of the Commission on Macroeconomics and Health.* Geneva: Author.

CHAPTER TWO

FUNDAMENTAL DETERMINANTS OF POPULATION HEALTH

Kathryn M. Cardarelli, Janet S. de Moor,
M. David Low, Barbara J. Low

Chapter Highlights

- The fundamental determinants of population health are grounded in the social, genetic, and physical environments and may influence multiple risk factors and health outcomes by directly shaping individual health behaviors as well as shaping access to living conditions, lifestyles, and goods and services such as health care and social resources.
- The population health perspective recognizes the entire spectrum of fundamental determinants and their interrelationships with health. As an approach it addresses both those factors that have been traditionally addressed as influencing health, such as individual health behavior, and those that are more distal from one's immediate environment, such as social capital or socioeconomic position.
- The outcomes of population health strategies extend beyond improved health status to include wider social, economic, and environmental benefits.
- Effective population health policy must affect an individual's social and economic circumstances over the course of a lifetime.

• **Although the U.S. health policy community is still struggling with major inequalities of access to health care and there is almost no emergent population health policy at the national level, other industrialized nations, such as Australia, Canada, Sweden, and the United Kingdom, have taken a more holistic approach to the development of health policy.**

The idea that social and environmental factors may have profound influences on human health is not new. As early as 400 BCE, Hippocrates (*On Airs, Waters and Places*) instructed would-be physicians to consider their patients' living environment and way of life as necessary components in taking a medical history.

Louis Villermé, a French statistician who pioneered many of the basic methods of what we now think of as epidemiology, carried out a remarkable series of studies on mortality in Paris in the early 19th century. He documented significant differences in mortality rates between neighborhoods (*arrondissements*) that were not due to differences in environmental factors such as quality of water, air, soil, and seasonal temperature or humidity, all of which had been thought to be causes of disease. Another newly emerging field, sociology, had begun to examine the relationship of social factors such as wealth and poverty to health and well-being; and by borrowing concepts from that new discipline, Villermé was able to demonstrate a nearly perfect fit between neighborhood mortality rates and relative poverty or wealth. He concluded that because both poverty and wealth were factors amenable to social policy, social or public policy could be important determinants of the health of populations. In her description of Villermé's work, Krieger (1992, p. 417) pointedly observed that his findings about the nature of disease "did not depend on technological or biomedical breakthroughs, but upon broadening the natural discourse of science with explicitly political concepts." This insight nicely frames the field of study of population health and related policies addressed in this chapter.

A 20th-century landmark event in the history of population health is directly attributable to the fields of policy and politics. After the government of Canada had enacted the legislation that provided for generous federal sharing in the cost of medical and hospital care delivered by the provinces, the federal minister of health published a monograph titled *A New Perspective on the Health of Canadians* (Lalonde, 1974) in which he asserted that the health of the population did not depend primarily on medical care but on nonmedical factors such as sociodemographic, geographic, and environmental influences. The publication had an impact on public health thinking around the world, and was an important factor in the 1980 decision of Julius Richmond, then the U.S. surgeon general, to establish new health goals for the United States based on knowledge of health disparities and the expectation of reducing them through broad-based, government-sponsored health promotion programs.

Canadian and British researchers have made important new contributions to the field of population health. Researchers at the Canadian Institute for Advanced Research Program in Population Health have labored for over 20 years, with active participation from researchers in the United States and the United Kingdom, to conduct, evaluate, and synthesize research from relevant fields such as economics, sociology, political science, demography, public health, and medicine in order to understand more fully why some people are healthy and others not (Evans, Barer, & Marmor, 1994). Their work has made defining contributions to illuminating the influence of social hierarchies on population health and health disparities. These Canadian researchers made no claim to inventing a new field of science or even of public health, but their ability to see common ground in the published works of so many different disciplines and their discovery of the ubiquity of the socioeconomic gradient in health represent landmark contributions to the field. British researchers Richard Wilkinson (1996) and Michael Marmot and his colleagues (1984, 2001, 2004) have similarly conducted innovative research, particularly in the United Kingdom and the United States, that has stimulated serious and creative inquiry into the role of occupational hierarchies, income, and income inequalities in health.

Notwithstanding the existing and growing knowledge of the importance of population-level social, economic, and environmental factors to health over the last forty years, public health in general and epidemiology in particular have continued to focus on identifying individual-level risk factors in preventing disease. In her critique of modern epidemiology, Krieger (1994) summarized how the field is guided by the tenet of multiple causation, in the expectation of finding the "web of causation." Krieger argues that epidemiologic research is predominantly occupied with delineating the interrelated risk factors responsible for patterns of health and disease. The dominant framework fails to distinguish between determinants of individual health and determinants of population health and does not fully address why or how diseases occur. The web-of-causation interpretation of disease causality gives prominence to biomedical risk factors and implies that populations are the sum of their individual parts, subordinating or even ignoring contextual factors that influence the prevalence and distribution of risk factors in a given population (Krieger, 1994; Shy, 1997).

British epidemiologist Geoffrey Rose (1985) suggested that public health should shift its attention away from individuals and begin to study the characteristics of populations. One of the key tenets of his argument was that "A large number of people exposed to a small risk may generate many more cases than a small number exposed to a high risk" (p. 37). That is, the small number of individuals at high risk for heart disease, for example, represents only a small proportion of all deaths from the condition (McKinlay & Marceau, 1999), yet the dominant prevention strategy in the United States devotes huge efforts to the identification of those individuals who are at highest risk for a disease, the modification of risk factors in this small population, and ultimately to their treatment. A shift in prevention perspective according to Rose's suggestion would have profound implications for public health policy. We would no longer continue to funnel finite resources only to those who are at highest risk for a disease by targeting expensive interventions that may be appropriate for particular individuals (e.g., screening); instead, we would use those resources more efficiently to reduce the entire burden of a disease within a population. Rose noted that focusing on population-level variables such as socioeconomic position or environmental pollution would have greater utility in prevention strategies, because removal of such factors would potentially decrease the incidence of disease. Despite the potential to significantly affect the burden of disease in a population, an important limitation of Rose's strategy is that "a preventive measure which brings much benefit to the population offers little to each participating individual" (Rose, 1985, p. 38).

Rose's second insight is that the causes of individual cases may not be the same as the causes of population rates of disease. This observation has important implications for population health. Although most chronic diseases in industrialized countries are associated with individual health behaviors, social and cultural forces at the population level may influence individual behavioral choices. That is, we may think of behavior as a proximal determinant of some disease, whereas social and physical factors act as more distal or fundamental determinants in a chain of causation. For example, cigarette smoking is a proximal determinant of emphysema, but media advertising practices that influence smoking habits may be a more distal factor in the causal pathway to emphysema. Rose (1985) did not suggest ignoring proximal causes of disease altogether but urged that the public health community place greater priority on identifying and modifying those causes of disease that exist at the population level. These factors may facilitate the expression of the individual-level risks or may act directly on the distribution of the individual-level risks themselves (Schwartz & Diez-Roux, 2001).

This broad view of the origins of good and bad health, as distinct from focus on the mechanisms of disease, is slowly gaining attention in the United States (McKinlay & Marceau, 2000). Air and water quality, social and economic conditions, education policies, adequate housing, and the availability of safe transportation affect whole populations, not just specific individuals; and the growing concern over health disparities that are systematically related to these factors is one of the drivers of this shift in attention. The population health approach is a response to the need for broader and more effective frameworks to guide research and public policy.

In summary, we may define *population health* as "the health of a population as measured by health status indicators and as influenced by social, economic, and physical environments, personal health practices, individual capacity and coping skills, human biology, early childhood development, and health services" (Dunn & Hayes, 1999, p. S7). Improving population health therefore requires understanding the ecology of health and the interrelationships among contextual factors and health outcomes. We may conceptualize these contextual factors as the fundamental determinants of population health, which represent critical resources that serve to improve health and well-being (Link & Phelan, 1995). This chapter provides an overview of the research related to the fundamental determinants of health as well as efforts to address such evidence in population health policy.

Conceptual Model

Although scholars have developed many models to explain the interconnectedness among the fundamental determinants, including the biological, social, and political environments and health outcomes, we have chosen to use the framework of Evans and Stoddart (1990, 2003), because it captures the broad range of proximate and distal determinants of population health and depicts the direction and dynamic nature of the relationship between the fundamental determinants and health (see Figure 2.1).

Evans and Stoddart's framework (1990, 2003) grounds the fundamental determinants in the social, biological/genetic, and physical environments and modifies them to reflect the relationship of population health to the model's principal components. Specifically, we subsume the concepts of well-being and prosperity into the concept of population health. We made this change in order to reflect the comprehensive definition of population health emerging within the field and defined by Dunn and Hayes (1999). We have also modified the original model (Evans & Stoddart, 1990) to reflect recent research on the potential influence of socioeconomic and environmental factors on genetic expression. The core of the original model remains, as do the fundamental concepts that guide the framework.

The physical and socioeconomic environments and genetic and other biological endowments can interact along dynamic pathways to affect the development of disease directly or indirectly, as in the case of the social environment, through their effects on an individual's behavioral (e.g., smoking, drinking, exercise) and biological (e.g., suppressed immune function, neuroendocrine response, autonomic nervous system dysregulation) response to the external stressors. A person's behavioral or biological response to environmental stressors directly affects health, functional capacity, and the development of disease.

FIGURE 2.1.   CONCEPTUAL FRAMEWORK OF FUNDAMENTAL DETERMINANTS OF POPULATION HEALTH.

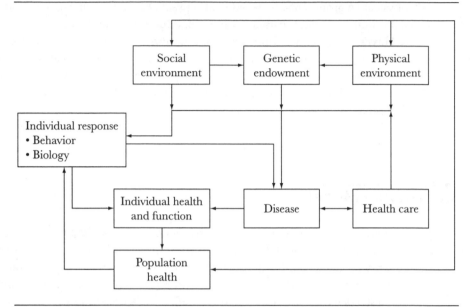

Note. Adapted and reprinted from "Producing Health, Consuming Health Care," by R. G. Evans & G. L. Stoddart, 1990, *Social Science and Medicine, 31*, p. 1359, fig. 5. Used with permission from Elsevier. See also Evans & Stoddart (2003).

Evans and Stoddart (1990) depicted disease and health care in the context of a feedback loop, in which the level of disease is positively related to health care intervention, which is then negatively related to the level of disease. The receipt of health care is determined by a person's perceived need and the level of access afforded to that person, and the effectiveness of the health care intervention is determined by the degree to which it decreases the level of disease and improves health. In this model, health care resources do not directly affect population health. This is important to note because it contrasts with the prevailing biomedical approach to improving the health of populations by providing additional resources for medical care. The only factors that have a direct influence on population health are the social and physical environment (otherwise known as fundamental determinants) and individual health and function. The social and physical environment may also indirectly affect population health through individual behavior, which influences individual health and function.

The framework shown in Figure 2.1 is unique in that it differentiates between disease as the health care system defines it, a definition that is driven by the state of knowledge and technology; health as the individual defines it, a definition driven by one's perceived sense of health and functional capacity; and health as one can measure it within a population.

The framework on which we base our conceptual model (Evans & Stoddart, 1990) is widely used in the field of population health, although some criticized it for lacking breadth and depth and for simplifying the relationships between the different components of the model. Coburn and colleagues (2003) argued that the Evans and Stoddart model of the determinants of population health is too simplistic and does not address a more complex reality. In other words, the model may not clearly depict the dynamic nature of the relationships among the fundamental determinants, one's genetic makeup, the health care system, and health outcomes. Similarly, Poland, Coburn, Robertson, and Eakin (1998) suggested that the model oversimplifies the relationship between wealth and health.

Although we believe that one of the greatest strengths of Evans and Stoddart's framework (1990, 2003) is its simplicity, we have modified it here by adding the concept of population health; and we wish to emphasize that the factors influencing health status exist at both the individual and population levels. We also emphasize that readers should understand all variables, and the interrelationships among them, as acting over time in a social, cultural, and geographical context. Policies of all kinds and at all levels of administration have the potential to affect each of the depicted factors and the ways in which they interact with one another. Finally, we do not intend the model to be an exhaustive catalog of the fundamental determinants of health. The relative importance of each of the broad factors in the model depends on the health outcome of interest, as well as on factors such as the life stage of the individual in question (see Chapter Four) and the type and magnitude of specific exposures within each factor.

Coburn and colleagues (2003) also charged that the model fails to include a vision for agency and action, that is, the means through which situations can change, especially through social and political struggles to bring about improved living conditions and better health care. We acknowledge the value in this political economy perspective on the fundamental determinants of population health that economic and political factors "create, enforce and perpetuate economic and social privilege and inequality" (Krieger, 2001, p. 670). One may interpret the model to include the change that may result from social movements, such as social cohesion, and the political environment, within the factor of social environment. This implicit agency factor can be a strength of the model because it can serve as a guide to classes of indicators, kinds of evidence, and their interrelationships to inform the design and implementation of effective policy interventions.

Although the model lacks an explicit time variable, it inherently recognizes the dynamic state of the depicted relationships, as well as the effect of time, including both the accumulation of exposures over time and any possible differences in the interrelationships at any one point in the life course.

Some also criticized the Evans and Stoddart framework (1990, 2003) for its apparent de-emphasis of the importance of health care. Poland et al. (1998) suggested that the model unfairly minimizes the contribution of health care to alleviating certain illnesses or to improving quality of life. But as Evans and Stoddart (2003, p. 375) pointed out, the model sees clinical medicine as central for those who are currently ill, and primary care that "exploits" the potential for preventive interventions and coordinates the care for those with multiple co-morbid conditions can affect population health. Although clinical interventions undoubtedly do save lives and improve quality of life at the individual level, they cannot fully explain why some populations are healthier than others. It follows that simply increasing investments in health care is not an efficient way of improving the health of the population.

In sum, we believe that although critics (Coburn et al., 2003; Poland et al., 1998) have raised important issues about the Evans and Stoddart framework, we also believe that the framework as we have modified it provides a comprehensive and illustrative model of the fundamental determinants of population health, a model that has the potential for broad application in population health–oriented research and policy development. We will use the framework in a later section of this chapter that organizes and presents the evidence regarding the fundamental determinants of population health.

Measuring Population Health

No consensus exists as to the most appropriate measure of population health, although researchers have recently made advances in measuring it (Institute of Medicine, Committee on Summary Measures of Population Health, 1998; Murray, Salomon, & Mathers, 2000; World Health Organization, 2002). There are many measures of mortality, morbidity, and corresponding perceptions of well-being. One should tailor the choice of measure to the intended purpose, whether in policy development or research. For example, if a program planner in a large metropolitan region wishes to evaluate the effectiveness of maternal and child health clinics, she may examine whether there is a significant association between the number and location of maternal and child health clinics and low–birth weight deliveries. In this case, she might select an area-based measure of population health, such as the prevalence of low birth weight in the different census tracts, and use the findings to make a decision about moving clinics or creating new ones. An example from a research perspective that is grounded in the fundamental determinants of health is the association between levels of civic participation in a community and the health of those who live in the community. Depending on the hypothesized pathways through which one believes social factors to influence health, an appropriate measure of population health might be one that reflects the quality of life of the community members, such as self-rated health.

Morgenstern (1995) has proposed three categories of population health measures: aggregate, environmental, and global. Aggregate measures involve combining information from individuals, such as population morbidity rates. Environmental measures focus on factors that are external to the individual, such as air quality, but may have a corresponding measure at the individual level. Global measures do not have a corresponding measure at the individual level and include contextual factors such as social policies.

Although most approaches to population health currently use aggregate measures, McDowell, Spasoff, and Kristjansson (2004) suggest that measuring the health status of a population using a single indicator such as health-adjusted life expectancy is too limiting and that researchers should use a more comprehensive approach that includes environmental- and global-level measures. They argue that along with measures of morbidity and mortality, it would be useful to include measures of health processes within the population, such as the degree of commitment to reducing social disparities in population health (measured, for example, as consistent promulgation of evidence-based social and health policy to reduce disparities). Equity, effectiveness, and efficiency may be applied as criteria for evaluating the impact of such policies. (The definition, indicators, and applications of these criteria for evaluating policies are elaborated in Table 1.4 in Chapter One.)

Often neglected in discussions regarding the best measures of population health are the ethical and policy implications of using different measurement strategies. Certainly, the choice of measure for population health can affect policy decisions. Some have suggested that traditional measures of population health may be insensitive to important questions of distributive justice (Daniels, 1998). This is the case when public health officials advocate for laws requiring seat-belt usage and immunization of all children. These efforts offer modest benefits to individual drivers or children in the short term but may offer tremendous benefits to the population as a whole through reductions in the loss of life and injury and associated direct and indirect costs. As the Institute of Medicine report (Committee on Summary Measures, 1998) pointed out, although it is unlikely that a single, universally accepted measure of population health should be determined, it would be useful for policy purposes to increase consensus on which measures to use for which purposes.

Research on the Fundamental Determinants of Health

Research on the influence of fundamental determinants on health has proliferated over the last twenty years, aimed at explaining and addressing the widening social inequalities in health. The evidence stems from diverse fields including epidemiology, medicine, psychology, public health, economics, and sociology. Sir Michael Marmot (2004) and many others have noted that the distribution of health within a population appears to follow a social gradient: the higher one's position in the social hierarchy, the lower the risk of ill health. Although the slope of the gradient may vary between countries and regions, and over time within a given country's population, the gradient appears to have existed in all societies and at all times in history. Although the finding is robust, the explanations for such a strong relationship between social position and health are not yet clear. According to the conceptual model in Figure 2.1, the major determining factors are most likely to be in the social environment and the physical environment.

Although the chapters that follow will discuss in further detail the empiric findings in these areas, we present a brief overview of the key findings on the fundamental determinants of population health.

Social Environment

Much of the research into the causes of health inequalities has centered on the influence of socioeconomic position (SEP). SEP reflects social stratification; research studies usually define it operationally by measures of income, occupation, and/or education. The mechanisms through which SEP is associated with morbidity and mortality are not clear, but elucidating the pathways will depend in part on determining the relative contribution of each of the major indicators of SEP—income, occupation, and education—and distinguishing the construct that each of the factors represents.

Income reflects spending power and access to nutrition, housing, transportation, and health care. Some suggest that the relationship between income and health is explained by physiologic effects of a person's relative social and economic circumstances (Marmot & Wilkinson, 2001), and others argue that the explanation lies in differential access to material resources (Lynch, Smith, Kaplan, &

House, 2000). Chapter Five further details this debate. Occupation or employment status may represent varying degrees of physical activity, prestige, responsibility, exposure to toxic substances, and other working conditions, all of which may increase one's risk of morbidity and/or mortality (Leigh, 1983; Mackenbach et al., 1997; Ross & Mirowsky, 1995). Occupation also serves as a major link between education and income (Lynch & Kaplan, 2000).

Finally, education represents an accumulation of knowledge, skills, and abilities learned in school and through experience (Mirowsky & Ross, 2003). Education shapes employment opportunities and earning potential (Ross & Van Willigen, 1997; Ross & Wu, 1995); confers psychosocial resources such as a sense of control and social support; and engenders health-promoting behaviors such as exercising, eating a healthy diet, and refraining from smoking, drinking, and substance use (Ross & Wu, 1995). Chapter Four will discuss in further detail the pathways through which the work environment and education may influence health.

SEP may influence health through differential exposure to social forces that may have a more direct impact on health (Adler & Newman, 2002). For example, individuals of low SEP are more likely to be socially isolated, a characteristic that some have linked to increased risk of mortality (Berkman & Glass, 2000). Specifically, individuals who are socially isolated or who have little engagement in social networks have an increased risk of all-cause mortality (Berkman & Syme, 1979; Blazer, 1982; House, Robbins, & Metzner, 1982; Kaplan et al., 1988; Orth-Gomer & Johnson, 1987; Penninx et al., 1997; Schoenbach, Kaplan, Fredman, & Kleinbaum, 1986; Seeman et al., 1993; Seeman, Kaplan, Knudsen, Cohen, & Guralnik, 1987; Sugisawa, Liang, & Liu, 1994; Vogt, Mullooly, Ernst, Pope, & Hollis, 1992; Welin et al., 1985). Again, there is no consensus on the pathways through which this occurs, although scholars have suggested a few. Social support may prevent a stressful or threatening appraisal of a difficult life event or may affect physical health by facilitating or hindering health behaviors such as eating a healthy diet, exercising, smoking, or consuming alcohol (Cohen, 1988; Cohen & Wills, 1985). Social support can also increase immune competence or suppress the neuroendocrine and hemodynamic response, both of which can impede the development of coronary artery disease (Cohen, 1988; Cohen & Wills, 1985). Moreover, social isolation may affect the rate of aging (Berkman, 1988).

We can distinguish *social capital*, a term that denotes those features of social structures that serve as resources for individuals and that facilitate collective action (Coleman, 1990; Putnam, 1993), from social networks or social support by its level of measurement. Social capital and social cohesion are collective or group-level dimensions of the social environment, whereas social networks or social support is measured at the individual level (Kawachi & Berkman, 2000). Epidemiologic studies have found that social capital is inversely associated with overall mortality at the state level (Kawachi, Kennedy, Lochner, & Prothrow-Stith, 1997) and with individual-level self-rated health (Kawachi, Kennedy, & Glass, 1999). Proposed pathways through which social capital may influence health outcomes include exposure to health behaviors of neighborhood residents (Rogers, 2003); differential access to services and amenities (Sampson, Raudenbush, & Earls, 1997); and psychosocial processes, by boosting interpersonal trust (Kawachi et al., 1997) or by building self esteem (Wilkinson, 1996). Chapter Six provides a fuller discussion of social capital as it relates to community development.

Discrimination, conceptualized as forms of expressing dominance and oppression among social relationships (Krieger, 2000), is another exposure in the social environment that may be related to health. Groups to which discrimination may be directed include those based on gender, sexual orientation, race or ethnicity, age, or disability. Evidence of the impact of discrimination on mental health suggests that self-reported experiences of discrimination are associated with poorer health; potential pathways through which this may occur include exposure to noxious substances or hazardous work conditions, inadequate health care, economic or social deprivation, or direct mental or physical trauma (Krieger, 2000). Social isolation resulting from discrimination and racial segregation has been proposed as a mechanism through which poverty is perpetuated among African Americans living in inner-city areas (Wilson, 1996). An exploratory study found that the experience of racial discrimination by low-income African American mothers was associated with very low birth weight of their infants (Collins et al., 2000). Researchers are now developing new approaches and refining methodology related to measuring the experience of discrimination to better examine the influence of discrimination on health outcomes (Institute of Medicine, Committee on Understanding and Eliminating Racial and Ethnic Disparities in Health Care, 2003).

Physical Environment

Physical environments that result in exposure to harmful agents have direct health consequences. Lead, asbestos, carbon dioxide, and industrial waste are a few of these noxious agents. Scholars have consistently linked outdoor air pollution to asthma morbidity and mortality (Wong & Lai, 2004), and studies have identified household crowding as a significant risk factor for respiratory illness in children (Bulkow, Singleton, Karron, Harrison, & Alaska RSV Study Group, 2002; Holberg et al., 1991).

The widening of social disparities in health may be directly linked to conditions in neighborhoods. The geography of a neighborhood has the potential to influence the infrastructure that will develop, which in turn may influence the resident population and ultimately the social contacts among residents (Macintyre & Ellaway, 2003). For example, certain industries may choose a location based on availability of transportation such as a major waterway. A concentration of petrochemical facilities in one community may result in higher levels of ambient air pollution or lower property values and a subsequent decline in quality of life in the neighborhood. Equally, the physical characteristics of an environment may exist for reasons associated with the social environment. For example, government agencies may locate toxic waste dumps in places that are predominantly home to a population less likely to resist the construction of such an entity in its neighborhood. The environmental justice movement seeks to eliminate such situations by achieving the same degree of protection from environmental and health hazards and equal access to decision-making processes regardless of race, culture, or income (U.S. Environmental Protection Agency, 2004). Chapter Three discusses issues of environmental justice more fully.

Evidence to date suggests that there may be a moderate association between neighborhood conditions (including both physical and social conditions) and health outcomes, after controlling for individual SEP and other characteristics (Kawachi & Berkman, 2003). For example, older adults who reside in deteriorated neighborhoods experience more physical health problems than do elderly people who dwell in more favorable living environments (Krause, 1993, 1998). Adolescents who live in dangerous neighborhoods marked by graffiti, low residential stability, and low SEP have higher levels of depression, anxiety, oppositional defiant disorder, and conduct disorder (Aneshensel & Sucoff, 1996). Noise pollution may be associated with increased levels of hypertension and cardiovascular disease (Stansfeld & Matheson, 2003). However, most of the studies that found these associations have relied on cross-sectional data, and the results are therefore subject to various interpretations including reverse causation (in which the outcome may have caused the exposure rather than the other way around). An example of bias is the suggestion that cognitive or emotional processes, such as beliefs about how the environment and health are related, may lead to reporting bias—that is, research subjects may selectively disclose or conceal information that distorts the true relationship between neighborhood characteristics and health (Macintyre & Ellaway, 2003).

How neighborhood characteristics operate to affect health is still not completely clear, but it may involve cognitive or emotional processes in addition to physical effects. A neighborhood's physical conditions, including architectural design and boarded-up housing, as well as the ambient hazards, such as graffiti, crime, violence, and drug dealing, shape the opportunities for social interaction and physical activity and residents may perceive them as threatening (Aneshensel & Sucoff, 1996; Cohen et al., 2003). This may in turn trigger certain emotional processes or influence health-risk behavior. Further, physical structures may influence criminal behavior by increasing opportunities to commit crime or by limiting informal social controls (Cohen et al., 2003). Figure 1.3 in Chapter One traces the intervening and downstream health consequences of race-based residential segregation, for example.

Based on data gathered in the 1960s and 1970s, British epidemiologist David Barker suggested that characteristics of the physical environment that influence child development may have consequences for adult mortality. A study of three small neighboring towns in Britain found varying standardized mortality ratios for all-cause mortality and for ischemic heart disease and cerebrovascular disease (Barker & Osmond, 1987). Compared to the British average, one town had 21% greater mortality; another was 10% above the average; the third was the same as the national average. To explain these differences, investigators looked to historical information from the turn of the century about living and working conditions. They concluded that in addition to poor maternal health and infant-feeding practices, poor housing and dampness were largely responsible for the differences in mortality.

One of the challenges in understanding the impact of neighborhood conditions on health is that it involves simultaneously studying the influence of individual-level characteristics and the influence of characteristics at the group or contextual level. Recent advances in statistics offer considerable promise for identifying the impact of neighborhood characteristics on population health. Multi-level analysis allows investigators to examine data at each of these levels simultaneously (Duncan, Jones, & Moon, 1998; Subramanian, Jones, & Duncan, 2003). This allows for improved efficiency of estimation and more sensitive evaluation of the influence of contextual factors on population health, while controlling for individual-level factors (Reise & Duan, 2003).

Individual Response: Behavior and Biology

Many of the exposures described earlier affect health by influencing health behaviors, which in turn shape exposure to physiologic risk factors, ultimately leading to disease. For example, education, a commonly used indicator of SEP, might lead to a greater sense of personal control or optimism about the future (Pincus & Callahan, 1994). A *sense of control* is the belief that one can and does master, control, and shape one's own life (Mirowsky & Ross, 1998). This might empower people to embody health-promoting behaviors, thereby altering health behaviors or adherence to medical treatments or the ability to self-manage chronic illnesses (Mirowsky & Ross, 1998).

What is less clear is which biologic mechanisms may be acting in the pathways linking the fundamental determinants and health, although investigators have proposed a few (Brunner, 2000). One pathway is *biologic embedding* (Hertzman, 1999a, 1999b; Hertzman & Wiens, 1996), the mechanism through which early experiences affect the structural development and the chemistry of the central nervous system, thereby shaping cognitive and emotional development, subsequent academic performance, and primary and secondary coping behavior.

A second pathway through which the determinants of health are experienced and exert their effects is grounded in a life-course perspective. According to this perspective, the accumulation of exposures to adverse environments over the life course may affect one's risk for disease. Environmental exposures experienced during certain critical periods of growth may influence chronic disease risk later in life by programming the structure or function of organs, tissues, or body systems (Brunner, 2000; Kuh & Ben-Shlomo, 2004; Kuh, Ben-Shlomo, Lynch, Hallqvist, & Power, 2003). Chapter Four will fully describe these two frameworks.

The third major proposed pathway linking the fundamental determinants and health is *allostatic load*, operationally defined as the impact of chronic stress on the neuroendocrine and physiological functioning that exerts an influence on health (McEwen, 1998; Taylor, Repetti, & Seeman, 1997). One consequence of stress is an immediate increase in the amount of cortisol circulating in the body (Selye, 1976). Chronic or frequently experienced stress results in chronically high levels of circulating cortisol, which may produce fatigue, immune suppression, insulin resistance, and even structural damage to neurons (Sapolsky, 1998). Some have suggested that social or environmental stressors may influence allostatic load by altering the balance between protective and damaging effects of stress mediators (McEwen, 1998).

Further elucidation of the pathways through which the fundamental determinants affect health should be firmly grounded in appropriate theory. One such theory involves an ecosocial perspective. Krieger (1994; 2001, p. 672) defined an ecosocial approach as one that takes into account "a social production of disease perspective while aiming to bring in a comparably rich biological and ecological analysis." This perspective accounts for simultaneous pathways incorporating social and environmental factors at multiple levels into our biology. It further acknowledges an accumulation of exposures occurring from the time of conception to death (Krieger, 2001). Other guiding theories for research investigating the pathways linking fundamental determinants and health include psychosocial theory (Cassel, 1976; McEwen, 1998) and the social production of disease–political economy of health (Link & Phelan, 1995, 2002). Psychosocial theory asserts that human interactions may result in an adverse biological response, whereas the social production of disease–political economy of health framework does not address biology but suggests that social, political, and economic factors essentially influence health. Finally, we should emphasize that despite a recent increase in research on biologic mechanisms that may explain part of the association between social and environmental exposures and health, researchers should exercise caution when trying to draw conclusions from this limited and evolving body of empirical evidence.

Future Research

The population health research agenda in the United States is still in its infancy, and the majority of studies reflect the prevailing biomedical view of health. Much of the research has focused on identifying and intervening with risk factors among population subgroups and the environments that may explain observed health disparities. Because of the unique history of the United States with respect to slavery and discrimination, population health research in this country is often considered to be synonymous with research on racial and ethnic health disparities. For the most part, in such studies, researchers pay too little attention to larger sociopolitical and macroenvironmental factors (for example, a history of discrimination and blocked social and economic opportunity) that may explain why certain subgroups of people such as racial and ethnic minorities have certain risk factors to begin with or why there are such great variations in health status within particular ethnic or racial subgroups.

It is notable that in 2003, the National Institutes of Health awarded grants to establish eight Centers for Population Health and Health Disparities. Ironically, the focus of the centers' activities was predominantly on the more proximal determinants of health. For example, the centers propose to identify risk factors that might explain disease incidence and prevalence: biological (e.g., the effect of psychosocial factors on tumor development, growth, and response to treatment in animal models) (Gehlert, 2003), behavioral (e.g., determinants of treatment-seeking behavior, screening behavior, and general health behaviors) (Paskett, 2003; Rebbeck, 2003), and psychological (e.g., relationship between psychosocial stressors and allostatic load, identifying salient sources of stress) (Tucker, 2003). The centers had a secondary focus on upstream factors, with projects designed to evaluate the effect of neighborhood-level factors on health (Goodwin, 2003; Lurie, 2003).

To date, research findings on the fundamental determinants of health have come from short- and long-term observational and longitudinal empiric and theoretical studies. These studies employed a variety of study populations, used many different estimation techniques, and controlled for a multitude of factors. Each study's findings add to the body of evidence and should be integrated when used for purposes of developing policy. Of particular concern is the choice of study design based on a carefully specified causal model. Because of the lack of practicality and ethical constraints to randomizing individuals to many types of social and physical factors, the field will continue to rely primarily on observational studies. The complex interrelationships among multiple levels of factors should be considered, and the importance of the different levels should be underscored to aid in policy development and program design. That is, investigators should not only consider how to measure the fundamental determinants (such as race-based residential segregation) but also bear in mind the broader societal meaning and policy import of the resulting findings.

As well as needing sound research design, future studies should employ analytic techniques that measure the association between multiple social and environmental factors and disease. For example, studies that include contextual factors may employ the use of multilevel modeling, which allows an investigator to examine the factors that might affect health at a variety of levels, such as the individual, family, and neighborhood levels (Raudenbush & Bryk, 2002). Another technique that may be of value is structural equation modeling, which allows the investigator to empirically measure the causal relationships between variables— to, for example, specify the precise means through which various determinants (such as income) may ultimately affect health (Kaplan, 2000; MacCallum & Austin, 2000). Selected applications of structural equation modeling allow these effects to be estimated at a variety of levels (Muthen, 1994). These statistical tools have proved useful in the fields of economics, sociology, and psychology and may deserve greater consideration for etiologic research.

Participatory action research may play a role in elucidating the social and political issues related to population health, particularly as it concerns the identification of priority concerns and issues in effective population health policy and in the development, research, and dissemination of solutions to issues. . . . *Community-based participatory research* (CBPR) may be defined as

> a collaborative process that equitably involves all partners in the research
> process and recognizes the strengths that each brings. CBPR begins with a re-
> search topic of importance to the community with the aim of combining knowl-
> edge and action for social change to improve community health and eliminate
> health disparities (Minkler, Blackwell, Thompson, & Tamir, 2003, p. 1210).

Chapter Six will provide greater detail of the role of communities in illuminating issues associated with population health.

Current Policies That Attempt
to Address Fundamental Determinants

Because the population health perspective recognizes the entire spectrum of fundamental determinants and their interrelationships with health, the approach addresses both those factors that investigators have traditionally considered—such as health behavior—and those that are more distal from one's immediate environment—such as social capital or socioeconomic position. Furthermore, the outcomes of population health–oriented strategies extend beyond improved health status to wider social, economic, and environmental benefits (Public Health Agency of Canada, 2002). Lastly, the population health approach is grounded in evidence-based decision making at each stage of policy development and supports research that covers the range of factors that affect health and well-being (Public Health Agency of Canada, 2002).

Investigators have demonstrated repeatedly that social and economic circumstances affect health throughout the life course. It follows, therefore, that effective health policy must affect people's social and economic circumstances over their lifetimes (Marmot, 2004). National-level public policies explicitly based on population health research are in various stages of development in several Western nations, including the United Kingdom (Harrison, 1998; La Parra & Alvarez-Dardet, 2001; Scottish Council Foundation, Healthy Public Policy Network, 1999). In Canada the Canadian Institute for Advanced Research (CIAR) has labored for nearly two decades as a policy enterprise (Hayes & Dunn, 1998; Huynh, 2002; Legowski & McKay, 2000); other efforts are taking place in Australia (Oldenburg, McGuffog, & Turrell, 2000) and Sweden (Ågren, 2003). In this section we briefly describe some of the domestic and international efforts to address population health.

Contrasting Policy Perspectives

As Nijhuis and van der Maesen (1994) suggested, a nation's philosophical orientation toward the public and health drives policymakers' views of the causes of health and disease, which in turn shape both the scope of public health activities and the level of public health intervention. The social philosophy can view the public either as individualistic, with unique individuals as the primary focus, or collectivist, focusing on the social relationships and networks of which individuals are members (Nijhuis & van der Maesen, 1994).

Moreover, as is usually the case in the United States, health can be viewed from a mechanistic orientation, seeing the individual as the sum of his or her biophysiologic and neurophysiologic parts and disease as arising from dysfunction in one or more of these parts. This perspective sees a dichotomy of disease or nondisease and attributes the restoration of health or nondisease to causal mechanisms. Health can also be viewed, according to Nijhuis & van der Maesen, from a holistic perspective, which sees health as an expression of the degree to which an individual is capable of achieving an existential equilibrium within a given set of environments and resources. Disturbance of this equilibrium is interpreted as multilevel and multifactorial, and the focus is on health promotion. Using the latter of these perspectives, McKinlay and Marceau (2000) categorize public health activities that are downstream, such as primary and secondary prevention, as reflecting individualistic and mechanistic ideology and public health activities that are upstream, such as public health policies, as reflecting a collective and holistic ideology.

Policy Examples: United States. The United States is probably the most extreme example of a society that sees health and health care, for the most part, as the responsibility of the individual. The United States is the only country in the Organisation for Economic Co-operation and Development (OECD) that does not have a national health care system. Because of the very high cost of medical care in the United States, where health services are largely treated like consumer goods, access, in particular to primary and preventive care, is often restricted to people with health insurance. The majority of working-age citizens and their dependents have health insurance through their employers. Older individuals and certain people who are disabled receive health insurance from Medicare; and Medicaid covers poor families with children, certain disabled people, and low-income elderly. Some uninsured children living in low-income families are also eligible for health insurance through the State Children's Health Insurance Program (Docteur, Suppanz, & Woo, 2003). Despite these programs, around 16% of the population is uninsured (U.S. Census Bureau, 2004); and low-wage and unskilled workers, people working in the service industry, small business employees, minorities, and immigrants disproportionately bear the burden of not having health insurance (Docteur et al., 2003).

U.S. health policy largely subscribes to a mechanistic view of health and spends the bulk of its resources on downstream approaches, treating people who are already sick or who are at increased risk of becoming sick, rather than on upstream approaches, intervening to keep the total population healthy. The business of biomedicine subsumes most health care specialties including public health. In 2002 the United States spent 14.6% of its gross domestic product (GDP) and $5,267 per capita on health care; by contrast, Switzerland, which has the next most expensive system, spent 11.2% of its GDP and $4,219 per capita on health care (OECD, 2004). Some of the factors responsible for burgeoning health care costs include the early adoption and rapid diffusion of technologically sophisticated interventions and the use of expensive pharmaceuticals (Docteur et al., 2003). A study of health care quality in individual states (Baicker & Chandra, 2004) showed a clear inverse relationship between the amount spent for Medicare services and the quality of care that the patient received. The authors attributed this finding to excessive use of specialist services and too little primary and preventive care. Consistent with these findings is the absence of a direct relationship between overall spending on health care and health status. For example, despite the United States spending far more than any other country in the OECD, its people's life expectancy ranked 21st among the member OECD countries and 24th in infant mortality in 2001 (OECD, 2004).

In the United States, where the health policy community is still struggling with major inequalities of access to health care, there is almost no distinct and coherent population health policy at the national level. The National Policy Association has reviewed the evidence for social determinants of health in the United States and summarized its members' views on desirable policy directions (Auerbach, Krimgold, & Lefkowitz, 2000), concluding that work focusing on the fundamental determinants of health provides a wealth of policy options for future exploration.

On the state level, the Kansas Health Foundation sponsored a conference in 1998 with the intention of designing a blueprint for improving population health in Kansas. The conference resulted in a publication (Tarlov & St. Peter, 2000), but little specific policy change has evolved in that state. In Minnesota public, private, and nonprofit constituencies came together to create the Minnesota Health Improvement Partnership (MHIP), which identified health as a shared responsibility. MHIP continues to leverage the resources of its partner organizations toward achieving jointly developed health improvement goals, and influencing policy directions is an explicit goal (MHIP Social Conditions and Health Action Team, 2001). However, like its counterpart in Kansas, this new enterprise has yet to demonstrate marked policy change.

An Institute of Medicine report (Committee on Understanding, 2003) amply documented important initiatives that have been introduced in the United States to address the disparities in racial and ethnic health care. These include the surgeon general's Healthy People goal of eliminating the differences in health status between minorities, the poor, and the majority white population; the Minority Health and Health Disparities Research Act of 2000; the HealthCare Equality and Accountability Act of 2003; and the Closing the Health Care Gap Act of 2004, among others. In addition to these congressional initiatives, there are several existing reports and studies like the *National Healthcare Disparities Report* (Agency for Healthcare Research & Quality, 2003) and *Making Cancer Health Disparities History* (National Cancer Institute, 2004). As we pointed out earlier, these initiatives focus either on improving access to care for individuals or on attempting to elucidate the reasons for specific kinds of health disparities, tracking, for example, differences in breast cancer survival rates between white and African American women. Their primary focus is not on the fundamental social-structural and economic determinants of racial and ethnic health disparities, such as residential segregation and related social, economic, and environmental health risks.

Policy Examples: Other Countries in the OECD. We shall next examine some policy initiatives that have been undertaken in other OECD countries.

Australia. Just as the social philosophy and orientation toward health drives the biomedical, public health, and population health enterprise in the United States, cultural ideology shapes the face of population health in other countries. For example, to address social disparities in health, Australia has taken a more collective and holistic approach. To improve its population's health, Australia concentrates on social, physical, and economic environments as potential targets for interventions to reduce health disparities, and the nation's plans emphasize collaboration between different social sectors (i.e., housing, education, and employment) to improve the health of disadvantaged groups. National targets for future intervention in Australia include both upstream and downstream approaches designed to change macrolevel social and economic policies to reduce poverty and income inequality, improve living and working conditions, reduce behavioral risk factors in disadvantaged groups, and improve the equity of the health care system by maintaining an accessible universal health care system publicly funded through taxation and by redistributing resources within the health care system to support public health and health promotion (Oldenburg et al., 2000).

United Kingdom. The United Kingdom has been a leader in population health research. From the Whitehall studies (Marmot, Shipley, & Rose, 1984; North et al., 1993), which demonstrated that morbidity and mortality rates were inversely associated with employment grade in the British civil service, to the 1998 *Independent Inquiry into Inequalities in Health Report* (Acheson, 1998), the United Kingdom has demonstrated a commitment to understanding and minimizing social inequalities in health. The recommendations made in the Acheson report are good examples of upstream initiatives intended to reduce health inequalities. The flavor of the recommendations also illustrates a more collective social philosophy and more holistic orientation to health than those of the United States. The Acheson report (p. 120) recommended that "all policies likely to have a direct or indirect effect on health should be evaluated in terms of their impact on health inequalities, and should be formulated in such a way that by favoring the less well off they will, wherever possible, reduce such inequalities." The report also made specific recommendations to improve health disparities stemming from structural factors (i.e., income, education, employment, housing, mobility and pollution, nutrition and agricultural policy, and the national health service) and to improve the health of different population subgroups (that is, mothers, children, and families; young people and working adults; older people; ethnic groups; and men and women).

More recently the United Kingdom drafted a document (Department of Health, 2003) that summarized the national plan to reduce inequalities in infant mortality, overall mortality, and life expectancy. The plan proposes supporting families and children (e.g., mainstreaming Sure Start, a government program that offers early education, child care, health, and family support to all children), engaging communities and individuals (e.g., the National Strategy for Neighborhood Renewal), encouraging prevention and effective health care (e.g., initiatives to reduce smoking, obesity, and injuries and to improve immunization rates), and addressing the underlying determinants of health (e.g., initiatives to improve the social and structural environment). Generally speaking, the United Kingdom has embraced an integrated plan of upstream and downstream approaches to reduce social disparities in health.

Canada. Canada embraces population health as its public health agenda and recognizes the importance of factors external to the medical care system in shaping the public's health (Public Health Agency of Canada, 2002). Several noteworthy contributions identifying nonmedical determinants of health have shaped the present-day face of population health in Canada. For example, in 1974 Lalonde suggested that Canada could achieve greater improvements in health by bettering the social, political, and physical environment rather than increasing resources in the medical care system alone (Lalonde, 1974). In 1986 Epp presented a report at the Ottawa Charter for Health Promotion, which elaborated on Lalonde's ideas by focusing on social and economic determinants of health such as income and education. In 1989 the CIAR coined the term *population health* and posited that social and economic determinants of health interact in a dynamic fashion to affect health status. A report by the Federal, Provincial, and Territorial Advisory Committee on Population Health (1994) illustrated a national commitment to population health and summarized the state of knowledge about social and economic determinants of health and provided a framework to guide population health efforts (Public Health Agency of Canada, 2002). Specifically, this framework for action on population health emphasized the need for policy to address social and economic factors (i.e., income, employment, workplace characteristics), the physical environment (i.e., physical aspects of the workplace, the built environment), personal health practices, individual capacity and coping skills (i.e., coping resources, biological endowment), and health services. In particular, the report emphasized the need to address the dynamic interactions between these factors.

Sweden. Sweden is the most collectively oriented country discussed thus far, and its national public health policy, which functions to generate social conditions to ensure population health, with particular attention to vulnerable population subgroups, illustrates well the nation's comprehensive view of health (Ågren, 2003). This approach evolved from the realization of the limits of medical care and the awareness of growing social disparities in health. National objectives in Sweden are based on influencing the fundamental determinants of health rather than specific diseases because public policy can modify such determinants. Sweden's public health policy outlines 11 objectives that address important determinants of health:

- Strengthen public participation and influence
- Promote economic and social security
- Provide secure and favorable conditions during childhood and adolescence
- Facilitate a healthier working life
- Create a healthy and safe environment and products
- Provide preventive health care and health promotion
- Protect against communicable diseases
- Promote safe sexuality and reproductive health
- Increase physical activity
- Encourage good eating habits and provide safe food
- Reduce alcohol and tobacco use and eliminate illicit drugs and excessive gambling

According to Ågren (2003, p. 6), the breadth of public health objectives in Sweden underscores that "the vast majority of public health work must take place outside the medical care service."

In summary, the population health approach and subsequent policy initiatives of different developed countries reflect both their social philosophy and their beliefs and value systems regarding health and its determinants. As such, the business of population health must be understood and evaluated in context. Indeed, in many ways the business of population health *is* the context in which people live and work. Given the breadth and complexity of fundamental health determinants (see Chapters Three through Six), policy initiatives that are intended to improve the health of the population must also be based on the potential efficiency, effectiveness, and equity of the initiatives. They must have an identifiable scope, act on the determinants of health and their interactions, implement strategies to reduce inequities in health status, apply the appropriate mix of interventions, address health issues in an integrated way, work across the life span, act in multiple settings, establish a coordinating mechanism to facilitate intersectoral action, have a process of continuing evaluation and assessment, and assign accountability for outcomes (Public Health Agency of Canada, 2002).

As McKinlay and Marceau (2000, p. 26) acknowledged, "discussion can advance from a consideration of the advantages and disadvantages of different approaches, or from futile discussion of the 'best' approach, to appreciation of the underlying philosophies and views of health that manifest themselves in everyday health programs and the measurement of their effectiveness and efficiency." From all of the work done in this field to date, one thing is abundantly clear: Allocating more resources to acute care in the form of doctors and hospitals is not the most efficient or effective way to improve population health.

Chapter Three introduces the concept of sustainable development and elaborates the role of the physical environment in influencing human health (see Figure 2.1), particularly the environmental consequences of conventional corporate decision making.

References

Acheson, D. (1998). *Independent inquiry into inequalities in health report.* London: Stationery Office.

Adler, N. E., & Newman, K. (2002). Socioeconomic disparities in health: Pathways and policies. *Health Affairs, 21*(2), 60–76.

Agency for Healthcare Research & Quality. (2003). *National healthcare disparities report, 2003* (AHRQ Publication No. 04–0035). Rockville, MD: Author.

Ågren, G. (2003). *Sweden's new public health policy: National public health objectives for Sweden.* Stockholm: Swedish National Institute of Public Health.

Aneshensel, C. S., & Sucoff, C. A. (1996). The neighborhood context of adolescent mental health. *Journal of Health and Social Behavior, 37*, 293–310.

Auerbach, J. A., Krimgold, B. K., & Lefkowitz, B. (2000). *Improving health: It doesn't take a revolution.* Washington, DC: National Policy Association/Academy for Health Services Research and Health Policy.

Baicker, K., & Chandra, A. (2004). Medicare spending, the physician workforce, and beneficiaries' quality of care. *Health Affairs, 23*(3), W4-184–W4-197.

Barker, D.J.P., & Osmond, C. (1987). Inequalities in health in Britain: Specific explanations in three Lancashire towns. *British Medical Journal, 294*, 749–752.

Berkman, L. F. (1988). The changing and heterogeneous nature of aging and longevity: A social and biomedical perspective. *Annual Review of Gerontology and Geriatrics, 8*, 37–68.

Berkman, L. F., & Glass, T. (2000). Social integration, social networks, social support, and health. In L. F. Berkman & I. Kawachi (Eds.), *Social epidemiology* (pp. 137–173). New York: Oxford University Press.

Berkman, L. F., & Syme, S. L. (1979). Social networks, host-resistance, and mortality: A nine-year follow-up study of Alameda County residents. *American Journal of Epidemiology, 109,* 186–204.

Blazer, D. G. (1982). Social support and mortality in an elderly community population. *American Journal of Epidemiology, 115,* 684–694.

Brunner, E. J. (2000). Toward a new social biology. In L. F. Berkman & I. Kawachi (Eds.), *Social epidemiology* (pp. 306–331). New York: Oxford University Press.

Bulkow, L. R., Singleton, R. J., Karron, R. A., Harrison, L. H., & Alaska RSV Study Group. (2002). Risk factors for severe respiratory syncytial virus infection among Alaska Native children. *Pediatrics, 109,* 210–216.

Cassel, J. (1976). Contribution of social environment to host resistance: Fourth Wade Hampton Frost Lecture. *American Journal of Epidemiology, 104,* 107–123.

Coburn, D., Denny, K., Mykhalovskiy, E., McDonough, P., Robertson, A., & Love, R. (2003). Population health in Canada: A brief critique. *American Journal of Public Health, 93,* 392–396.

Cohen, D. A., Mason, K., Bedimo, A., Scribner, R., Basolo, V., & Farley, T. A. (2003). Neighborhood physical conditions and health. *American Journal of Public Health, 93,* 467–471.

Cohen, S. (1988). Psychosocial models of the role of social support in the etiology of physical disease. *Health Psychology, 7,* 269–297.

Cohen, S., & Wills, T. A. (1985). Stress, social support, and the buffering hypothesis. *Psychological Bulletin, 98,* 310–357.

Coleman, J. S. (1990). *Foundations of social theory.* Cambridge, MA: Harvard University Press.

Collins, J. W., David, R. J., Symons, R., Handler, A., Wall, S. N., & Dwyer, L. (2000). Low-income African-American mothers' perception of exposure to racial discrimination and infant birth weight. *Epidemiology, 11,* 337–339.

Daniels, N. (1998). Distributive justice and the use of summary measures of population health status. In Institute of Medicine, Committee on Summary Measures of Population Health (Ed.), *Summarizing population health: Directions for the development and application of population metrics* (pp. 58–71). Washington, DC: National Academy Press.

Department of Health. (2003). *Tackling health inequalities: A programme for action.* London: Author.

Docteur, E., Suppanz, H., & Woo, J. (2003). *The US health system: An assessment and prospective directions for reform* (OECD Economics Working Paper 350). Paris: Organisation for Economic Co-operation and Development.

Duncan, C., Jones, K., & Moon, G. (1998). Context, composition and heterogeneity: Using multilevel models in health research. *Social Science and Medicine, 46,* 97–117.

Dunn, J. R., & Hayes, M. V. (1999). Toward a lexicon of population health. *Canadian Journal of Public Health—Revue Canadienne de Santé Publique, 90*(Suppl. 1), 7–10.

Epp, J. (1986). *Achieving health for all: A framework for health promotion.* Ottawa, Ontario: Health and Welfare Canada.

Evans, R. G., Barer, M. L., & Marmor, T. R. (Eds.). (1994). *Why are some people healthy and others not? The determinants of health of populations.* New York: Aldine de Gruyter.

Evans, R. G., & Stoddart, G. L. (1990). Producing health, consuming health care. *Social Science and Medicine, 31,* 1347–1363.

Evans, R. G., & Stoddart, G. L. (2003). Consuming research, producing policy? *American Journal of Public Health, 93,* 371–379.

Federal, Provincial and Territorial Advisory Committee on Population Health (Canada). (1994). *Strategies for population health: Investing in the health of Canadians.* Ottawa, Ontario: Health Canada.

Gehlert, S. (2003). *Center for Interdisciplinary Health Disparities Research.* Retrieved April 16, 2004, from Computer Retrieval of Information on Scientific Projects, http://crisp.cit.nih.gov

Goodwin, J. S. (2003). *UTMB Center for Population Health and Health Disparities.* Retrieved April 16, 2004, from Computer Retrieval of Information on Scientific Projects, http://crisp. cit.nih.gov

Harrison, D. (1998). *Integrating health sector action on the social and economic determinants of health: The UK response under New Labour.* Retrieved November 15, 2004, from http://www.rhpeo. org/ijhp-articles/e-proceedings/verona/1/index.htm

Hayes, M. V., & Dunn, J. R. (1998). *Population health in Canada: A systematic review* (Canadian Population Research Networks [CPRN] Study No. H 01). Ottawa, Ontario, Canada: CPRN.

Hertzman, C. (1999a). The biological embedding of early experience and its effects on health in adulthood. *Annals of the New York Academy of Sciences, 896,* 85–95.

Hertzman, C. (1999b). Population health and human development. In D. P. Keating & C. Hertzman (Eds.), *Developmental health and the wealth of nations: Social, biological, and educational dynamics* (pp. 21–40). New York: Guilford Press.

Hertzman, C., & Wiens, M. (1996). Child development and long-term outcomes: A population health perspective and summary of successful interventions. *Social Science and Medicine, 43,* 1083–1095.

Holberg, C. J., Wright, A. L., Martinez, F. D., Ray, C. G., Taussig, L. M., & Lebowitz, M. D. (1991). Risk factors for respiratory syncytial virus–associated lower respiratory illnesses in the first year of life. *American Journal of Epidemiology, 133,* 1135–1151.

House, J. S., Robbins, C., & Metzner, H. L. (1982). The association of social relationships and activities with mortality: Prospective evidence from the Tecumseh Community Health Study. *American Journal of Epidemiology, 116,* 123–140.

Huynh, P. (2002). *The emergence of a population perspective within Canada: The influence of a research organization on the public policy process.* Unpublished doctoral dissertation, University of Texas Health Science Center at Houston School of Public Health.

Institute of Medicine, Committee on Summary Measures of Population Health. (1998). *Summarizing population health: Directions for the development and application of population metrics.* Washington, DC: National Academies Press.

Institute of Medicine, Committee on Understanding and Eliminating Racial and Ethnic Disparities in Health Care. (2003). *Unequal treatment: Confronting racial and ethnic disparities in health care.* Washington, DC: National Academies Press.

Kaplan, D. (2000). *Structural equation modeling: Foundations and extensions.* Thousand Oaks, CA: Sage.

Kaplan, G. A., Salonen, J. T., Cohen, R. D., Brand, R. J., Syme, S. L., & Puska, P. (1988). Social connections and mortality from all causes and from cardiovascular disease: Prospective evidence from Eastern Finland. *American Journal of Epidemiology, 128,* 370–380.

Kawachi, I., & Berkman, L. F. (2000). Social cohesion, social capital, and health. In L. F. Berkman & I. Kawachi (Eds.), *Social epidemiology* (pp. 174–190). New York: Oxford University Press.

Kawachi, I., & Berkman, L. F. (Eds.). (2003). *Neighborhoods and health.* New York: Oxford University Press.

Kawachi, I., Kennedy, B. P., & Glass, R. (1999). Social capital and self-rated health: A contextual analysis. *American Journal of Public Health, 89,* 1187–1193.

Kawachi, I., Kennedy, B. P., Lochner, K., & Prothrow-Stith, D. (1997). Social capital, income inequality, and mortality. *American Journal of Public Health, 87,* 1491–1498.

Krause, N. (1993). Neighborhood deterioration and social isolation in later life. *International Journal of Aging and Human Development, 36,* 9–38.

Krause, N. (1998). Neighborhood deterioration, religious coping, and changes in health during late life. *Gerontologist, 38,* 653–664.

Krieger, N. (1992). The making of public health data: Paradigms, politics and policy. *Journal of Public Health Policy, 13,* 412–427.

Krieger, N. (1994). Epidemiology and the web of causation: Has anyone seen the spider? *Social Science and Medicine, 39,* 887–903.

Krieger, N. (2000). Discrimination and health. In L. F. Berkman & I. Kawachi (Eds.), *Social epidemiology* (pp. 36–75). New York: Oxford University Press.

Krieger, N. (2001). Theories for social epidemiology in the 21st century: An ecosocial perspective. *International Journal of Epidemiology, 30,* 668–677.

Kuh, D., & Ben-Shlomo, Y. (Eds.). (2004). *A life course approach to chronic disease epidemiology* (2nd ed.). New York: Oxford University Press.

Kuh, D., Ben-Shlomo, Y., Lynch, J., Hallqvist, J., & Power, C. (2003). Life course epidemiology. *Journal of Epidemiology and Community Health, 57,* 778–783.

La Parra, D., & Alvarez-Dardet, C. (2001). The new UK health inequalities targets. *Journal of Epidemiology and Community Health, 55,* 289.

Lalonde, M. (1974). *A new perspective on the health of Canadians: A working document.* Ottawa, Ontario, Canada: Department of National Health and Welfare.

Legowski, B., & McKay, L. (2000). *Health beyond health care: Twenty-five years of federal policy development* (Canadian Population Research Networks [CPRN] Discussion Paper No. H 04). Ottawa, Ontario, Canada: CPRN.

Leigh, J. P. (1983). Direct and indirect effects of education on health. *Social Science and Medicine, 17,* 227–234.

Link, B. G., & Phelan, J. C. (1995). Social conditions as fundamental causes of disease. *Journal of Health and Social Behavior* [Special issue], 80–94.

Link, B. G., & Phelan, J. C. (2002). McKeown and the idea that social conditions are fundamental causes of disease. *American Journal of Public Health, 92,* 730–732.

Lurie, N. (2003). *Understanding neighborhood impacts of health.* Retrieved April 16, 2004, from Computer Retrieval of Information on Scientific Projects, http://crisp.cit.nih.gov

Lynch, J. W., & Kaplan, G. A. (2000). Socioeconomic position. In L. F. Berkman & I. Kawachi (Eds.), *Social epidemiology* (pp. 13–35). New York: Oxford University Press.

Lynch, J. W., Smith, G. D., Kaplan, G. A., & House, J. S. (2000). Income inequality and mortality: Importance to health of individual income, psychosocial environment, or material conditions. *British Medical Journal, 320,* 1200–1204.

MacCallum, R. C., & Austin, J. T. (2000). Applications of structural equation modeling in psychological research. *Annual Review of Psychology, 51,* 201–226.

Macintyre, S., & Ellaway, A. (2003). Neighborhoods and health: An overview. In I. Kawachi & L. F. Berkman (Eds.), *Neighborhoods and health* (pp. 20–43). New York: Oxford University Press.

Mackenbach, J. P., Kunst, A. E., Cavelaars, A.E.J.M., Groenhof, F., Geurts, J.J.M., Andersen, O., et al. (1997). Socioeconomic inequalities in morbidity and mortality in Western Europe. *Lancet, 349,* 1655–1659.

Marmot, M. G. (2004). Tackling health inequalities since the Acheson Inquiry. *Journal of Epidemiology and Community Health, 58,* 262–263.

Marmot, M. G., Shipley, M. J., & Rose, G. (1984). Inequalities in death: Specific explanations of a general pattern. *Lancet, 1,* 1003–1006.

Marmot, M. G., & Wilkinson, R. G. (2001). Psychosocial and material pathways in the relation between income and health: A response to Lynch et al. *British Medical Journal, 322,* 1233–1236.

McDowell, I., Spasoff, R. A., & Kristjansson, B. (2004). On the classification of population health measurements. *American Journal of Public Health, 94,* 388–393.

McEwen, B. S. (1998). Stress, adaptation, and disease: Allostasis and allostatic load. *Annals of the New York Academy of Sciences, 840,* 33–44.

McKinlay, J. B., & Marceau, L. D. (1999). A tale of three tails. *American Journal of Public Health, 89,* 295–298.

McKinlay, J. B., & Marceau, L. D. (2000). To boldly go . . . *American Journal of Public Health, 90,* 25–33.

Minkler, M., Blackwell, A. G., Thompson, M., & Tamir, H. (2003). Community-based participatory research: Implications for public health funding. *American Journal of Public Health, 93,* 1210–1213.

Minnesota Health Improvement Partnership Social Conditions and Health Action Team. (2001). *A call to action: Advancing health for all through social and economic change.* St. Paul, MN: Division of Community Health Services.

Mirowsky, J., & Ross, C. E. (1998). Education, personal control, lifestyle and health: A human capital hypothesis. *Research on Aging, 20,* 415–449.

Mirowsky, J., & Ross, C. E. (2003). Education as learned effectiveness. In J. Mirowsky & C. E. Ross (Eds.), *Education, social status and health* (pp. 25–31). New York: Aldine de Gruyter.

Morgenstern, H. (1995). Ecologic studies in epidemiology: Concepts, principles, and methods. *Annual Review of Public Health, 16,* 61–81.

Murray, C.J.L., Salomon, J. A., & Mathers, C. (2000). A critical examination of summary measures of population health. *Bulletin of the World Health Organization, 78,* 981–994.

Muthen, B. O. (1994). Multilevel covariance structure analysis. *Sociological Methods and Research, 22,* 376–398.

National Cancer Institute. (2004). *Making cancer health disparities history: Report of the trans-HHS cancer health disparities progress review group.* Washington, DC: Author.

Nijhuis, H.G.J., & van der Maesen, L. J. (1994). The philosophical foundations of public health: An invitation to debate. *Journal of Epidemiology and Community Health, 48,* 1–3.

North, F., Syme, S. L., Feeney, A., Head, J., Shipley, M. J., & Marmot, M. G. (1993). Explaining socioeconomic differences in sickness absence: The Whitehall II study. *British Medical Journal, 306,* 361–366.

Oldenburg, B., McGuffog, I. D., & Turrell, G. (2000). Socioeconomic determinants of health in Australia: Policy responses and intervention options. *Medical Journal of Australia, 172,* 489–492.

Organisation for Economic Co-operation and Development. (2004). *OECD health data (including second and final Internet update).* Paris: Author.

Orth-Gomer, K., & Johnson, J. V. (1987). Social network interaction and mortality: A six-year follow-up study of a random sample of the Swedish population. *Journal of Chronic Diseases, 40,* 949–957.

Paskett, E. D. (2003). *Reducing cervical cancer in Appalachia.* Retrieved April 16, 2004, from Computer Retrieval of Information on Scientific Projects, http://crisp.cit.nih.gov

Penninx, B.W.J.H., van Tilburg, T., Kriegsman, D.M.W., Deeg, D.J.H., Boeke, A.J.P., & van Eijk, J.T.M. (1997). Effects of social support and personal coping resources on mortality in older age: The Longitudinal Aging Study Amsterdam. *American Journal of Epidemiology, 146,* 510–519.

Pincus, T., & Callahan, L. F. (1994). Associations of low formal education level and poor health status: Behavioral, in addition to demographic and medical, explanations. *Journal of Clinical Epidemiology, 47,* 355–361.

Poland, B., Coburn, D., Robertson, A., & Eakin, J. (1998). Wealth, equity and health care: A critique of a "population health" perspective on the determinants of health. *Social Science and Medicine, 46,* 785–798.

Public Health Agency of Canada. (2002). *Population health approach.* Retrieved January 14, 2005, from http://www.phac-aspc.gc.ca/ph-sp/phdd/

Putnam, R. D. (1993). *Making democracy work: Civic traditions in modern Italy.* Princeton, NJ: Princeton University Press.

Raudenbush, S. W., & Bryk, A. S. (2002). *Hierarchical linear models: Applications and data analysis methods* (2nd ed.). Thousand Oaks, CA: Sage.

Rebbeck, T. (2003). *Determinants of disparity in prostate cancer outcomes.* Retrieved April 16, 2004, from Computer Retrieval of Information on Scientific Projects, http://crisp.cit.nih.gov

Reise, S. P., & Duan, N. (Eds.). (2003). *Multilevel modeling: Methodological advances, issues, and applications.* Mahwah, NJ: Erlbaum.

Rogers, E. M. (2003). *Diffusion of innovations* (5th ed.). New York: Free Press.

Rose, G. (1985). Sick individuals and sick populations. *International Journal of Epidemiology, 14,* 32–38.

Ross, C. E., & Mirowsky, J. (1995). Does employment affect health? *Journal of Health and Social Behavior, 36,* 230–243.

Ross, C. E., & Van Willigen, M. (1997). Education and the subjective quality of life. *Journal of Health and Social Behavior, 38,* 275–297.

Ross, C. E., & Wu, C. L. (1995). The links between education and health. *American Sociological Review, 60,* 719–745.

Sampson, R. J., Raudenbush, S. W., & Earls, F. (1997, August 15). Neighborhoods and violent crime: A multilevel study of collective efficacy. *Science, 277,* 918–924.

Sapolsky, R. M. (1998). *Why zebras don't get ulcers: An updated guide to stress, stress-related diseases, and coping.* New York: Freeman.

Schoenbach, V. J., Kaplan, B. H., Fredman, L., & Kleinbaum, D. G. (1986). Social ties and mortality in Evans County, Georgia. *American Journal of Epidemiology, 123,* 577–591.

Schwartz, S., & Diez-Roux, R. (2001). Commentary: Causes of incidence and causes of cases: A Durkheimian perspective on Rose. *International Journal of Epidemiology, 30,* 435–439.

Scottish Council Foundation, Healthy Public Policy Network. (1999). *The possible Scot: Making healthy public policy.* Retrieved January 3, 2005, from http://www.scottishcouncilfoundation. org/pubs_more.php?p=34

Seeman, T. E., Berkman, L. F., Kohout, F., Lacroix, A., Glynn, R., & Blazer, D. (1993). Intercommunity variations in the association between social ties and mortality in the elderly: A comparative analysis of three communities. *Annals of Epidemiology, 3,* 325–335.

Seeman, T. E., Kaplan, G. A., Knudsen, L., Cohen, R., & Guralnik, J. (1987). Social network ties and mortality among the elderly in the Alameda County Study. *American Journal of Epidemiology, 126,* 714–723.

Selye, H. (1976). *The stress of life* (Rev. ed.). New York: McGraw-Hill.

Shy, C. M. (1997). The failure of academic epidemiology: Witness for the prosecution. *American Journal of Epidemiology, 145,* 479–484.

Stansfeld, S. A., & Matheson, M. P. (2003). Noise pollution: Non-auditory effects on health. *British Medical Bulletin, 68,* 243–257.

Subramanian, S. V., Jones, K., & Duncan, C. (2003). Multilevel methods for public health research. In I. Kawachi & L. F. Berkman (Eds.), *Neighborhoods and health* (pp. 65–111). New York: Oxford University Press.

Sugisawa, H., Liang, J., & Liu, X. (1994). Social networks, social support, and mortality among older people in Japan. *Journals of Gerontology, 49,* S3–S13.

Tarlov, A. R., & St. Peter, R. F. (Eds.). (2000). *The society and population health reader: Vol. 2. A state and community perspective.* New York: New Press.

Taylor, S. E., Repetti, R. L., & Seeman, T. (1997). Health psychology: What is an unhealthy environment and how does it get under the skin? *Annual Review of Psychology, 48,* 411–447.

Tucker, K. (2003). *Center for Research/Nutrition and Health Among the Elderly.* Retrieved April 16, 2004, from Computer Retrieval of Information on Scientific Projects, http://crisp.cit.nih.gov

U.S. Census Bureau. (2004, August 2). *Income, poverty, and health insurance in the United States: 2003* (Current Population Reports P60–226). Washington, DC: Author.

U.S. Environmental Protection Agency. (2004, June 17). *Environmental justice.* Retrieved August 25, 2004, from http://www.epa.gov/compliance/environmentaljustice/

Vogt, T. M., Mullooly, J. P., Ernst, D., Pope, C. R., & Hollis, J. F. (1992). Social networks as predictors of ischemic heart disease, cancer, stroke and hypertension: Incidence, survival and mortality. *Journal of Clinical Epidemiology, 45,* 659–666.

Welin, L., Svardsudd, K., Anderpeciva, S., Tibblin, G., Tibblin, B., Larsson, B., et al. (1985). Prospective study of social influences on mortality: The study of men born in 1913 and 1923. *Lancet, 1,* 915–918.

Wilkinson, R. G. (1996). *Unhealthy societies: The afflictions of inequality.* New York: Routledge.

Wilson, W. J. (1996). *When work disappears: The world of the new urban poor.* New York: Knopf.

Wong, G.W.K., & Lai, C.K.W. (2004). Outdoor air pollution and asthma. *Current Opinion in Pulmonary Medicine, 10,* 62–66.

World Health Organization. (2002). *Summary measures of population health: Concepts, ethics, measurement and applications.* Geneva: Author.

CHAPTER THREE

SUSTAINABLE DEVELOPMENT

Sondip K. Mathur, Carl S. Hacker, Lu Ann Aday

Chapter Highlights

- *Sustainable development* refers to development that creates economic vitality while assuring the stewardship of natural resources.
- The epidemiology of the marketplace examines how and why economic activity may be causing ecosystem change and explores corporate policy initiatives for corrective or ameliorative strategies.
- When routine business decision making ignores defining principles of ecosystem behavior, ecosystems may be persistently stressed, which could ultimately lead to adverse consequences for population health.
- Sustainable business practices make ecological effectiveness and economic profitability the foundation for socially responsible business practice.
- Public health strategies grounded in the sustainable development perspective would broaden the focus from a hazard to a habitat dimension, look beyond sick individuals to stressed ecosystems, and generate corporate strategies to assure the health of populations and communities.

- **Principles from the fields of economics and ecology can contribute to a better understanding of health and population health policy.**

Introduction

This chapter presents evidence regarding the impact of ecosystem change and related ecological determinants on population health, and it introduces an innovative framework to analyze the role of corporate decision making and associated economic activity in exacerbating or ameliorating these impacts. With its focus on the natural environment and ecosystems as fundamental determinants of health, the chapter examines the interaction of the economic system with the ecosystem, associated unintended ecosystem change, related health consequences, and the implications for corporate policy.

The discussion acknowledges the important role of market institutions for resolving the three fundamental questions that all societies must confront:

- What goods and services should be produced and in what quantities?
- How should these goods and services be produced?
- For whom should these goods and services be produced?

Most significantly, these questions are resolved in the marketplace by decentralized economic entities (e.g., businesses and corporations as they respond to business goals to maximize profits in the context of market demand and supply).

The ecological evidence and discussions presented in later sections and summarized in Tables 3.1a to 3.1c. compel an examination of the population health perspective, as conceptualized in recent policy debates by health economists and social epidemiologists (Evans & Stoddart, 2003), which often argued that income and wealth are the fundamental determinants of health. This perspective contends that policies directed toward creating income and wealth, in terms of a health production function, may be considered more efficient than additional investment in curative health care services. Although the evidence on ecological determinants confirms that the health of populations is determined by many factors outside of the formal health care system, we disagree with the assumption that unqualified wealth creation produces population health. The disagreement arises because, when we create economic wealth at the expense of ecosystem function, the ecological determinants of health will counter the welfare gains from economic growth. From an ecological determinants perspective, although society should pay more attention to the wealth-producing aspects of the economy, wealth production must not be premised solely on the assumed positive relationship between wealth and health. The process of wealth creation, when disconnected from ecosystem behavior, may trigger ecological and what might be adverse determinants of population health.

The incidence and distribution of environmental hazards in turn may account for health disparities because the global spread of the impacts of ecosystem change is uneven. Therefore, our interest in the process of wealth creation goes beyond observing the inequities of wealth and socioeconomic status to focus on the inequities in the distribution of environmental risks resulting from economic activity. Finally, although we are sympathetic to recommendations that additional funding for the curative health care system may not always represent a sound investment in population health, our argument includes the notion that the health care system may be treating the symptoms of ecological dysfunction rather than addressing fundamental causes. In the wake of the impact of economic activity on ecosystem function, society may reduce conventional health care costs and promote population health if policies and practices address the ecological correlates of poor health.

Overview

We introduce the concept of an *epidemiology of the marketplace,* which both examines how and why economic activity may be causing ecosystem change with adverse population health implications and explores corporate policy initiatives for corrective or ameliorative strategies. This requires identifying evidence on normal ecosystem function, the ecological determinants of population health, and the economic determinants of ecosystem change.

We use the terms *ecosystem change* and *ecosystem modification* interchangeably, and we avoid using the term *ecosystem degradation* because of its normative content. Furthermore, we recognize the difference between intended and unintended impacts of economic activity. For example, economic development and medical and health care services seek to improve life expectancy and quality of life. Therefore, we consider ecosystem modifications and related adverse population health impacts as among the *unintended* outcomes of economic activity. For example, land transformations and dust accumulations due to mining activities may have unintended human health outcomes such as lung diseases or exposure to toxic materials like mercury.

One should not confuse the epidemiology of the marketplace with ecological epidemiology, a branch of epidemiology that views disease as a result of the ecological interactions between populations of hosts and parasites and environmental factors. In our examination of the epidemiology of the marketplace, we will review the literature that links the impacts on human health due to the modification of the ecosystem connected with economic activity.

Public health is "what we, as a society, do collectively to assure the conditions in which people can be healthy" (Institute of Medicine, Committee for the Study of the Future of Public Health, 1988, p. 1). Our discussions and recommendations extend beyond the governmental model of public health to highlight the relevance and significance of business decision making and corporate policies in the service of population health. We view the policies and actions of corporations as a public health concern. Collective action is manifested in the marketplace, as various market organizations, whether public or private, for profit or not for profit, resolve basic social and economic questions on what, how, and for whom to produce.

Fields of Study

Sustainable development policy refers to development that creates economic vitality while assuring the stewardship of natural resources. Corporate business practices can have important impacts on the environment and human health. Consequently, we identify principles from the fields of economics and ecology to understand population health, and we discuss how the two fields can contribute to a better understanding of population health policy.

Economics is the science of making decisions in the presence of scarce resources. *Resources* are simply anything used to produce a good or service or generally to achieve a goal. In particular, we will be interested in *managerial economics,* which studies how to direct scarce resources in the way that most efficiently achieves a managerial or corporate goal. This is grounded in the principles of microeconomics, which focuses on the behavior of firms, in contrast to macroeconomics, which addresses the issues of local, national, and international economies. Macroeconomics underlies the discussion of the role of economic policies on population health in Chapter Five.

On the other hand, *ecology* is the study of the relationship of living things to one another and to their environment. In particular, we are interested in *ecosystems,* the functioning ecological units characterized by the cycling of matter and the flow of energy (Raven & Berg, 2004). Ecosystems vary in size. A vast tall-grass prairie is an ecosystem, as is a small pothole filled with water. The boundaries of an ecosystem are rarely clear and never rigid. Ecosystems tend to blend into each other. Depending on the scale, our natural environment can be seen as a single ecosystem, or a lake can be divided into several ecosystems.

In the same vein, we define economic systems to be composed of functioning economic units characterized by matter and energy flows. Interactions between functioning economic units (e.g., corporations) and ecological units (i.e., ecosystems) will structure our review of market-related ecological determinants of population health.

This chapter's approach has a starting point somewhat different from conventional economic models, even though it will draw on concepts and principles from that discipline. Rather than attempting a monetary valuation of complex issues such as global warming, species loss, and ecosystem change, the discussion will take an approach that recognizes the biophysical realities underlying the operations of the economic system. The full explication of the causal mechanisms and documentation of related scientific certainty of the ecological impact of economic activity is beyond the scope of this chapter. Given that humans lack both the knowledge and the ability to substitute for the functions of ecosystems and natural cycles, we will argue that policy formulation must either consider the precautionary principle (which we will define shortly) or, at a minimum, be willing to take environmental impacts into account in corporate decision making.

The precautionary principle, adopted by the European Union and by the Rio Declaration from the United Nations Conference on Environment and Development held in 1992 (Grandjean, 2005), recommends that entities should not use the absence of full scientific certainty as a reason to postpone decisions where there is a risk of serious or irreversible ecological harm. In the United States, the principle has inspired legislative mandates aimed at reducing public health risks from exposure to harmful environmental contaminants (Daly & Farley, 2004; Soule, 2004). For example, the Food Quality Protection Act and the Amendment to the Safe Drinking Water Act of 1996 mandate the U.S. Environmental Protection Agency to develop a screening and testing program for endocrine-disrupting chemicals. In this context we conceive corporate responsiveness to imply a strategic approach to avoid unnecessary intrusions into normal ecosystem functions and natural cycles. The strategic approach has two distinct elements: proaction and cost-effectiveness of action.

Proaction refers to a readiness to take action in advance of scientific proof or beyond legal compliance. *Cost-effectiveness* refers to conformance with the goal to achieve economic efficiency. For example, we consider business practices that require use of substances and materials that are easily broken down in ecosystems to be ecologically responsive. These practices, however, are expected to be profitable. This chapter further elaborates and illustrates this strategy in the final section, through a case study of a corporate strategy.

In order to draw out the ecological determinants of population health, we compare and contrast how economic units and ecosystems cycle materials and resources in support of their respective productive activities. Investigators have observed that human health consequences are one consequence of the ecosystem change resulting from economic activities. Market practice is considered ecologically consequential when the economic cycling of resources among competing economic ends may be in opposition, mostly unintentionally, with natural cycles that support normal ecosystem function. This chapter explores the potential for corporate policy to both maximize business profits and promote population health through environmentally responsible business practices.

Epidemiology of the Marketplace

The analytical dimensions of this chapter are outlined in the concept of the epidemiology of the marketplace and illustrated in Figure 3.1. We present evidence on normal ecosystem function, the ecological determinants of population health, and the economic determinants of ecosystem change.

The first set of evidence comprises basic scientific principles and understandings from ecology that define the *function* of ecosystems and identify what natural systems do and do not do as they go about their business of cycling resources and materials around its various components. We present a simple ecological model of a normally functioning ecosystem. We also explain the concept of an ecosystem and define ecosystem modification or change. Examples of ecosystem modification include changes in the nutritional resources in the system; depletion

FIGURE 3.1.   EPIDEMIOLOGY OF THE MARKETPLACE.

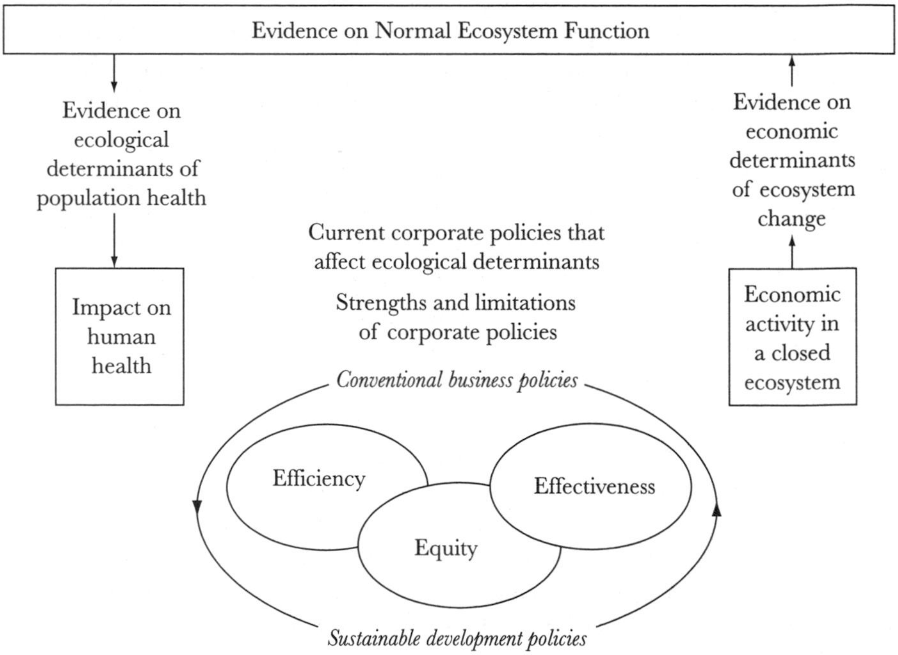

of the atmospheric ozone; climate change; and change in species size, distribution, and diversity. These ecosystem changes may include effects internal to ecosystems or due to external causes.

The second set of evidence on the ecological determinants of population health reviews literature to present selected data regarding a host of threats to human health as a consequence of ecological imbalance and environmental change. Although the data highlight the relevance of ecological factors for population health, they also serve to identify certain external stimuli that may cause changes in ecosystems. In this regard, note that ecosystems often depend on selected natural stimuli for their persistence and stability (Rapport, Regier, & Hutchinson, 1985). For example, natural fires in forests release minerals stored in the soils and in tree biomass to create space and reduce competition for moisture, nutrients, heat, and light. Likewise, some species depend on fire for seed release from cones and have numerous adaptations that ensure their survival after a fire. Such events, repetitive and expected, are part of natural systems.

The third set of evidence on the economic determinants of ecosystem change examines how economic activity may be causing ecological and environmental change, in order to point toward remedial corporate practices and strategies. We perceive the economic allocation of raw materials in the production of goods and services and the ecological movement of basic resources among the biotic (living) and abiotic (nonliving) components of an ecosystem as a cycle because neither process can create or destroy matter or energy. In other words, both economic and natural systems, without exception, are subject to the law of conservation of matter and energy (the first law of thermodynamics). The two systems merely shift resources through time and space.

We are interested in those ecosystem changes that are a product of economic activity and corporate decision making as they reflect the ecological determinants of population health. Examples of economic actions include excessive rates of harvesting of renewable resources and discharge of pollutants at rates greater than ecosystems can metabolize them. We review only those types of ecological modifications or changes that are likely to have been directly, indirectly, or partly caused by routine corporate and business policies and practices. In other words, we are interested in those economic determinants that affect ecosystems systematically and persistently. We do not view the impacts of noneconomic stressors, such as human conflicts and wars, even if driven by economic pressures, to be systematic, expected, or anticipated.

Furthermore, we will link the evidence on threats to human health to ecosystem change only as a by-product of economic activity. Conventional economic models recognize that under certain conditions an economic entity's pursuit of self-interest results in costs and benefits to others. Such a cost or benefit is called an *externality* in economics. A common example of an externality is a factory's emission of smoke as a by-product of production. If the factory is able to avoid responsibility for the consequences of its smoke, such as the expenses of painting soot-covered buildings nearby or laundering sooty clothes, others in society must bear the costs. This example illustrates a *negative externality*, a situation in which production entails costs for others, such as those living near a factory.

An externality may be deemed relevant when it creates sufficient demand on the part of those whom it affects to change the situation. Economic theory suggests several approaches to correcting relevant externalities. In general, these can be categorized as defining property rights, taxing negative externalities or subsidizing positive ones, selling rights to create an externality, and establishing regulatory controls. However, the concept of externality has rarely been extended to costs and benefits accruing to noneconomic entities such as ecosystems or their components. Although not trivial or irrelevant, ecosystem impacts of economic activity have largely remained outside conventional economics policymaking, partly because markets do not fully capture the demand for corrective actions.

Economic systems have long relied on ecosystems for resources and materials, but the relationship is increasingly one of mutual dependency. This is because global, regional, and local economic markets have become so large that related economic cycling of materials resources affects local, regional, and global ecosystem function. Given that market economies dominate our economic and cultural landscapes, the laws of demand and supply have become omnipresent and almost as inviolable as the laws of thermodynamics. Therefore, this chapter's authors will view the corporate profit motive and corporate environmental and ecological responsibility not as conflicting accountabilities but as interdependent and mutually reinforcing.

We argue that internalization of ecological concerns does not of necessity impose additional costs on corporations. In this context North (1990, pp. 80–81) identifies the concept of *adaptive efficiency*, which concerns a readiness of "a society to acquire knowledge and learning, to induce innovation, to undertake risks and creative activity of all sorts, as well as to resolve problems and bottlenecks of the society through time" in decentralized decision-making environments (such as the market system) that "allow societies to maximize the efforts required to explore alternate ways of solving problems." This notion of adaptive efficiency implies that corporations typically operate under informational uncertainty (Furubotn, 1999). Although the corporation may be making a profit, it may do so without knowing whether it has reached its best possible position, and it may desire to experiment further as resources become available. In support of this argument, the final section of this chapter will present a case study in ecologically responsible business practices.

Policy Domains

Corporate policy, with its goal to maximize profitability or firm value, is the policy domain of interest. Within the domain of corporate policy, we identify alternate business and managerial strategies in terms of their impact on the ecological determinants of population health. Sustainable development policies attempt to balance economic efficiency with environmental effectiveness and social equity; conventional business policies are primarily directed at economic efficiency (or profit maximization).

Sustainable development refers to development that simultaneously creates economic vitality, environmental stewardship, and social equity (Roseland, 2000; Weinberg, 2000). In this broad perspective, sustainable development attempts to reconcile two fundamental societal questions: What is to be developed? What is to be sustained? (Mathur & Aday, 2002). For example, an emphasis on what to develop may focus on human development, economic development, and community development. Human development may include aspects such as life expectancy, education, and equal opportunity. Economic development would include growth of wealth and the productive and consumptive sectors, whereas community development may encompass development of social institutions and social capital. On the other hand, what to sustain focuses on community sustainability and maintenance of nature's life support systems. Community sustainability would refer to maintaining cultures, places, and social groups. Maintaining nature's life supports would include sustaining ecosystem services, environmental resources, and biodiversity. The fundamental determinants of population health, as described in Chapter One, may thus be related to various dimensions of sustainable development.

Although we recognize the comprehensiveness of the concept of sustainable development, this chapter examines the interdependence between ecological productivity and economic productivity as a determinant of population health. In particular, we use the concept of sustainable development policy to reconcile the social goals of profit maximization and population health. In this context we define three policy evaluation criteria: effectiveness, efficiency, and equity.

Corporate policy that seeks to maximize profit or net benefits will imply pursuit of economic efficiency, whereas a business strategy's ecological responsiveness will indicate its effectiveness in the service of population health. Ecological effectiveness, in turn, may also serve dimensions of equity because it implies stewardship of resources for continuing a lifestyle without diminishing existing resources for future generations. For example, ecological effectiveness serves intergenerational justice, defined as the maintenance of (natural) resources and benefits across generations. Another dimension of equity that may be relevant relates to the notion of environmental justice. Environmental justice is concerned with the inequities in the distribution of environmental risks that may account for health disparities. Ecological effectiveness may serve the environmental justice dimension because it may contribute to minimizing the incidence of regional, local, and global population health consequences associated with ecosystem change.

Finally, we appraise the strengths and limitations of corporate policies in the service of population health and ecological responsiveness. However, we consider the goal to earn (and maximize) profits as one that business requires. The business organization was established as an economic agency to provide goods and services to society, and the profit motive is the principal incentive for free enterprise. All other business responsibilities are predicated on the economic responsibility of the corporation. Corporate social responsibility (CSR) is a concept that studies business and societal relations (Carroll, 1991). We do not frame our adaptation of ecological responsiveness as a component of CSR, unlike the original CSR models from business administration and strategy literature, as a moral or ethical element. We conceptualize ecological responsiveness as an economically efficient corporate strategy that is relatively more effective for population health and thereby represents a business strategy that is both prudent and socially responsible.

Building on these ideas, we suggest applying a framework of CSR to evaluate corporate strategies that seek to maximize economic efficiency and environmental effectiveness. A modified model for illustrating CSR assesses business policy performance in terms of sustainable development's three E's: efficiency (economic), effectiveness (ecological), and equity (environmental) (Figure 3.5).

Evidence Regarding Research on Fundamental Determinants

As highlighted in Figure 3.1, this chapter will present three types of evidence to illuminate the role of environmental factors and related business activity in influencing population health:

- Normal ecosystem function
- Ecological determinants of population health
- Economic determinants of ecosystem change

Evidence on Normal Ecosystem Function

Ecosystems are the ecological units (sets of organisms) living in an area, their physical environment, and the interactions between them (Daily, 1997; Rapport, 1989). They are complex open systems with linkages to neighboring ecosystems through energy transfers and matter (nutrient) flows. Ecosystems are functioning units of nature that cycle materials and resources among both biotic (living) and abiotic (nonliving) environments. This characterization identifies ecosystem functions.

Figure 3.2 (Harvey & Hallet, 1977) displays these ecosystem functions. Figure 3.2 illustrates a local as well as a regional or global ecosystem, because the global natural environment is a continuum of local ecosystems. Metaphorically, ecosystems are like economic markets: Although essentially local, they are also regional, national, and global. Just as local market forces link up with other similar market forces to form a global continuum, physical, chemical, and biological processes mediate nutrient flows and the linkages across and among local ecosystems.

The Natural Cycle: A General Model of Ecosystem Function. The living organisms that compose the biosphere support natural cycles that largely function to pass chemicals and nutrients among these organisms, the lithosphere, hydrosphere, and atmosphere. The biosphere encompasses all living beings, together with their environment. The lithosphere is the outer part of the solid earth (such as the earth's crust) in contrast to its fluid envelopes, the hydrosphere and the atmosphere. The hydrosphere comprises the watery layer on the earth's surface (including water vapor). The atmosphere consists of the envelope of gases surrounding the planet. The lithosphere undergoes change through gradual transfer of material by volcanic eruption, the circulation of ground water, and the process of erosion and deposition. Therefore, it is the third mobile envelope, comparable with the hydrosphere and the atmosphere. These natural cycles sustain themselves with energy from the sun.

The evolutionary processes that gave rise to the assemblage of biotic communities continue today, along with their abiotic components, as ecosystems. The results of these adaptive processes are biotic communities that tend to perpetuate themselves through mechanisms of natural checks and balances such as predator-prey interactions and hormonal control of reproductive rates (e.g., population density increases stimulate hormonal release in rodents to regulate ovulation and thus population).

Appendix 3.1 highlights a case study of ecosystem function and change in the Iowa Prairie. The case study serves to explain the relationship among the components of the ecosystem as illustrated in Figure 3.2.

Ecosystem Services. Normally functioning ecosystems often provide a whole suite of economic services to human society. These services range from renewal services such as purification of water and availability of clean air to control and mitigation activities such as pest control (Daily, 1997). In general, the nature and value of earth's life-support systems have been highlighted primarily through their disruption and loss of ecological services. Costanza and colleagues (1997) estimated the value of

FIGURE 3.2.   GENERAL MODEL OF ECOSYSTEM FUNCTION: THE NATURAL CYCLE.

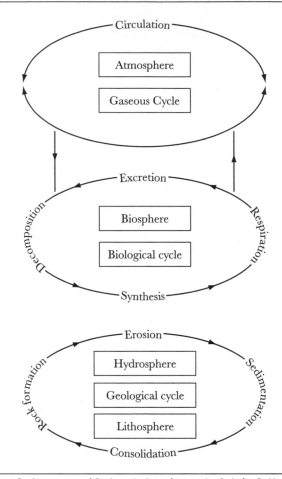

Note. Adapted from *Environment and Society: An Introductory Analysis,* by B. Harvey & J. D. Hallet (Cambridge, MA: MIT Press, 1977), p. 11, fig. 3. Used with permission of Palgrave Macmillan.

various ecosystem services to be about $33 trillion. They included ecosystem services such as climate and weather pattern regulation, water supply management, erosion control and soil formation, nutrient cycling and waste treatment, pollination and food production, and biological control and genetic resources.

Following are a few ecosystem services that society values:

- Purification of water and availability of clean air
- Detoxification and decomposition of wastes

- Generation and renewal of soil and soil fertility
- Mitigation of floods and droughts
- Natural pest control
- Pollination of crops and natural vegetation
- Dispersion of seeds and translocation of nutrients
- Elements for agricultural, medicinal, and industrial enterprise
- Protection from the sun's harmful ultraviolet rays
- Support of diverse human cultures
- Providing of aesthetic beauty
- Intellectual stimulation

The services that natural systems provide obtain from the normal ecosystem function we described earlier. When ecosystems change, the changes affect many of its services. When society perceives the impacts of the ecosystem change as diminishing the scope and level of such services, it may view such ecosystem modifications as degradations.

Ecosystem Change. The only thing constant about ecosystems is change. But even though they are forever transforming and evolving, pristine ecosystems preserve their resilience and productive biodiversity (see Appendix 3.1). Rapport (1989) notes three approaches used to assess the well-being or health of an ecosystem, all of which parallel the practice of human medicine. The first identifies critical characteristics that differentiate healthy from sick ecosystems. The second measures the counteractive capacity to handle burdens. This refers to the ability of ecosystems to bounce back, or recover their equilibrium, after perturbations, whether from endogenous (internal) or exogenous (external) sources. The third identifies risk factors. Just as the health of individuals may be at risk from certain stressors (e.g., diet, overeating, and stress in relation to risks of coronary disease), so may exposure to certain sources of stress from economic activity (such as the contamination of aquatic systems with industrial wastes, naval operations, and sewage discharges) affect the sustainability and well-being of ecosystems. This last approach is most directly related to the formulation and assessment of population health policy.

Principles Governing Ecosystem Behavior. The following three observations are drawn from the simple ecological model summarized in Figure 3.2 and the case study in Appendix 3.1. First, populations in a normally functioning ecosystem have evolved so that materials, such as nutrients and chemical flows in the ecological part of a natural cycle, remain largely localized. This tempers interactions among neighboring ecosystems, keeps local ecosystems self-sustaining, and prevents concentrations of metals, minerals, and fossil fuel fumes from building up in the biosphere.

In contrast, economic systems transport matter and energy through time and space in a manner that may not be consistent with natural cycles.

Secondly, populations in a normally functioning ecosystem have evolved so that the natural cycle's metabolic rate to absorb and exude nutrients keeps the food chain in balance. The food chain is calibrated and regulated by trophic levels. For example, plants, lowest on the food chain, are autotrophs: They can transform energy from an inanimate source (solar radiation). All other living organisms are heterotrophs and are higher up on the food chain. Heterotrophs derive the energy they require for growth and maintenance by ingesting tissue from another organism. Heterotrophs release energy from compounds such as carbohydrates and use this energy to synthesize the proteins, nucleic acids, and other chemical compounds that they require for growth.

The first and second observations imply a third conclusion: that the natural cycling of materials does not compromise an ecosystem's biodiversity or its capacity for production. Ecosystems use natural resources at a rate that is not greater than the rate at which resources can be recreated or renewed.

In summary, we can conclude that natural cycles in pristine ecosystems *do not* do the following:

- Persistently and regularly increase the amount of natural substances extracted from the earth's lithosphere
- Persistently and regularly produce substances faster than they can be broken down and reintegrated into ecosystems or deposited in the lithosphere
- Persistently and regularly erode the physical basis for the productivity and diversity of the ecosystem

The three observations describe how ecosystems behave as they go about their business of cycling raw materials and natural resources. The interpretation of these ecosystem norms as policy variables then transforms the ecological model into a behavioral model for economic entities. To the extent that businesses make routine decisions that ignore these guidelines, they persistently modify ecosystems and may ultimately affect population health. The observations of ecosystem behavior provide a basis for evaluating corporate policies and decision makers as they go about their business of cycling raw materials and natural resources (Robèrt, 2002).

Evidence on the Ecological Determinants of Population Health

Based on the concept of the epidemiology of the marketplace, this section presents evidence that links ecosystem change with adverse population health in a manner that highlights how economic activity may modify ecosystems.

Economic Activity, Ecosystem Change, and Population Health. Although a significant body of literature documents intensified impact on the biosphere from economic activity, for example, due to overharvesting of natural resources and prolific transport of exotic species that modify local ecosystems (Rapport, 2000), the focus is almost always on the scale or excessiveness of economic activities. However, instead of targeting economic activities per se, we focus on unintended market outcomes (market externalities) as inconsistencies between economic activity and ecosystem function.

The previous section identified three defining market externalities or unintended market outcomes that are displayed in Figure 3.3 as stimulants of the ecological determinants of population health.

Tables 3.1a through 3.1c categorize economic activities in terms of the three ecological determinants. Each table identifies a component of the ecosystem that is affected, for example, the atmosphere, aquatic systems, and terrestrial ecosystem. Almost all economic activities could be grouped, in general terms, to contributing to an ecological event that may modify the ecosystem.

FIGURE 3.3.   THE ECOLOGICAL DETERMINANTS
OF POPULATION HEALTH.

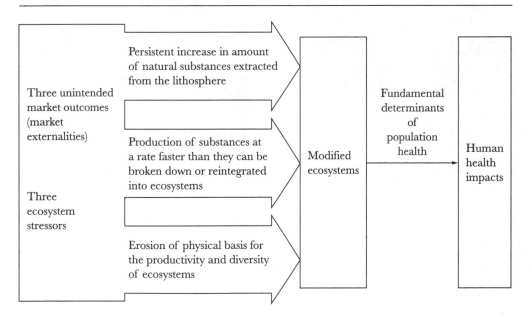

TABLE 3.1a. EXAMPLES OF ATMOSPHERIC CHANGES
AND POTENTIAL HEALTH IMPACTS.

Ecological Events/Ecosystem Determinant	Economic Activity/Driving Force	Ecosystem Change (Ecosystem Response/Change)	Potential Human Health Impacts
Persistently and regularly extract substances from the earth's lithosphere	Increased extraction and burning of fossil fuel (for transporta- tion, manufacturing, animal husbandry, and cement produc- tion) and deforesta- tion for land use, resulting in increased concentration of atmospheric green- house gases	Global climate change characterized by extreme variations in temperature, pre- cipitation, humidity, or drought	Malaria (Argentina), dengue (Australia), hantavirus (south- western United States), mortality due to heat waves (United States)
Persistently and regularly produce substances faster than they can be broken down and reintegrated into the cycles of ecosystems or deposited in the lithosphere	Pollution from power plants, metallurgy, the coal industry, the chemical industry, and vehicular emissions	Lower visibility	Respiratory disease is a leading cause of death (large number of countries)
	Radioactive contamination	Accumulation of radioactive elements in different parts of the ecosystem	Birth defects, mental anomalies, immune disorders (former Soviet Union)
Persistently and regularly erode the productivity and diversity of ecosystems	Deforestation for industrial, domestic fuel, and human habitat uses	Global climate change characterized by extreme variations in temperature, precipitation, humidity, or drought	Disease epidemics (Chad, Ethiopia, Mali, Senegal, Togo, Uganda)

Note. Adapted from *An Assessment of Risks and Threats to Human Health Associated with the Degradation of Ecosystems,* by L. Kochtcheeva and A. Singh (Sioux Falls, SD: United Nations Environmental Programme, Division of Environmental Information, Assessment and Early Warning—North America, 1999), pp. 11–16, tab. 1. Used with permission.

TABLE 3.1b. EXAMPLES OF AQUATIC SYSTEM CHANGES AND POTENTIAL HEALTH IMPACTS.

Ecological Events/Ecosystem Determinant	Economic Activity/Driving Force	Ecosystem Change (Ecosystem Response/Change)	Potential Human Health Impacts
Persistently and regularly extract substances from the earth's lithosphere	Contamination with heavy metals (cadmium)	Accumulation of biochains (Japan)	Progressive irreversible kidney damage
	Oil contamination, industrial pollution, and pollution from naval operations and sewage discharges, intensive navigation	Deterioration of marine ecosystems from a severe imbalance (Black Sea, Azov Sea, Caspian Sea)	Decrease in life expectancy; skin and eye diseases
Persistently and regularly produce substances faster than they can be broken down and reintegrated into the cycles of ecosystems or deposited in the lithosphere	Biological and chemical contamination	Harmful toxic and nontoxic algal blooms from the rapid reproduction and localized dominance of phytoplankton	Poisoning, diarrhea, dehydration, memory loss, weakness, gastroenteritis, bacterial infections, swimming-related illnesses, neurological diseases, deaths (coastal regions of U.S. and South America)
		Shellfish poisoning, wildlife mortalities, sunlight penetration prevention, oxygen shortages, reservoirs of bacteria	
Persistently and regularly erode the productivity and diversity of ecosystems	Rising levels of ecosystem destruction and pasture change; decrease in depth and amplitude of water fluctuations leading to reduction of wildlife habitats	Raised levels of hydrogen sulfide and petroleum products pollution (Volga River)	Skin and eye diseases

Note. Adapted from *An Assessment of Risks and Threats to Human Health Associated with the Degradation of Ecosystems,* by L. Kochtcheeva and A. Singh (Sioux Falls, SD: United Nations Environmental Programme, Division of Environmental Information, Assessment and Early Warning—North America, 1999), pp. 11–16, tab. 1. Used with permission.

TABLE 3.1c. EXAMPLES OF TERRESTRIAL ECOSYSTEM CHANGES AND POTENTIAL HEALTH IMPACTS.

Ecological Events/Ecosystem Determinant	Economic Activity/Driving Force	Ecosystem Change (Ecosystem Response/Change)	Potential Human Health Impacts
Persistently and regularly extract substances from the earth's lithosphere	Mining activities	Accumulation of mining dust and land transformation	Lung diseases (United States) Exposure to mercury (Brazil)
Persistently and regularly pro-duce substances faster than they can be broken down and re-integrated into the cycles of ecosystems or deposited in the lithosphere	Radioactive soil contamination	Contaminated vegetation and food growth (Siberian and Arctic regions)	Rising incidence of cancer, birth defects
	Soil contamination from fertilizers and organic manure contamination	High levels of nutrients in rivers due to increases in nitrate levels (Western Europe)	Bottle-fed babies at serious risk, possible carcinogenesis
Persistently and regularly erode the productivity and diversity of ecosystems	Conversion of forests into cotton or sugarcane culture and cattle pasture	Land-use changes leading to favorable habitats for rats and increase in infectious sources	Hemorrhagic fever (Venezuela)
		Alteration of hydrologic cycles	Malaria (Central America)
	Intensified agri-cultural irrigation schemes	Damage of local ecosystems and changes in insecti-cide resistance	Malaria (Central America)
	Agroecosystem development inundates land for rice growing	New breeding grounds for insects	Japanese encephalitis (Japan, China, India)

Note. Adapted from *An Assessment of Risks and Threats to Human Health Associated with the Degradation of Ecosystems,* by L. Kochtcheeva and A. Singh (Sioux Falls, SD: United Nations Environmental Programme, Division of Environmental Information, Assessment and Early Warning—North America, 1999), pp. 11–16, tab. 1. Used with permission.

Although the data presented in the tables is not exhaustive, it relies heavily on an assessment of risks and threats to human health associated with the degradation of ecosystems by Kotchtcheeva and Singh (1999). In related research, McMichael (1993) and Patz (2000) also report threats to public health as a consequence of ecological imbalance including mortality related to heat waves in the United States, hantavirus, malaria, dengue fever, water-borne cryptosporidiosis, and cholera—all due to global climate change. Burnett, Jessiman, Stieb, and Krewski (2000) and Wilson (2000) conducted epidemiological studies in a number of countries to demonstrate associations between concentrations of ambient air pollution and adverse human health outcomes, including premature mortality, cardiorespiratory hospitalizations, emergency department visits for respiratory diseases, asthma attacks, respiratory symptoms, and restricted activity.

The potential impact on human health due to the modification of the ecosystem is an outcome of several simultaneous processes such as deforestation, pollution, global climate change, and other mutually linked changes. Linking potential impacts on human health to ecosystem modification is confounded by an absence of direct, strong, connective mechanisms and scientific certainty. New epidemiological research challenges include developing predictive models that link climatogical and ecological change as determinants of health (Patz, 2000), linking population health to the environment's carrying capacity (Kochtcheeva & Singh, 1999), and offering decision makers the best available judgments based on existing empirical evidence on health impacts (McMichael, 1993, 2001). As indicated earlier, this chapter focuses on the epidemiology of the marketplace and not on ecological or clinical epidemiology.

In this context, even if the scientific credibility of existing studies may be debatable, the evidence in this section, in conjunction with the precautionary principle, highlights ecosystem change as a factor that corporate decision makers may take into account in formulating socially responsible corporate policy.

Evidence on the Economic Determinants of Ecosystem Change

From a policy perspective, a compelling question is to understand why the economic system conducts its business in a manner that may conflict with ecosystem function. In other words, why do we observe the three unintended market outcomes illustrated in Figure 3.3? The answer lies in the way that society confronts three basic economic questions:

- What goods should be produced and in what quantities?
- How should these goods and services be produced?
- For whom should these goods and services be produced?

In general, a society or nation can answer these questions in three ways. First, the market process uses supply and demand and material incentives to answer the questions. The other two ways use political command-and-control processes or customs and traditions to resolve the resource use and allocation decisions. The market process is the predominant resource allocation mechanism, whereas the latter two temper the decision process. Therefore, the way that business resolves these questions in the marketplace is what determines the epidemiology of economic activity. Whether for profit or for population health, the resolution of resource allocation and use is the central issue.

Standard economics models decisions regarding resource allocation in a closed economic system (Daly & Farley, 2004). Figure 3.4 illustrates a closed system as a circular flow diagram containing a business and a household sector (Ekelund & Tollison, 2000). The inner loop is the physical flow of output and corresponding dollar expenditures on final output (i.e., the GDP). The outer loop is the flow of services of production inputs (e.g., labor and capital) and the return flow of their respective incomes (e.g., wages and interest). By definition, the part of a loop that is above the boxes must equal the part of the loop that is below the boxes. For example, expenditures by economic entities correspond to their income flows. Conventional economics models the simple two-sector closed domestic economy as being open when it includes the international and government sectors. Economics conceptualizes the flow of goods and services between households and firms and the government and international markets as leakages and injections with respect to the domestic private (two-sector) economy. Examples of leakages would

FIGURE 3.4.   CLOSED MODEL OF ECONOMIC SYSTEM: THE ECONOMIC CYCLE.

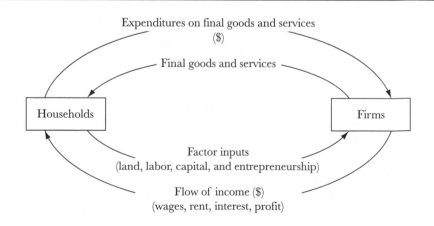

be household savings, government taxation, and imports; injections include public or private investment, government purchases, and international exports.

The point to note is that economic models do not explicitly incorporate ecosystem injections and leakages (i.e., the natural sector is missing in Figure 3.4. and its usual extensions). This conceptual limitation is also reflected in conventional business economics practice and corporate decision making. Recognition of the disconnection between economic systems and natural systems serves to ground our understanding of the tensions between economic activity and ecosystems.

One way to explicitly connect the economic system and ecosystem is to visualize the circular flow of raw materials, resources, and goods, as illustrated in Figure 3.4, as being contained within the larger flow of basic raw materials depicted in the natural cycles in Figure 3.2. Economic systems share and depend on the productivity of the ecosystem and its natural cycles. Alternately, we can state that the economic cycle of production and consumption is an open system and the ecosystem functions as a closed system, because nothing of significance escapes the earth's gravitational field.

The essential point is that conventional economic principles that model the economic system as closed and disconnected from the natural cycle present themselves as evidence that economic activity may be unintentionally causing ecosystem changes. A strong potential exists to modify ecosystem functions when injections and leakages from the economic system to the ecosystem conflict with the rates of assimilation and production of the natural cycles. The sets of evidence that we present in this section argue for a need to assess and reformulate policies in a way that forges consistency between the functions of business corporations and the ecosystem.

Current Policies That Address Fundamental Determinants

The evidence regarding how and why unintended market outcomes stimulate the ecological determinants of population health suggests that business objectives (such as profit maximization) and the public health objectives (for population health) must be reconciled in the marketplace. Therefore, the policy domain relevant for addressing the ecological determinants of population health is corporate policy.

Conventional Corporate Policy and Managerial Strategies

Corporate policy, with its objective to earn profits (or increase firm value), is the primary policy goal. Note that we will use the terms *firm, company,* and *corporations* interchangeably. The traditional (neoclassical) theory of economics defines the *firm* as a collection of resources that is transformed into products that consumers demand. The costs at which the firm produces are governed by the available technology, and the amount it produces and the prices at which it sells are influenced by the structure of the markets in which it operates. The difference between the revenue it receives and the cost it incurs is *profit*. If a firm does not seek to increase (or maximize) its value over time, it will be in danger of either going out of business, being taken over by competitors, or having its stockholders elect to replace management.

A responsible company must be aware of its shareholders, the quality of its goods and services, the effectiveness of its research and development, social values and attitudes, and employee welfare concerns. But it must align these concerns with management's primary responsibility to increase profits. Firms often reach this goal by trying to achieve intermediate targets. For example, an intermediate objective may be to maximize market share and may require lowering prices in the short run. Likewise, in order to provide a technologically advanced product, a corporation might decide to allocate more resources to research and development. The strategy to lower prices or add research and development expenses may reduce the amount of profit that the corporation earns in the short run. Both strategies, however, would likely result in increased profits over time as the corporation increases market share and its technological lead over its competitors. Although a corporation can select from a number of other goals, the assumption of profit maximization provides a clear-cut model for explaining how corporations can use economic concepts and tools of analyses to make optimal decisions.

Sustainable Development Policy: Strategy to Reconcile Profit Maximization and Population Health

The policy challenge is to conceptualize a strategy that will eliminate conflicts among policy goals (i.e., profit maximization and population health). Sustainable development, however, offers promise as a policy strategy to anchor corporate decision making at the intersection of economic, environmental, and social responsibilities.

Sustainable business policy refers to practices that simultaneously create economic vitality, environmental stewardship, and social equity (Roseland, 2000; Weinberg, 2000). Mathur and Aday (2002, p. 53) note that "decision making in this context must deliberately internalize various societal concerns—social costs and benefits (i.e., market externalities) that may otherwise not be fully accounted for in market outcomes."

Mathur and Aday (2002, p. 56) emphasize that "in sustainable development, the operative conjunctive is *and*—to sustain *and* to develop," for example, to sustain the environment and develop the . . . economy. They continue: "However, when the focus shifts to economic development mostly, conflicts arise among the various social goals related to economics, equity, and environment." We propose viewing corporate policy through the lens of sustainable development; integrating the goal of population health in business economics structures decision making at the intersection of economics, equity, and the environment.

Again, we argue that the responsibility for sustainable development rests with various participants in the market process. Although approaches to sustainable development leave it to some set of decision makers who must balance what to sustain and what to develop, there seems to be a misplaced perception that planners and planning will play a significant role in a community's transition toward sustainable development. Mathur and Aday (2002, p. 57) contend that

> the path to sustainable development lies largely with local businesses and other market participants, while planners and planning models can only ineffectively control decentralized economic market decisions. In large-scale market economies characterizing U.S. society and communities, businesses and corporations, public and private organizations, for-profits and not-for profits represent decentralized decision making environments that determine *what* is to be produced for *whom, where* and *how.* In their dual roles as consumers and producers, it is they *who* largely resolve what to develop and what to sustain.

Economic Efficiency, Ecological Effectiveness, and Environmental Equity

Economic theory of the corporation defines *economic efficiency* as the allocation of the corporation's resources that results in maximum benefit at minimum cost (i.e., maximization of net benefits or profits). Corporate policies are deemed efficient if they maximize performance on the goal to earn profits. In short, the firm has one goal and one criterion: to earn and maximize profits. Economics would then consider corporate policies that aim to promote alternate goals (e.g., promoting population health) at the expense of profit, by definition, inefficient.

However, the concept of sustainable development indicates the inadequacy of profits as a general measure of socioeconomic performance and highlights how sustainable development precepts can provide opportunities for corrective action. Although economic health, ecological health, and population health appear to be issues that are distinct and apart, sustainable development can provide the bridge that connects these systems.

A commonly understood expectation of sustainable development is that humanity has the ability to ensure that it meets the needs of the present without compromising the ability of future generations to meet their own needs (World

Commission on Environment and Development, 1987). This implies that a major premise of sustainable development is that conscious human decision and action can resolve contemporary problems (Mathur & Aday, 2002). Therefore, we propose the use of the concept of sustainable development as a mechanism that facilitates a deliberate internalization of various societal concerns in decision making.

Corrective measures would require businesses to view sustainable development as a nexus of excellent managerial and production systems, aligning with and restoring natural systems, and in optimal service of population health and economic efficiency. In this formulation the goals of profit maximization and ecological effectiveness coalesce to motivate the search for production methods that optimize individual and public welfare.

Figure 3.5 illustrates this conceptualization. It nests the policy domain (corporate policy) within the traditional (two-sector) economic model presented in Figure 3.4. Conventional corporate policies are distinct from ecologically responsive corporate policies (sustainable business practices). The latter explicitly address the defining principles of natural ecosystem functioning. In either case, whether firms formulate corporate policies in the context of a closed economic model (i.e., disconnected from the natural cycles of an ecosystem) or in accordance with ecological responsiveness, the policies first and foremost must meet the required corporate policy goal to maximize profits.

The concept of sustainable development also helps to frame our evaluation of corporate policies in terms of the three E's (i.e., economic efficiency, ecological effectiveness, and environmental equity). Corporate policies are categorized as conventional strategies when they follow the closed economic model. Sustainable business practices accommodate norms of ecosystem behavior. Both strategic variations of corporate policy seek economic efficiency. But they differ in their emphasis and performance on the criteria of ecological effectiveness and environmental equity.

Figure 3.5 illustrates that the economic efficiency criteria can be met using alternate strategies. The decision to use alternate strategies to further business goals is an issue of corporate leadership and managerial choice. Conventional business or managerial strategies may affect the ecological determinants (i.e., potentially modify the ecosystem) because they are not conceived as ecologically responsive strategies. On the other hand, strategies that are formulated, to the extent possible, with regard to the norms of ecosystem behavior (as derived from the ecological model in Figure 3.2) are ecologically responsive. Such business practices are expected to be responsive to preserving ecosystem function and thus avoiding potential negative population health impacts.

In this context, a second policy evaluation criterion, effectiveness, assesses the extent to which strategies seek to minimize the impact of the economic system on

FIGURE 3.5.   CURRENT POLICIES THAT AFFECT ECOLOGICAL DETERMINANTS.

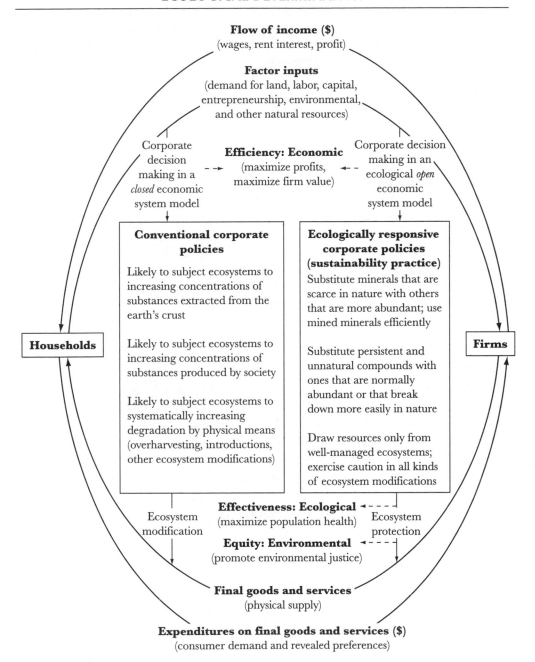

Flow of income ($)
(wages, rent interest, profit)

Factor inputs
(demand for land, labor, capital, entrepreneurship, environmental, and other natural resources)

Corporate decision making in a *closed* economic system model

Efficiency: Economic
(maximize profits, maximize firm value)

Corporate decision making in an ecological *open* economic system model

Conventional corporate policies

Likely to subject ecosystems to increasing concentrations of substances extracted from the earth's crust

Likely to subject ecosystems to increasing concentrations of substances produced by society

Likely to subject ecosystems to systematically increasing degradation by physical means (overharvesting, introductions, other ecosystem modifications)

Ecologically responsive corporate policies (sustainability practice)
Substitute minerals that are scarce in nature with others that are more abundant; use mined minerals efficiently

Substitute persistent and unnatural compounds with ones that are normally abundant or that break down more easily in nature

Draw resources only from well-managed ecosystems; exercise caution in all kinds of ecosystem modifications

Households

Firms

Ecosystem modification

Effectiveness: Ecological
(maximize population health)

Ecosystem protection

Equity: Environmental
(promote environmental justice)

Final goods and services
(physical supply)

Expenditures on final goods and services ($)
(consumer demand and revealed preferences)

ecological determinants of population health. Ecological effectiveness will serve dimensions of equity related to environmental protection and natural system changes. It may minimize the incidence of regional, local, and global population health consequences associated with ecosystem change in the interest of environmental justice. Environmental justice concerns relate to the inequitable distribution of ecological hazards and health risks, emanating primarily from economic activities, among underrepresented, disenfranchised populations in their workplaces and their communities. Further, it will promote intergenerational equity, because ecological effectiveness implies responsible stewardship of natural resources.

Strengths and Limitations of Current Policies

The discussion that follows examines alternate corporate strategies in terms of their perspectives on the ecological determinants of population health. This section will illustrate contrasting perspectives outlined in Figure 3.5 using a case study of business practice distinguished by its ecological responsiveness. The illustration views sustainability practice or ecological responsiveness as a component of CSR. The CSR concept frames sustainable development precepts as CSR components facilitating sustainability practice.

Pyramid of CSR

Carroll's original conception (1991) of a pyramid of social responsibility (see Figure 3.6) organizes multiple CSRs into four components: economic, legal, ethical, and charitable responsibilities. The CSR components reflect different levels of legitimacy or codification. Accordingly, economic and legal responsibilities are required; ethical responsibilities are socially expected; and philanthropy is socially desired. In Figure 3.6, economic responsibility appears as economic efficiency and philanthropy appears as corporate interests in charity or equity. The conceptualization orders the CSR components with economic responsibilities as the foundation and philanthropy as the apex. In other words, the firm that does not achieve economic performance (production of goods and services, creation of jobs, and generation of profits) cannot achieve other responsibilities either.

We have already discussed economic responsibility in detail. Just as society legitimizes and requires that businesses operate with economic responsibility, society requires businesses to meet their legal responsibilities. Society expects business to comply with federal, state, and local laws and regulations that are the ground rules under which it must operate. Therefore, legal responsibilities are the next

FIGURE 3.6.   FRAMEWORK FOR CORPORATE SOCIAL RESPONSIBILITY FOR POPULATION HEALTH.

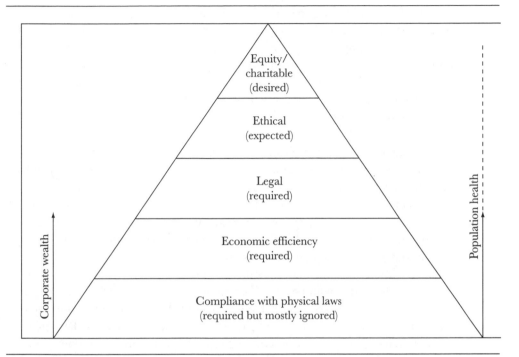

Note. Adapted from "The Pyramid of Corporate Social Responsibility: Toward the Moral Management of Organizational Stakeholders—Balancing Economic, Legal, and Social Responsibilities," by A. B. Carroll, 1991, *Business Horizons, 34,* p. 42, fig. 3. Used with permission of Elsevier.

layer on the pyramid to portray their historical development. They coexist with economic responsibilities as fundamental precepts of the free enterprise system.

The next component is ethical responsibility. This CSR includes those activities and practices that society expects or prohibits but has not yet codified into law. Responsiveness to environmental issues, civil rights, and consumer movements fall in the ethical component. Note that the layers of the CSR pyramid are porous and temporal. Changing ethics and social values precede and motivate establishment of new laws or regulations.

The final layer in the pyramid comprises desired responsibilities. These include, for example, that corporate actions be responsive to society's expectation that businesses be good corporate citizens. Such actions are discretionary or voluntary (e.g., philanthropy, charity, and humanitarian programs).

Modifying the CSR Pyramid and Defining Ecological Responsiveness

The CSR pyramid recognizes the dynamic interplay between and among the various CSR components. For example, environmental concerns, typically included in the ethical component, not only push into the category of legal responsibility but raise the prospect that businesses will operate at levels beyond legal requirements. We modify the original CSR pyramid (Carroll, 1991) to explicitly include compliance with physical laws, as a requirement for an ecologically responsive corporate business strategy.

Unlike Carroll (1991), we do not propose using the pyramid to move toward a moral management of organizational stakeholders wherein moral business behavior may involve voluntary acceptance of material loss (Windsor, 2001). Rather than advocating for corporate morality, we make a case for corporate leadership to ensure continuance of a lifestyle and interaction without lessening ecosystem function. Leadership may manifest entrepreneurial experimentation that keeps a corporation moving down a path of economic efficiency and environmental effectiveness.

Based on the arguments and evidence, we add the fifth responsibility, compliance with physical laws, as the foundation of the CSR pyramid. This responsibility is foundational and required because humans are hardly in a position to negotiate with the laws of nature. Unlike the laws of the legal system, natural laws cannot be altered. Everyone is subject to natural laws such as the laws of thermodynamics, gravity, or ecosystem function. One can only ignore them in decision making. Whereas violators of legal laws may or may not be brought to justice, ignorance of natural system laws will result in a response (e.g., ecosystem responses modeled in Figure 3.3 and listed in Tables 3.1a–3.1c as adverse population health consequences).

Symmetric with Carroll's definitions (1991) of the original four components of CSR, ecological responsibility requires that businesses perform in a manner consistent with ecosystem behavioral norms and that defines a successful corporation as one that fulfills its ecological obligations. In particular, ecologically responsible business practice would imply that economic activities minimize the following environmental impacts: persistently and regularly increasing natural substances extracted from the earth's lithosphere; persistently and regularly producing substances faster than they can be broken down and reintegrated into ecosystems or deposited in the lithosphere; and persistently and regularly eroding the physical basis for the productivity and diversity of ecosystem (see Figures 3.3 and 3.5).

Also, recognizing our goal to maximize population health, we add the dimension of population health in Figure 3.6 (to parallel or complement the goal to maximize corporate wealth). Corporate policy and related strategies can thus be evaluated on two dimensions: (economic) efficiency as it implies profit maximization and (ecological) effectiveness in the service of population health.

Figure 3.6 suggests that a corporation's economic obligations can coexist with other responsibilities. Friedman (1970) argued against simple altruism on the part of corporate decision makers but accepted strategic altruism grounded in sound business practices. Considerations of CSR do not contradict the principle of profit maximization. If companies were maximizers in the past, when conditions were less restrictive, they are still maximizers today but have to operate within the requirements of current standards and the costs and benefits that accompany them. In this context, the case study of the IKEA Corporation presented later in this chapter presents a compelling case that a firm does not have to compromise growth in profits and business competitiveness when it makes corporate ecological responsiveness part of a socially responsible business strategy.

Sustainability practice or ecological responsiveness can be grounded in North's notion of adaptive efficiency (1990). North conceptualized *adaptive efficiency* as a process of learning, enterprise, and technical innovation, undertaken in decentralized decision environments, to solve various societal problems. In this context, sustainable business practices can be viewed as efforts to explore alternate ways of solving ecological and other social issues in the decentralized market environment. Successful exploration of alternate solutions implies that, while making positive profits, the business manager does not know whether the firm has reached its best possible position. Toward that end, corporations may desire to experiment further as resources become available (Furubotn, 1999). When corporations operate under such informational uncertainty, there is potential for profitable research and development.

Case Study of Ecologically Responsive Corporate Policy:
The IKEA Corporation "Poisonous Bookshelves" Controversy

A case study of the IKEA Corporation illustrates how population health concerns motivate a company to perceive ecological responsiveness as a required responsibility. In addition, the case study demonstrates corporate strategies that put the business at the intersection of economic efficiency, environmental effectiveness, and social equity.

Background. IKEA, a profitable multinational company with annual revenues of over $7 billion (Nattrass & Altomare, 1999), is an internationally renowned home furnishings brand with more than 200 stores employing more than 85,000 workers in more than 30 countries. The company reports a steady and satisfactory rise in its corporate earnings (IKEA Systems, 1999). Therefore, the issue of compromising economic responsibility or economic efficiency does not arise.

Business Model. IKEA combines conventional business policy goals with a unique business strategy. Like other market participants, it seeks to increase market share, maximize revenues and profits, and maintain market competitiveness. What is unique is that IKEA seeks to obtain good results with minimum inputs. IKEA's business strategy focuses on resource efficiency and considers wastage of resources as unacceptable (Nattrass & Altomare, 1999). The managerial goal for efficient use of the corporation's scarce resources coincides with the social goals of stewardship of natural resources.

Another corporate core value at IKEA requires that employees support each other, act creatively and freely, and take the responsibility that comes with that freedom. These values spring from the company's concern that the fear of making mistakes impedes creativity and business evolution. Accordingly, IKEA views the challenges of a rapidly changing world and expanding markets as opportunities and regards unsuccessful initiatives (strategic mistakes) as what it calls "learnings" (Nattrass & Altomare, 1999, p. 48). This reflects a belief that entrepreneurship feeds on lessons learned. This business philosophy captures North's concept (1990) of adaptive efficiency and Furubotn's notion (1999) of experimentation to achieve economic efficiency.

IKEA and Corporate Social Performance. In the 1980s through the 1990s, IKEA started in the legal component of CSR and ended up in the ecological component. In both instances the social issue was population health. This section will highlight IKEA's strategic journey from reaction and accommodation to proaction and sustainability practice in response to this crisis.

In 1981 Denmark established a new law regulating the maximum emissions allowed from formaldehyde off-gassing in particleboard (a core component of many IKEA products). Subsequently, government tests of IKEA products revealed that some had formaldehyde emissions above the legislated limit; and media coverage drew dramatic attention to the issue. Legal fines were minor compared to the drop in IKEA's sales and image.

In the mid-1980s, customers, especially in Germany, IKEA's largest market, began to ask new questions that indicated their increasing concern about the environmental and health effects of products. Consumers raised questions about the source of the wood for the bookshelves and the toxicity of the lacquers on them. In the late 1980s, according to Nattrass and Altomare (1999), IKEA was criticized for packaging and paper wastage. IKEA's famous catalog was criticized for placing excessive demand for paper, pulp, and timber. Also, the catalog's production and disposal were considered wasteful; and the chlorine bleach used allegedly released residues in various aquatic environments (particularly in the Baltic Sea) that endangered marine life. Furthermore, the company was also criticized for the use of PVC plastic. A large fire in the plastic industry revealed the release of dioxins during the combustion of PVC.

In 1992 in Germany, the company faced yet another crisis. Its internationally popular product, the Billy bookshelf, was found in violation of legislated requirements for environmental formaldehyde. The source was not the particleboard that was actually regulated by law but the lacquer on the bookshelves. A large German newspaper and television station conducted an investigation for formaldehyde offgassing. Extensive media coverage called the IKEA product "Deadly Poisoned Bookshelves" (Nattrass and Altomare, 1999, p. 52). The regulatory details did not matter to the press. IKEA began to recognize that environmental concern was a new market reality. IKEA had to put a stop to the sales and worldwide production of Billy bookcases.

Moving Toward Sustainability Practices. Since the company's inception, IKEA's founders have stated that its mission was to create a better everyday life for the majority of the people. The company leadership realized that a company built on such a mission must take environmental and population health issues seriously.

In 1990 IKEA adopted its first environmental policy for a one-year trial period. In early 1992 it developed an action plan. Its task force provided IKEA's top management with recommendations regarding how IKEA works, how other companies work, and how society works. They advised the company's leaders that they were actually transforming resources into waste. The conversion process was measured at the cash register as *turnover*, which the task force characterized as the rate at which resources are transformed into waste. After the task force presented its analysis, IKEA began discussions about redesigning the company's relationship with the natural environment.

Although IKEA's environmental concerns are clearly connected to signals the firm received from a changing marketplace, they go beyond that. Its vision to "provide a better everyday life for a majority of people, originally meant that the majority of people should be able to afford attractive and durable home furnishings," but IKEA "now embraces a path that will help achieve a sustainable society in ecological balance" (Nattrass & Altomare, 1999, p. 63).

Corporate Strategy for Sustainability Practice. It must be noted that IKEA's recognition of a need for integrating environmental concerns into business thinking did not resolve the challenge of implementing the integration. IKEA's desire for strategic experimentation showed the way. The firm initially considered a strategy to introduce a new line of products called Eco-Plus. The environmentally responsive product line was expected to be relatively more expensive than its conventional products but priced lower than its market competition. The company, however, realized that creating an Eco-Plus line would imply that its other products were of inferior quality; besides, the double standard would contradict the company's vision.

IKEA recognized that it was not being forced to produce products beyond legal standards. It perceived that it had time both to experiment and to learn. Accordingly, the company conceived a new product development strategy, one that was not focused on making a portion of the company's product range environmentally robust but instead focused on improving the whole range incrementally. For example, IKEA has introduced low-energy light bulbs in its markets; experimented with powering its stores with solar energy; eliminated potentially toxic materials like lead, cadmium, and chrome from its products; and developed a line of children's furniture that is filled with inexhaustible and environmentally friendly materials (Nattrass &Altomare, 1999, p. 72). This strategic insight heralded IKEA's evolutionary shift toward ecological sustainability.

IKEA's new business strategy puts it squarely on the right side of Figure 3.5 (labeled ecologically responsive corporate policies, sustainability practice). Also, in terms of the CSR pyramid (Figure 3.6), IKEA clearly deemed ecological responsibilities a required responsibility, coexisting with the company's legal and economic responsibilities. The company's strategic responses proceed from reaction and defense during the 1980s, to accommodation and proaction in the 1990s, and finally toward a philosophy of sustainability practice today.

The movement affects how the company conducts its daily work, designs its product, analyzes the environmental effects of a product through its life cycle, chooses its suppliers, and makes decisions that involve its large global workforce. The philosophic change and movement along the CSR and strategic dimensions was gradual but persistent. The practice of sustainability required IKEA to systematically integrate in its daily operations changes in technology, knowledge, social values, tastes, and preferences. Environmental thinking is now an integral part of how IKEA's coworkers conduct the company's business.

A number of examples illustrate that IKEA is oriented toward the pursuit of ecologically responsive strategies (Nattrass & Altomare, 1999). IKEA's product design and development seeks to change over to renewable raw materials and energy sources. It uses substances and materials that are easily broken down in ecosystems and converted into new resources. It constructs products so that customers can easily separate the constituent materials for recycling.

IKEA's cost-cutting strategies are aligned at the corporate and societal levels. The firm seeks products with a long useful life, which can be repaired if they break. It plans use of materials, energy, technology, and transport to achieve maximum benefit for minimum expenditure of resources. It reuses the same product several times or recycles it as raw material for a new product.

IKEA fosters a policy that avoids intrusions into ecosystems. For example, it incinerates materials for heating purposes only if the gases emitted are such that natural ecosystems can deal with them. It recognizes that dumping waste or garbage or pumping it into rivers, lakes, and seas is not an alternative in a sustainable society. IKEA "ensures that its textile products are tested in internationally recognized laboratories to verify compliance with IKEA's basic requirements. This assures that there are no harmful substances in the products and that the customer can feel safe using them" (Nattrass & Altomare, 1999, p. 61).

Distinguishing Sustainability Practice from Other Practices for Public Health.
We chose the IKEA experience as a case study to illustrate the strengths and limitations of corporate strategies in the service of population health. Although other cases may illustrate how firms can accommodate public health without compromising economic efficiency, the IKEA example is distinguished by its ecological responsiveness.

For example, Carroll (1979) discusses a business case: Anheuser-Busch introduced a new adult beverage, Chelsea, containing more alcohol than the average drink. Consumer groups protested on the grounds that the company was targeting youth, who would find the higher alcohol content appealing. In protest, the consumer group deemed the marketing of Chelsea as socially irresponsible and called the drink Kiddie Beer.

Anheuser-Busch was defensive at first. The company maintained that the drink was safe and would not entice youngsters to a stronger drink. However, the criticism from consumer groups persisted. The company concluded that the socially responsible action would be to withdraw the product and redevelop it so that it would not be considered to adversely affect population health.

Anheuser-Busch responded to what consumer groups saw as its ethical responsibility. The product being introduced was strictly legal because it was within the maximum allowable alcoholic content standards. As the company realized that the public outcry might transform an ethical responsibility into an economic one, Anheuser-Busch reformulated its strategy.

By contrast, the IKEA case study, which also illustrates responsiveness to public health concerns, presents a business strategy that is comprehensive, proactive, and ecologically effective. The case reflects a corporate philosophy of social responsiveness that has the potential for balancing and satisfying the effectiveness, efficiency, and equity criteria.

Recommendations

The chapter highlights the need for a new strategy for public health, one that broadens the perspective from a hazard to a habitat dimension, one that looks beyond sick individuals to stressed ecosystems, and one that generates corporate strategies to assure the health of populations and communities (Beaglehole & McMichael, 1999; Mathur & Aday, 2002; McMichael, 1999; Rapport, 2000; Rose, 1985; Shea, 1992). It supports the contention that medical care within the health care system, supported by prudent individual behavior and regulatory protection, will no longer be enough to preserve or promote population health.

Look Beyond Hazards to Habitats

Even as the Intergovernmental Panel on Climate Change (McMichael, 1993) noted that sustaining the integrity of the earth's ecosystems is a requirement for population health, ecosystem integrity remains a rather unusual determinant of health. The unfamiliarity arises because modern epidemiological research has mostly focused on proximate and tangible risk-factor behaviors and influences on personal health (McMichael, 1999). In the United States, agencies such as the Environmental Protection Agency, the Occupational Health and Safety Agency, the Food and Drug Administration, and the Consumer Product Safety Commission often codify related public health concerns.

The evidence on the ecological determinants of health, however, points to the inadequacy of the existing regulatory system, which is dominated by actions directed at one chemical, one health risk, or one medium (air, water, food, soil) at a time (Omenn, 1996).

Look Beyond Sick People to Stressed Ecosystems

Conventional health sector policies are limited by their focus on health services. For example, they are often designed to increase access or redistribute net benefits to some group of individuals distinct from another (Longest, 2002). The most common examples of such policies are the Medicare and Medicaid programs.

Current public policies, as well as the health and medical care services of the curative sector, do not satisfactorily address toxic exposures in our environment; neither do they sufficiently widen the spectrum of health protection to include health-endangering environmental problems related to ecological change (McMichael, 1993).

The ecological determinants evidence suggests that the curative sector may in some cases be treating the symptoms and not the causes of ill health. Therefore, reallocation of resources and extension of health promotion and disease prevention research and practices in the area of environmental protection and ecosystem maintenance may constitute a more efficient use of scarce economic resources.

Look Beyond Conventional Corporate Policies Toward Sustainable Development

Due to the potential for damage to life support systems at the local, regional, and global levels, public health researchers have argued that we may be on the threshold of an epidemiological change in which the determinants of human health will increasingly be ecological (McMichael, 1993; Rapport, 2000). Although efforts that focus on prevention (e.g., sanitation, vaccines) must continue, emerging classes of ecological threats require a new strategy—a strategy that must bear on our past, present, and future decisions as producers and consumers.

In order to alleviate ecological modifications and related adverse impacts on humans, an effective strategy must do three things:

- Focus on restoring and sustaining ecological balance
- Involve those who make decisions about what to produce, how to produce, and for whom to produce
- Evolve in related decision-making environments—most fundamentally, in the marketplace

This chapter has set the stage for the chapters that follow by introducing a broad, interdependent, innovative, and long-term perspective on the environmental underpinnings of population health. Chapter Four focuses on the microcosm of the essential human impacts of the fundamental environmental and other determinants of population health—the development of productive potential throughout the life course.

References

Beaglehole, R., & McMichael, A. (1999). The future of public health in a changing global context. *Development, 42,* 12–16.

Burnett, R. T., Jessiman, B., Stieb, D., & Krewski, D. (2000). Population health issues in the management of air quality. *Ecosystem Health, 6,* 67–78.

Carroll, A. B. (1979). A three-dimensional conceptual model of corporate performance. *Academy of Management Review, 4,* 497–505.

Carroll, A. B. (1991). The pyramid of corporate social responsibility: Toward the moral management of organizational stakeholders—balancing economic, legal, and social responsibilities. *Business Horizons, 34,* 39–48.

Costanza, R., d'Arge, R., de Groot, R., Farber, S., Grasso, M., Hannon, B., et al. (1997). The value of the world's ecosystem services and natural capital. *Nature, 387,* 253–260.

Daily, G. C. (Ed.). (1997). *Nature's services: Societal dependence on natural ecosystems.* Washington, DC: Island Press.

Daly, H., & Farley, J. (2004). *Ecological economics: Principles and applications.* Washington, DC: Island Press.

Ekelund, R. B., Jr., & Tollison, R. D. (2000). *Economics: Private markets and public choice* (6th ed.). Reading, MA: Addison-Wesley.

Evans, R. G., & Stoddart, G. L. (2003). Consuming research, producing policy? *American Journal of Public Health, 93,* 371–379.

Friedman, M. (1970, September 13). The social responsibility of business is to increase its profits. *The New York Times Magazine,* pp. 122–126.

Furubotn, E. G. (1999). Economic efficiency in a world of frictions. *European Journal of Law and Economics, 8,* 179–197.

Grandjean, P. (2005). Implications of the precautionary principle for public health practice and research. *Human and Ecological Risk Assessment, 11,* 13–15.

Harvey, B., & Hallet, J. D. (1977). *Environment and society: An introductory analysis.* Cambridge, MA: MIT Press.

IKEA Systems. (1999). *Ikea home page.* Retrieved September 2, 2004, from http://www.ikea.com

Institute of Medicine, Committee for the Study of the Future of Public Health. (1988). *The future of public health.* Washington, DC: National Academies Press.

Kochtcheeva, L., & Singh, A. (1999). *An assessment of risks and threats to human health associated with the degradation of ecosystems.* Sioux Falls, SD: United Nations Environmental Programme, Division of Environmental Information, Assessment and Early Warning—North America.

Longest, B. B., Jr. (2002). *Health policymaking in the United States* (3rd ed.). Chicago: Health Administration Press.

Mathur, S. K., & Aday, L. A. (2002). Decision-making for rural community sustainability: The role of social capital in mediating the limitations of market and planning models. *Texas Journal of Rural Health, 20,* 52–61.

McMichael, A. J. (1993). Global environmental change and human population health: A conceptual and scientific challenge for epidemiology. *International Journal of Epidemiology, 22,* 1–8.

McMichael, A. J. (1999). From hazard to habitat: Rethinking environment and health. *Epidemiology, 10,* 460–464.

McMichael, A. J. (2001). Global environmental change as "risk factor": Can epidemiology cope? *American Journal of Public Health, 91,* 1172–1174.

Nattrass, B. F., & Altomare, M. (1999). *The natural step story for business: Wealth, ecology, and the evolutionary corporation.* Gabriola Island, BC, Canada: New Society.

North, D. C. (1990). *Institutions, institutional change, and economic performance.* New York: Cambridge University Press.

Omenn, G. S. (1996). Putting environmental risks in a public health context. *Public Health Reports, 111,* 514–516.

Patz, J. A. (2000). Climate change and health: New research challenges. *Ecosystem Health, 6,* 52–58.

Rapport, D. J. (1989). What constitutes ecosystem health? *Perspectives in Biology and Medicine, 33,* 120–132.

Rapport, D. J. (2000). A new strategy for public health. *Ecosystem Health, 6,* 1–2.

Rapport, D. J., Regier, H. A., & Hutchinson, T. C. (1985). Ecosystem behavior under stress. *American Naturalist, 125,* 617–640.

Raven, P. H., & Berg, L. R. (2004). *Environment* (4th ed.). Hoboken, NJ: Wiley.

Robèrt, K.-H. (2002). *The natural step story: Seeding a quiet revolution.* Gabriola Island, BC, Canada: New Society.

Rose, G. (1985). Sick individuals and sick populations. *International Journal of Epidemiology, 14,* 32–38.

Roseland, M. (2000). Sustainable community development: Integrating environmental, economic, and social objectives. *Progress in Planning, 54,* 73–132.

Shea, S. (1992). Community health, community risks, community action. *American Journal of Public Health, 82,* 785–787.

Soule, E. (2004). The precautionary principle and the regulation of U.S. food and drug safety. *Journal of Medicine and Philosophy, 29,* 333–350.

Weinberg, A. S. (2000). Sustainable economic development in rural America. *Annals of the American Academy of Political and Social Science, 570,* 173–185.

Wilson, M. E. (2000). Environmental change and infectious diseases. *Ecosystem Health, 6,* 7–12.

Windsor, D. (2001). The future of corporate social responsibility. *International Journal of Organizational Analysis, 9,* 225–256.

World Commission on Environment and Development. (1987). *Our common future.* New York: Oxford University Press.

Appendix 3.1

A Case Study of Ecosystem Function and Change: The Iowa Prairie

There are over 94 natural elements on earth. Matter is neither created nor destroyed; but biological, physical, and geochemical processes have resulted in these elements not being evenly distributed among the principal spheres of the earth, the biosphere, and the abiotic (nonliving) spheres—the geosphere and atmosphere. (See Figure 3.2.) The atoms and molecules that make up the organisms in the biotic community of an ecosystem are continually shifting among these organisms and the abiotic sphere.

A number of chemical elements are found in living tissue. Carbon, oxygen, hydrogen, nitrogen, phosphorus, and sulfur account for the bulk of elements in organisms. Other elements, even though present in lesser amounts, are essential for many living processes. These include iron, calcium, magnesium, manganese, and such curiosities as vanadium, along with others. Often these elements are found in combinations termed molecules. Examples include carbon dioxide, ammonia, phosphates, glucose, amino acids, and lipids. At any instant an atom might be either in an organism or a part of the abiotic environment. The shifting of elements between and among the biotic and abiotic spheres is termed *nutrient cycles.*

To demonstrate these principles, we first review a simplified model tall-grass ecosystem in Iowa and then describe how an atom of carbon, phosphorus, and nitrogen might move within this ecosystem and between this part of the biosphere, the atmosphere, and the geosphere. For an expanded and detailed description of ecosystems, see Raven and Berg (2004).

The Members of an Ecosystem on an Iowa Prairie

Our simplified ecosystem includes two primary producers, a stand of big bluestem grass and the prairie pea, a legume. A population of the prairie mouse, *Microtus,* and several populations of insects are the herbivores. A population of shrews and a population of sparrow hawks are the carnivores that feed on the mouse population. There is a host of decomposers, such as bacteria, fungi, nematodes, and insect larvae.

The Movement of Carbon in and Around an Iowa Prairie Ecosystem

The first cycle of carbon can begin with carbon dioxide from the atmosphere being drawn into the grass and peas; through the process of photosynthesis, the chloroplasts of the green cells of these green plants, using sunlight for energy, synthesize a molecule of glucose from this molecule of carbon dioxide and water. The metabolic pathways that create this molecule of glucose release a molecule of oxygen. (Actually, several molecules of carbon dioxide, water, and oxygen are involved in creating a balanced equation.) Chemically, glucose has a reduced chemical bond where energy is stored that can be released later through the process of respiration. This energy can be used later to drive other metabolic processes in the plant. Furthermore, this process releases gaseous oxygen that is added to the atmosphere. The energy released by respiration can drive the metabolic pathways that create and combine the amino acids, lipids, nucleic acids, and other materials that go into making a plant.

A prairie mouse and herbivore insects would forage on both the grass and peas. The carbon atoms incorporated in these plants in molecules of glucose, amino acids, lipids, and nucleic acids could become metabolized and incorporated into carbon-containing molecules of the mouse. The same process could happen in turn in the carnivores and decomposers. Once a carbon atom is fixed by a green plant from atmospheric carbon dioxide, that atom could cycle in this biological community indefinitely. When a molecule containing an atom of carbon becomes a gaseous molecule after it is metabolized through respiration, a molecule of carbon dioxide would leave an organism and enter the gaseous cycle (namely, the atmosphere), where it would likely become a part of a large pattern of circulation and could enter an ecosystem thousands of miles away. Indeed, this is largely what happens. Most materials stay locally in the biosphere.

Carbon Sinks

Here and there certain atoms and molecules are found on the lithosphere in large concentrations. These events are largely occurring over long geological periods and are typically termed *sinks,* to reflect their moving from the molecules that are turning over in the biosphere at a faster rate.

About 300 million years ago, a part of the biosphere in parts of the globe became entrapped such that the ordinary metabolic cycles that transformed carbon from the atmosphere through living tissue and back to the atmosphere slowed. The result was the formation of coal, oil, and natural gas deposits. These deposits can be considered sinks where carbon is now a part of the geosphere and no longer is available for circulation through the biosphere, other than through the intervention of humans. Of course, humans have been rapidly moving this sink from the geological cycle to the gaseous cycle with consequences that become more difficult to deny. Another carbon sink is where the carbonate shells of marine organisms have been laid down under the ocean. Here too, humans are moving this sink of carbon from the geological cycle to the atmosphere.

The Movement of Phosphorus in and Around an Iowa Prairie Ecosystem

An element important to organisms is phosphorus. A natural source for phosphorus on an Iowa prairie is weathered phosphate rock that underlies the soil of Iowa. This phosphorus likely will be in the form of a salt, potassium phosphate, which plants can readily absorb through their root hairs. Once absorbed, this salt would be incorporated into diverse organelles and chemical structures as cell membranes, nucleic acids, and phosphorolated compounds such as adenosine triphosphate. This atom would ordinarily stay in the ecosystem, passing among trophic levels until leached out.

The Movement of Nitrogen in and Around an Iowa Prairie Ecosystem

Carbon dioxide is 0.04% of the atmosphere, and nitrogen is over 78%. The nitrogen cycle can start when symbiotic bacteria associated with nodules of certain legumes (or prairie pea) fix nitrogen to nitrogen hydride. Other soil bacteria can nitrify this molecule to nitrates that plants can assimilate. Once a part of living cells, this nitrogen can be incorporated into amino acids and other molecules necessary for life. Denitrifying bacteria in soil return nitrogen gas to the atmosphere.

An Example of a Modified Ecosystem

Shortly after the arrival of Western Europeans to the prairies of Iowa, circumstances changed. Much of the tall-grass prairies were replaced with monocultures of corn, which is used to feed hogs. The phosphorus incorporated into corn and hogs is removed from the prairie's soil and biotic communities when these farmers ship these organisms to markets for distribution and sale. To replace this nutrient to grow more corn, phosphorus is mined in Florida, transported to Iowa, and placed on these fields. Furthermore, the biomass (such as animal waste) of these farms is removed to parts of the country other than Iowa, where it may be incorporated into the outfall of a sewage treatment plant that in turn may overload a small stream with phosphorus. This phosphorus can overwhelm the natural complex of species in the stream's ecosystem, leading to an explosive growth of algae. Even more surprisingly, this phosphorus from Florida (along with nitrogen fertilizers) is washing from the fields of the Midwest and accumulating in a region of the Gulf of Mexico off the Louisiana coast. This accumulation of phosphorus in a distant ecosystem is disrupting that ecosystem and producing barren areas in the Gulf of Mexico.

Of course, early arrivals from Western Europe increased economic activity. Migration brought motors to power engines to mine the phosphorus, process it, transport it, and spread it; to till the earth; to harvest the crop; and to deliver it. These motors typically are powered with fossil fuel that long ago was buried under the earth (yes, carbon that was part of an ecosystem that was not consumed) but now is accumulating in the atmosphere as carbon dioxide.

A Further Modification of an Ecosystem: Nonmetabolizable Compounds

The bulk of substances made by living organisms is the protoplasm that goes into the cells, tissues, and organism of their bodies. There is a surprising commonality in the molecular composition of organisms of quite divergent phylogenies. The DNA of cells of a nematode is made from the same kinds of molecules as that of a deer or a pine tree. All proteins are composed of a small number of amino acids. Even with this small array of metabolic building blocks, a large and diverse collection of adaptations has arisen. A consequence of this commonality of molecular composition is that when an organism at one trophic level is consumed by an organism at a subsequent trophic level, the biochemical pathways are in place that can rearrange even the larger molecules and atoms into the tissue of the subsequent level.

Yet with this molecular commonality, living organisms are capable of metabolically creating chemical compounds and crystalline structures of spectacular complexity and function. Even structurally simple organisms such as bacteria carry on processes that humans have yet to replicate. For example, soil bacteria and bacteria symbiotically associated with nodules of certain legumes are able to create molecules centered on nitrogen at ordinary pressures and temperatures that humans can do only with high pressures and temperatures. Spiders make fibers from the materials from the insects they consume that rival the steel that humans forge with high heat and much hammering. Some organisms also create compounds that repel or kill predators or competitors. Yet over sufficient periods of time, virtually every molecule of matter made by living organisms can be decomposed by some other organism to more elemental materials and returned to the biological cycles in the biosphere. Only humans have created compounds that some other organism cannot assimilate.

Humans have added a twist that is outside the chemistry of living organisms. Indeed, that is why it appears to achieve our ends. In very short order, we have learned how to synthesize compounds that living organisms do not yet have a way to decompose and return to living cycles. Two examples illustrate this point and some unforeseen and troubling consequences. These are persistent pesticides and plastics.

Pesticides are compounds that kill pests. Pests are organisms that are deemed to interfere with desired human activities, such as crop production, for example. (Other species have pests, but they have evolved mechanisms for this that allow the development of evolutionary equilibrium.) In the 1930s a Swiss chemist, Mueller, discovered the insecticidal properties of DDT. It became widely applied in the 1940s and appeared to provide a way to rid humanity of a large number of scourges. In short order, researchers discovered that many of the pests against which it was applied developed resistance to its effect. They further found that the chemical was not easily and routinely decomposed into basic molecules but instead was accumulating and amplifying in the biosphere. What seemed a simple way to provide a better environment became a blight on it.

A second example can be drawn from plastics. Over the past 90 years, we have found that we can remove hydrocarbon compounds from the earth, compounds that were deposited over 300 million years ago, and convert them into plastics such as nylon. This compound has made life more convenient and fashionable for many of us through such items as shirts and other articles of clothing. Yet we now have a compound that would take over 20 million years to reintegrate into an ecosystem. In contrast, cotton and wool, fibers that have been a part of natural ecosystems since time immemorial, can be recycled among living organisms with virtually no delay.

In a very short time, our society is now producing substances that systematically accumulate in ecosystems. There are no metabolic pathways through which these anthropogenic compounds can be integrated into natural ecosystems.

CHAPTER FOUR

HUMAN DEVELOPMENT

Barbara J. Low, M. David Low,
Kathryn M. Cardarelli, Janet S. de Moor

Chapter Highlights

- Whereas well-being and illness are influenced by biological, environmental, and social experiences that occur throughout the entire life span, the roots of learning, literacy, and the adaptive behaviors that sustain physical and mental health are established during the first few years of a child's life, exerting long-term influences on adult health and ultimately on community and societal function.
- Life-course epidemiology explores the factors that contribute to human development across the life course—including the home environment, early childhood care and experience, education, and the work environment.
- Human learning and education are potentially critical mediators of the relationship among political, economic, and social factors and health.
- One of the best ways to reduce health disparities and income inequalities while improving the health of the nation is to focus policies on optimizing both early childhood development and education, linking early child care, family support,

and developmental enrichment with K–12 education in a seamless continuum.

Introduction

Human development, health, and well-being are closely linked to one another, to socioeconomic status, and to educational attainment. Whereas well-being and avoidance of, or successful adaptation to, illness and stress are influenced by biological, environmental, and social experiences that occur throughout the entire life span, many researchers agree that the roots of learning, literacy, and the adaptive behaviors that sustain physical and mental health are established during the first few years of a child's life, exerting long-term influences on adult health and ultimately on community and societal function (Doherty, 1997; Hart & Risley, 1995; Keating & Hertzman, 1999; Montgomery, Bartley, & Wilkinson, 1997; Neuman & Dickinson, 2001).

Contextual factors influence health throughout an individual's life course. Among key determinants of population health such as social status, social affiliation, and stress (Wilkinson, 1999, 2002), *place* matters. "Place refers to both geographical location and to group membership in terms of family, friends or age, and on the basis of class, ethnicity, residence, and gender that arise out of the (political), social and economic structure of society" (Kuh, Ben-Shlomo, Lynch, Hallqvist, & Power, 2003, p. 780). Experiences related to conditions that define social class at an individual and neighborhood level (Osler & Prescott, 2003), including education (Ross & Mirowsky, 1999), exert a strong influence on health and adaptability over the life course (Krieger & Fee, 1994; Macintyre, 1986). The duration and quality of the educational experience also affect health and quality of life in adulthood through a variety of pathways (Ross & Mirowsky, 1999; Ross & Van Willigen, 1997; Ross & Wu, 1995, 1996).

Low socioeconomic status is one of the strongest predictors of poor health and development across the life course. Beyond and in addition to the serious effects of material deprivation that those living in poverty experience, psychosocial factors may mediate many of the negative effects of relatively low socioeconomic status that are influenced by the neuroendocrine mechanisms of the stress response (Kristenson, Eriksen, Sluiter, Starke, & Ursin, 2004). Such psychobiological adaptation occurs at home (Chandola, Kuper, Singh-Manoux, Bartley, & Marmot, 2004) and at work (Niedhammer, Tek, Starke, & Siegrist, 2004; Siegrist et al., 2004). Psychological factors, mediated through social interaction, may affect health, either directly through conscious individual-level processes or indirectly, by constraining behavior and lifestyle choices. Scholars do not yet clearly understand the interrelationships among these fundamentally significant processes (Martikainen, Bartley, & Lahelma, 2002).

Overview

Human development can be viewed as the product of all of the day-to-day processes, experiences, and events that influence the capabilities of individuals to lead healthy, satisfying, safe, responsible, and productive lives. Because the range of potential influences is so great, this chapter will focus primarily on those factors that appear to us to contribute most to human capital across the life course. *Human capital* is a conceptual measure of workforce economic capacity that combines individual, social, and information capital, directly determined by level of education, literacy, and psychosocial competence. The Organisation for Economic Co-operation and Development (OECD) defines *human capital* as "the knowledge, skills, competencies and attributes embodied in individuals that facilitate the creation of personal, social and economic well-being" (Healy et al., 2001, p. 18). Human capital encompasses individual development of skills, knowledge, and competence through social relationships, education, community participation, and individual behavioral choices such as tobacco smoking, and physical activity level (Becker, 1964, 1991; Coleman, 1988). Contributing factors include the home environment, early childhood care and experience, education, and the work environment.

As already noted, researchers (Thompson, 2001) now widely recognize the significance of the first few years of life for subsequent healthy development, although factors experienced later in life must also be considered (Greenough, 1997). This chapter therefore reviews life-course epidemiological evidence in detail, to assist in the creation of a framework for new policy recommendations based on criteria of effectiveness, efficiency, and equity.

Fields of Study

Developmental factors acting across the life course influence a broad range of outcomes, from general health to the ability to perform activities of daily living and to chronic disease (Keating & Hertzman, 1999; Kuh & Ben-Shlomo, 2004; Marmot & Wadsworth, 1997). Four key frameworks guide our examination of health and human development: the Evans and Stoddart model of population health (1990, 2003); the Hertzman model of life-course effects (Hertzman, Power, Matthews, & Manor, 2001); the developmental perspective of health as defined by Halfon and

Hochstein (2002); and the work of Kuh and colleagues (2003) on life-course epidemiology. These and other models describe determinants of health at multiple levels interacting and influencing individuals and populations over time.

The Evans and Stoddart model (1990, 2003) is presented in detail in Chapter Two (Figure 2.1) and provides general theoretical support for the content of this chapter. The concept of life-span development is elaborated by Hertzman et al. (2001) and supported by the work of Elder (1998), Leidy (1996), and Rutter (1989). Ben-Shlomo and Kuh (2002) provide a detailed overview of this approach in explaining the onset of chronic disease, with conceptual models that integrate biological, behavioral, and psychosocial pathways from gestation through childhood, adolescence, and young adulthood, operating both across an individual's life course and across generations.

The life-course approach integrates ecological and social factors into an ecosocial model of the determinants of population health (Krieger, 2001; Kuh & Ben-Shlomo, 2004). Similarly, Halfon and Hochstein's life-course human development framework (2002) involves key components of context, process, mechanism, and timing (see Figure 4.1). Adapted from Worthman (1999), this model illustrates the parallel and interacting nature of multiple developmental time frames: the stages of the life course; transitional periods and turning points; and crosscutting historical, economic, and political trends. The principal components of life-course human development influence health outcomes through the interplay among nested factors of health development. These include macrocontextual or environmental factors ("The Context of Health Development" in the figure) that interact and modify the microcontextual factors (2a in the figure), such as health developmental strategies and pathways (e.g., physiological, behavioral, and psychological).

At an individual level (2b), cumulative and programmed patterns mediate a complex array of regulatory processes such as psycho-neuroendocrine and immune function during critical and sensitive periods. The macro- and microcontexts are modified by specifically timed experiences over multiple time frames to affect developmental health outcomes (3 in the figure). Halfon and Hochstein (2002, p. 433) summarize their framework in several concepts presented in Figure 4.1 and by the following:

- Health is a consequence of multiple determinants operating in nested genetic, biological, behavioral, social, and economic contexts that change as a person develops;
- Health development is an adaptive process composed of multiple transactions between these contexts and the bio-behavioral regulatory systems that define human functions;

FIGURE 4.1.   PRINCIPAL COMPONENTS OF THE LIFE-COURSE HEALTH DEVELOPMENT FRAMEWORK AND THEIR INFLUENCE ON HEALTH OUTCOMES.

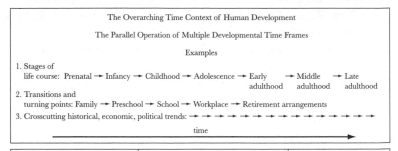

The Overarching Time Context of Human Development

The Parallel Operation of Multiple Developmental Time Frames

Examples

1. Stages of
   life course: Prenatal → Infancy → Childhood → Adolescence → Early → Middle → Late
                                                                        adulthood   adulthood   adulthood
2. Transitions and
   turning points: Family → Preschool → School → Workplace → Retirement arrangements
3. Crosscutting historical, economic, political trends: → → → → → → → → → → → → → → → → → →

time

---

1. The Context of Health Development

Macrocontexts/Environments

○ Genetic endowment of species
○ Physical environment
  • Availability of resources
  • Food, clean air, open space
  • Pathogen exposure
○ Social environment
  • Income, economic resources
  • Prosperity, disparities
  • Social conditions, connectedness
○ Family environment
  • Family structure, function, resources
  • Family life cycle and support
○ Psychological environment
  • Psychosocial stress
  • Behavioral response patterns
○ Culture and policy environment
  • Norms, values, policies
○ Health care system
  • Access, context, organization, quality of health services

2a. The Design and Process of Health Development

Microcontext

○ Design features and strategies
  • Selection of resources, optimization of function
  • Integration and coordination of biobehavioral processes
  • Growth, maturation, compensation
○ Health development processes
  • Physiological pathways and systems
  • Behavioral pathways and systems
  • Psychological pathways and systems

2b. The Mechanisms and Regulatory Processes of Health Development

Differences between individuals in the functioning mechanisms and processes account for variation in individual trajectories of health development.

○ Mechanisms/patterns
  • Cumulative
  • Programmed
○ Regulatory process
  • Critical and sensitive periods
  • Psychoneuro-endocrine regulation
  • Psychoneuro-immuno regulation
  • Setpoints, thresholds, feedback loops
  • Cross-system connectivity and circuits
  • Receptor populations, carrier proteins messengers

3. Developmental Health Outcomes

• Life expectancy
• Functional capacities (cognition, mood, physical activity, growth, fertility)
• Disease, disability, dysfunction
• School readiness and performance, job performance

Note. From "Life Course Health Development: An Integrated Framework for Developing Health, Policy, and Research," by N. Halfon and M. Hochstein, 2002, *Milbank Quarterly, 80,* p. 438, fig. 1. Used with permission of Blackwell Publishing. Adapted from "Epidemiology of Human Development," by C. M. Worthman, in C. Panter-Brick & C. M. Worthman (Eds.), *Hormones, Health, and Behavior: A Socio-ecological and Lifespan Perspective* (New York: Cambridge University Press, 1999), p. 91, fig. 1.

- Different health trajectories are the product of cumulative risk and protective factors and other influences that are programmed into biobehavioral regulatory systems during critical and sensitive periods; and
- The timing and sequence of biological, psychological, cultural, and historical events and experiences influence the health and development of both individuals and populations.

A life-course approach "offers an interdisciplinary framework for guiding research on health, human development, and aging" (Kuh et al., 2003, p. 778). Life-course causal models can follow four pathways leading from risk (e.g., potentially harmful biological, psychological, and social exposures) through (1) accumulation of independent risk, relative to time; (2) accumulation of clusters of risk, relative to time; (3) a chain of risk that involves additive effects (worsening effect after each exposure) over time, in which one adverse exposure or experience tends to lead to another through mediating factors (e.g., risk or protective factors that mediate the association between exposure and disease when it occurs after the exposure and is on the causal pathway), at least conceptually, and moderating factors (e.g., risk or protective factors that modify the association between an exposure or experience and disease or injury when the causal effect of the exposure of interest differs across levels of the modifying factor); or (4) a chain of risk that involves trigger effects (i.e., earlier exposures have no effect on disease or injury risk without the final link in the chain that precipitates disease or injury onset).

These pathways apply both to acute infectious disease (Hall, Yee, & Thomas, 2002) and to chronic behavior or psychosocial-related disease (Martikainen et al., 2002) through the life course, including biological incorporation or embedding of early experience into the structural and functional aspects of biological and behavioral systems (Hertzman, 1999) and its effects on adult health (Hertzman & Wiens, 1995). As infants develop, they interact with their environment and in turn shape the experiences to which they must adapt mentally, physically, and socially. Through this process the child's behavior itself influences genetic expression, and this is further reflected in altered behavior (National Research Council, Committee on Integrating the Science of Early Childhood Development, 2000; Siegel, 1999; Thompson, 2001).

As noted earlier, appropriate stimulation and positive early experience have profound impacts not only on the development of those neural systems subserving cognitive, emotional, neuroendocrine, and neuroimmune functions (Keating & Miller, 1999) but also on genetic expression of factors that modify the effects of stress hormone receptors, and therefore the individual's responses to stress, throughout life (Meaney et al., 1996). As a result of this biological embedding, Keating and Miller (1999) posit developmental trajectories characterized by human acquisition of competence and coping skills and by regulation of responses to new or challenging experiences. An example of the origin of such a trajectory is infant distress, integrating neurophysiological, behavioral, and social responses that help the infant to regulate its own emotion as well as to facilitate parental responses. Infants who are successfully able to regulate their attention, emotion, and social functions are better able to learn and to cope with challenges or novel experiences. The quality of interpersonal relationships and social environment strongly influences infant developmental trajectories involving self-regulation, competence, and coping. These experiences set the stage for future competence in learning, formal education, and prosocial behaviors (Keating & Miller, 1999), although the mature brain will continue to adapt to positive and negative environmental exposures throughout life (Nelson & Bloom, 1997).

To shift the traditional clinical paradigm of health during childhood and adolescence to a more encompassing epidemiological approach that includes adolescent developmental and behavioral factors, Garbarino and Ganzel (2000) formulated the human ecology of early risk. This ecological model emphasizes that the "habitat of the child at risk includes family, friends, neighborhood, church, and school, as well as immediate forces that constitute the social geography and climate (e.g., laws, institutions, and values), and the physical environment" (p. 76). Like Bronfenbrenner (1979) in his model of the ecology of human development, Garbarino has focused on the multisystem social environment in which the young person lives and develops. Using Bandura's model (1986b) of reciprocal determinism, it is important to consider the bidirectional interrelation among individual factors (cognitive, affective, and biological), as well as behavior and the external environments in which children and adolescents function. Although adolescence is a time of experimentation with risk taking (Irwin, 1993), intervention to prevent or reduce harm may be optimal at several specific transition points along the developmental pathway (Grzywacz & Fuqua, 2000). We provide a detailed discussion of lifecourse exposure to risk, including an explanation of the concepts of critical periods, latent effects, and cumulative effects, in the latter part of this chapter.

These and other conceptual frameworks previously described provide the foundation for measuring health, development, and well-being across the life course, as well as for creating policy designed to promote health.

Policy Domains

Despite incomplete data on how to change developmental trajectories and limited availability of measurement tools for early child development (Shonkoff, 2003), we submit that federal, state, and local policies in the domains of early childhood education, early child care and welfare, and health would best serve the needs of the most vulnerable as well as the more advantaged members of society by acting as early as possible in the life course *before* costly health and social problems are incurred. These policies would best serve children and their families if they were integrated at each level of government.

Evidence highlighting the health consequences of cumulative exposures in research on life-course dynamics can be linked to policies that amplify or moderate inequalities in socioeconomic position, education, and ultimately in health (Graham, 2004; Kamerman, Neuman, Waldfogel, & Brooks-Gunn, 2003). As well as the education, family, social welfare, and health-related policies outlined, other findings from Halfon and Hochstein (2002) and many examples of early childhood education research support new policy recommendations, such as those from UCLA's Center for Healthier Children, Families and Communities (2004).

The evidence of the need for a new approach to policies in the broad domain of human development is highlighted in statistics showing relatively poor health status within and significant health disparities across the population (National Institutes of Health [NIH], 2002; NIH Working Group on Health Disparities, n.d.; World Health Organization, 2000); very high health care costs nationally (American Medical Association [AMA], Ad Hoc Committee on Health Literacy for the Council on Scientific Affairs, 1999; U.S. Department of Health and Human Services [USDHHS], NIH, National Library of Medicine, 2000); and significant disparities in educational attainment across the population (U.S. Department of Education [USDE], National Center for Education Statistics [NCES], 1997, 2001a, 2001b). Also, a great deal of evidence shows that both inadequate income and income disparities are associated with poor health (Deaton, 2002; Marmot, 2002). In all of these areas, the United States, with its vast resources, could create and sustain more effective, efficient, and equitable policies.

Evidence Regarding Research on Fundamental Determinants

This section provides a broad overview of concepts related to healthy life-course development; ways to measure it at a population level; and ways that development of human capital is thought to affect health through various pathways, particularly through education. We describe important determinants for each major stage of life-course development, with a particular focus on its dynamic nature through variable types, exposure, and trajectories related to risk, as well as moderating factors, timing, and context of development.

Measures of Child Health and Human Development

The health and well-being of children is a clear indication of the general health and well-being of any community. Among many industrialized nations, indicators or measures of poor child health include child abuse and neglect, unsatisfactory child development (physical, cognitive, and socioemotional), poor school achievement, and child poverty (Micklewright & Stewart, 2000). Child poverty has profound effects on child health and development.

One of the most crucial transition points in the human life course occurs when children begin school, usually between ages four and six. Although there is little consensus on the definition of *school readiness* (Saluja, Scott-Little, & Clifford, 2000) beyond age at point of entry into formal schooling, most would agree that it involves a positive interaction between the individual child, the family, the school, and the surrounding community. At the individual level, school readiness encompasses the essential but not exhaustive level of child developmental characteristics (Meisels, 1999) likely to promote successful learning experiences, measured within five domains: health and physical development, emotional well-being and social competence, approaches to learning, communicative skills, and cognition and general knowledge (Kagan, 1999; National Education Goals Panel, Goal 1 Technical Planning Group, 1995). The adequacy of school preparation and services to help children to maximize their potential development in each of those domains is an essential component of school readiness. As well as providing educational resources, family support for school readiness involves providing adequate child care and nurturing, parental involvement in promoting reading and literacy promotion, and education and modeling to promote effective social and emotional competence (for example, through simple conflict resolution skills training and guidance to help children to follow basic rules at school).

Socioeconomic factors affect child development early in life, particularly in the United States. According to Gershoff at the National Center for Children in Poverty, "When low family incomes compromise child development, we all pay the price in higher costs for special education and mental and physical health services, lower levels of educational achievement, and a less prepared work force" (Gershoff, 2003, p. 8). The rate of child poverty is much higher in the United States than in most other Western industrialized nations (Luxembourg Income Study, 2004). Using nationally representative data on 21,255 U.S. kindergartners from the Early Childhood Longitudinal Study, kindergarten class of 1998–99, Gershoff (2003) examined academic, social, and physical indicators of child development at the end of the kindergarten year. She found significant disparity in school readiness between children from families with economic security and those from low-income families (that is, families with an annual income between $18,400 per year, the federal poverty-level marker for a family of four, and $36,800, which represents 200% of the federal poverty level) (USDHHS, Office of the Assistant Secretary for Planning and Evaluation, 2003a). Figure 4.2 depicts data from a nationally representative sample of children in 1998. These data indicate that most children from the poorest families achieved significantly lower test scores for reading, math, and general knowledge than did their peers from families with incomes of $55,200 or more (over 300% of federal poverty level), although 16% of the children from the lowest-income families scored in the upper range compared to half of the children from the highest-income families (Gershoff, 2003, p. 5).

Gershoff (2003) noted that the minimum economic security that families needed in order to realistically provide their children with basic housing, food, and

FIGURE 4.2. AVERAGE READING, MATH, AND GENERAL KNOWLEDGE STANDARDIZED TEST SCORES WITHIN INCOME-TO-NEEDS GROUPS, 1998.

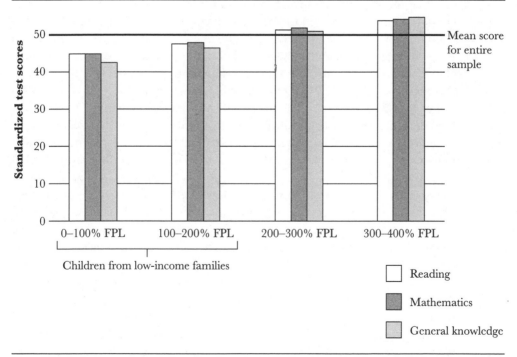

Note. FPL = federal poverty level. From *Low Income and the Development of America's Kindergartners* (Living at the Edge Research Brief No. 4), by E. Gershoff (New York: National Center for Children in Poverty, 2003), p. 5, fig. 2. Used with permission.

health care is actually about double the poverty-level income. She found a strong linear relationship between family-income level and children's developmental outcomes for social and emotional functioning, cognitive skills, and health: "the more income a family has, the better children do" (p. 7).

Several countries measure other child and adolescent health and developmental outcomes, such as infant mortality, teen pregnancy and parenting rates, school dropout rates, and social inclusion or exclusion (Micklewright & Stewart, 2000; United Nations Children's Fund International Child Development Centre, 2002). *Social exclusion* (Kahn & Kamerman, 2002), a term that French policy-makers adopted in the 1970s, is described as "what can happen when people or areas suffer from a combination of linked problems such as unemployment, poor skills, low incomes, unfair discrimination, poor housing, high crime, bad health and family breakdown" (Social Exclusion Unit, 2004, p. 4). Kamerman (2002b, p. 3) defines it as "the process by which individuals and groups are wholly or partly closed out from participation in their society, as a consequence of low income and constricted access to employment, social benefits and services, and to various aspects of cultural and community life."

The Australian Institute of Family Studies (2002) recommended monitoring child development through the use of indicators similar to those addressed in Canada. The Canadian Federal, Provincial and Territorial Early Childhood Development Agreement (Minister of Public Works and Government Services Canada, 2001) highlights four child developmental objectives to direct policies that promote the physical and emotional health, safety, learning success, and social engagement and responsibility of all its youngest residents. To help guide human development policy, the Canadian government has funded research to create a population-based measurement of early childhood development, now used in many school districts nationwide. The Early Development Instrument (EDI) is a psychometrically sound tool that encompasses the domains of cognitive, physical, social, emotional, and communication competence as well as general knowledge (Janus & Offord, 2000) previously described as individual developmental characteristics of school readiness. The EDI helps teachers to screen individual children at age four or five for readiness to learn and is used to predict future school performance among groups of children as well as to assess the efficacy of community support of its youngest residents and their families. Since 1998 more than 90,000 Canadian children in 40 communities have been evaluated with the EDI to promote healthy families and competent children throughout their early development. Figure 4.3 illustrates findings from initial research that show the gradient reflected by the percentage of children screened with the EDI who scored within the lowest 10% of children in their community, who were not ready to learn

FIGURE 4.3. READINESS TO LEARN AT SCHOOL BY FAMILY INCOME: NATIONAL LONGITUDINAL STUDY OF CANADIAN YOUTH, 2000.

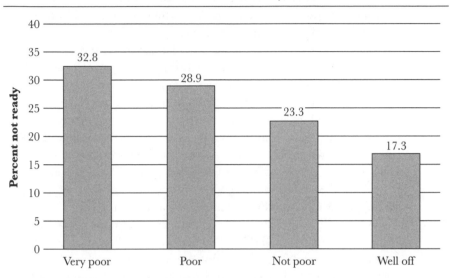

Note. N = 1,799. From *The School Readiness to Learn Project in Canada,* by D. R. Offord and M. Janus, 2002, http://www.offordcentre.com/readiness/files/PUB.6.2002_Offord-Janus.pdf, p. 18. Used with permission.

in kindergarten, by their family socioeconomic status (Edudata Canada, n.d.; Founder's Network, 2004).

In the United States, extensive measures of child and adolescent health and development also focus on the multidimensional assessment of physical, emotional, social, and mental status, including academic performance at the individual and population level (Riley et al., 1998). Systematic, regularly reported data collected nationally reflect child morbidity and mortality outcomes, as well as maternal prenatal care, maternal mortality, infant birth weight, nutrition, immunization history, experience of child abuse and neglect, hospitalizations, youth health-risk behavior, teen pregnancy, youth sexually transmitted disease prevalence, and health insurance status as part of the child health index (Annie E. Casey Foundation, 2004). Annual reports from the Federal Interagency Forum on Child and Family Statistics (2004) and USDHHS (2004) examine demographic factors such as fertility rates and out-of-wedlock births, economic well-being (including child poverty), family structure and composition, parental employment status, health conditions (including infant mortality rates and low birth weight), health care, health behavior (including alcohol and tobacco use, drug abuse, accidental mortality, suicide, and sexual activity), and education (including school readiness, early childhood education, literacy and numeracy skills, school problems and failure, school enrollment, and highest grade completed).

Since 1975 the Foundation for Child Development Index of Child Well-Being Project (2004) has generated an annual composite score of child well-being in the United States. The index of child well-being measures 28 key indicators of child and youth well-being within the domains of health, safety/behavioral, maternal well-being, productive activity, emotional/spiritual well-being, place in community, and social relationships. Notably, investigators reported a significant drop in composite scores linked to family and economic changes in the United States from 1981 to 1994. Despite gains since that time, the 2002 well-being status, as determined for U.S. children and youth from all race and ethnic groups, was only slightly better than that of the baseline measured in 1975.

Among all U.S. residents, the leading health indicators that are monitored by *Healthy People 2010* (USDHHS, 2000) include the following: physical activity, overweight and obesity, tobacco use, substance abuse, responsible sexual behavior, mental health, injury and violence, environmental quality, immunization, and access to health care. Surveillance of child well-being does not usually include child health–related behavior (Brown, 1997); however, the Youth Risk Behavior Surveillance Survey (Kolbe, 1990) does measure these behaviors annually among U.S. high school–age youth enrolled in school (Grunbaum et al., 2002). As part of the child health index, child morbidity and mortality outcomes are measured as well as individual and family health-related data. Inclusion of these contextual indices provides an informative picture of the range of development that U.S. children and youth experience (USDHHS, Health Resources and Services Administration, Maternal and Child Health Bureau, 2002).

In 1989 the National Institutes of Child Health and Development (NICHD) began an extensive longitudinal study of early childhood care and youth developmental outcomes through grade six in the Study of Early Child Care (NICHD Early Child Care Research Network, 1994). Researchers in Texas, California, and Alabama have been tracking child health and development among youth from age 10 (grade five) through age 20, using an extensive battery of child and family measures within the home, school, and neighborhood contexts. The Healthy Passages project, funded by the Centers for Disease Control and Prevention (CDC), is a community-based longitudinal study of the developmental trajectories of 1,750 youth to identify the etiological factors that predict health-risk behaviors and related health outcomes and to examine factors related to disparities in health outcomes across racially and ethnically diverse youth populations (Windle et al., 2004).

In general, measurement of individual and community health assets associated with positive development has its basis in the field of community development (McKnight, 1999). The national health objectives for *Healthy People 2010*, based on the *Healthy People 2000* objectives for national health promotion and disease prevention, provide a comprehensive preventive framework of child and youth priorities that include in-school health education and normative development programs (USDHHS, 1991; USDHHS, National Center for Health Statistics [NCHS], 2004).

Complementing these objectives for healthy child development are the national educational goals prescribed in *America 2000: An Education Strategy* (USDE, 1991) to promote school readiness, to prevent school failure and dropout, and to increase high school graduation rates. The Goals 2000: Educate America Act (1994), now archived, deemed that

> by the year 2000, all students would leave grades 4, 8, and 12 having demonstrated competency over a wide range of academic subjects ensuring that every school in America would prepare students for responsible citizenship, further learning, and productive employment.

Although this remains only a lofty aspiration, the public school system is in a position to make a unique and direct impact on both the education and health of many U.S. children (Simeonsson & Gray, 1994). However, research has shown that the environmental characteristics of schools, such as health and safety measures, nutrition services, and parental and community involvement, must be modified concurrently with promotion of behavior change at the levels of the individual and community in order to achieve lasting health-behavior changes (Kelder, Edmundson, & Lytle, 1997; Simons-Morton, Parcel, O'Hara, Blair, & Pate, 1988).

Stages of Life-Course Development

Physical, intellectual, emotional, and social development occurs throughout the life course. Although brain development, represented by neuronal growth, migration, connectivity, and neurosynaptic changes, occurs most dramatically during the first years of life, neurological function retains its plastic nature (Gazzaniga, Volpe, Smylie, Wilson, & LeDoux, 1979) to a great extent and continues to adapt to demands through adolescence and adulthood (Nelson & Bloom, 1997; Thompson & Nelson, 2001). This experience-dependent brain plasticity is most apparent in the cerebral cortex for higher functions involving thinking, memory, and learning (Dowling, 1998; Greenough, Withers, & Anderson, 1992). Each stage of human development is essential for healthy functioning, but the balance and relative timing of exposure to specific stimuli are linked to adaptation and plasticity, particularly during the perinatal period (DeWitt et al., 1997) and early childhood (Shore, 2003).

The effects of the early environment, both negative and positive, are long lasting (Carnegie Corporation of New York, 1994). The literature now contains a great deal of evidence for a close relationship between early life conditions, later performance in school, adult literacy, health status, and mortality (Evans, Barer, & Marmor, 1994; Keating & Hertzman, 1999).

Gestation. Beginning at the time of conception, human embryo development is influenced by biological programming in utero (Godfrey & Barker, 2001), which is in turn affected by the health and nutritional status of the mother (Ehrenberg, Dierker, Milluzzi, & Mercer, 2003) and by environmental influences such as toxins, for example, lead (Lanphear, Dietrich, Auinger, & Cox, 2000). The gestation period lasts on average about 266 days or 38 weeks, although the time between conception and birth is usually closer to 40 weeks (Grunfeld, 1995). Brain development begins about one month after conception, and early cognitive capability has been demonstrated as soon as six weeks prior to birth (DeCasper, Lecanuet, Busnel, Granier-Deferre, & Maugeais, 1994; Kisilevsky et al., 2003). We know from research in developmental neuroscience that learning starts at birth and that brain development in the first years of life is both rapid and extensive. Early sensory and emotional experience directly affects both the absolute number of mature, differentiated brain cells and the connections between them. The more numerous the connections, the greater will be the child's capacity for learning. Genes can and do specify the brain's basic "wiring," the common neural architecture, but there are not nearly enough genes to specify the trillions of connections that characterize the optimally functioning human brain. Most of those grow and become established as a direct consequence of sensory and emotional experience. Without the experience the connections either will not develop or will not be maintained (Huttenlocher, 1984; Rakic, Bourgeois, & Goldman-Rakic, 1994; Shore, 2003).

Not only is brain development before age three more rapid and important than we have previously thought, but early brain development is vulnerable to environmental influences such as stress and lack of nurturing. Chronic exposure to stress is linked to specific genetic changes that influence neuroendocrine function, for example, through dysregulation of forebrain glucocorticoid receptor gene expression (Meaney et al., 1996). During the neonatal period, cell growth and development of neurological, cardiopulmonary, endocrine, immunological, and musculoskeletal systems are particularly vulnerable to disruption by significant adverse events such as trauma, infection, nutritional deprivation, or toxic levels of certain drugs such as alcohol (Roccella & Testa, 2003).

Infancy. Neurosynaptic growth and refinement of brain function accelerates markedly after birth, particularly during the first six months. During this period general neurocognitive development and specific processes such as cerebral myelination (laying down of fatty material to form a sheath around the nerve cells) depend largely on the interaction between genetic endowment and environmental stimulation; in addition, as noted earlier, the child's brain development is driven by experience (Hockfield & Lombroso, 1998; Neville & Bavelier, 1999). Low birth weight poses a significant barrier to healthy infant development, but in the United States the incidence has been relatively unchanged for over three decades at a rate of 8% of all live births (NCHS, 2003a). "Babies born at low birth weight (less than 2500 grams, or 5.5 pounds) are most susceptible to physical disabilities, developmental delays, and infant death" (USDHHS, Health Resources, 2002, p. 7). The rate of low or very low birth weight for African American infants is the highest among race or ethnic groups at 13.4%; Hispanic babies experience the lowest such rate at 6.5% (NCHS, 2003a).

From birth through the first two years of life, many factors influence early human development and directly affect perceptual, cognitive, social, and emotional status (Muir & Slater, 2000; Siegel, 1999; Thompson, 1999). In addition to infant temperament and reactivity (Kagan, 1994), determination of later cognitive and emotional resiliency may depend on the quality and extent of early brain development experienced, particularly in the deep forebrain centers that support emotion and memory function (Dawson, 1994; Nelson, 1995). Animal studies indicate that important forebrain development and stimulation of receptor sites that promote spatial learning and memory function are strongly influenced by maternal-infant interaction and nurturing (Liu, Diorio, Day, Francis, & Meaney, 2000). In human development some of the key factors involve critical or sensitive periods that depend on the relative timing and balance of certain types of experience such as adequate nutrition (e.g., folic acid), sensory stimuli in the physical environment (e.g., visual and speech), parental nurturance and parent-child attachment (Thompson, 1999), protection from harm (Felitti et al., 1998), and the social environment including the broader influences of family and parenting (Daw, 1995; Lamb, Bornstein & Teti, 2002).

Concurrently, development of language and social function depends largely on the adequacy and type of positive, repetitive, and low-stress stimulation the child receives from the environment and the care providers, such as being exposed to spoken language, being read aloud to, interacting face-to-face, and practicing associating words with objects (Kuhl, 1993; Landry, Smith, Swank, & Miller-Loncar, 2000; Woodward & Markman, 1998). Cognitive development is continuous and incremental and persists at least through puberty or later (Kirby & Hurford, 1997). Neurological development and resultant cognitive capacity involve many complex processes, so that some authors have asserted that intelligence and brain development are neither simply nor directly related (Bruer, 1998).

Early Childhood or Preschool Years. The quality, amount, and consistency of nurturing, support, and stimulation that children receive depends largely on the socioeconomic, family, and neighborhood context in which they live (Gershoff, 2003). During the first five years of life, inequalities in child development appear as gradients that are shaped by the following factors: parent education level; parenting style; family income; neighborhood quality and cohesion; safety; and access to quality child care, developmental programs, and health care (Keating & Hertzman, 1999). Almost one quarter of children in the United States and Canada are estimated to be vulnerable and may be at risk for future developmentally related problems (Duncan & Brooks-Gunn, 1997; Willms, 2002).

The early childhood preschool period involves tremendous acceleration in physical, emotional, intellectual-cognitive, and social development. Unused neurological synapses that developed so exuberantly during infancy are selectively lost during childhood, depending on the type of stimulation and environmental input that the child experiences—a phenomenon called *synaptic pruning* (Chechik, Meilijson, & Ruppin, 1999). Brain development continues, forming the capacity for healthy emotional and intellectual function.

The preschool years encompass an important period of human development between ages two and six, before U.S. children begin compulsory education (from ages seven through fifteen). During this time children mature from toddlerhood until they are enrolled in preschool or prekindergarten, usually at four to five years of age. Depending on a child's place of residence, local policy, family resources, and preference, preschool may consist of a formal or informal program that provides supervision for interactive activity and peer play, social skills instruction, and often, but not always, early classroom activities that prepare the child for development of reading and language skills. Preschool influence on early child development is associated with later academic achievement (Ladd & Price, 1987). Some school districts offer kindergarten for five-year-olds to provide more teacher-led instruction and social skill development.

Whether in preschool or early childhood care, children may be supervised by biological or foster parents, trained caregivers, preschool educators, or untrained care providers or child minders. Caregiving involves a positive interaction between the child and the provider, ideally through developmentally appropriate promotion of the child's control over the learning experiences of interest. The caregiver must help to manage the learning environment to ensure child safety and to provide appropriate stimulation while interacting with the child in a responsive, nurturing, and socially supportive manner. Caregiver use of gestures, verbal communication, and play (Bergen, 2002) are crucial for early language and cognitive development (Bruner, Jolly, & Sylva, 1976; Nicolopoulou, 1993). Warm, effective parenting and close family relationships serve as protective factors to optimize early child social and emotional development (Werner, 1993), although the absence of these factors is not sufficient to cause later socioemotional or behavioral dysfunction (Flint & Kilgour, 1966; Winick, Meyer, & Harris, 1975). Parenting style (Darling & Steinberg, 1993), modeling (Bandura, 1986b), and family activities strongly influence short- and long-term adoption of health-related behaviors such as those involving nutrition and exercise or compliance with medical care (Baranowski & Nader, 1985; Campbell, 1986). It is now clear that the quality and adequacy of early care giving can influence future development through the life course (Brandtjen & Verny, 2001) and that socioeconomic factors that affect the quality of care giving as well as access to formal child care and preschool are strong determinants of health in an ecological sense. Children raised in deep poverty are most vulnerable to experiencing poor health (Hertzman, McLean, Kohen, Dunn, & Evans, 2002; NICHD Early Child Care Research Network, 2003; Werner & Smith, 1982).

In the 21st century, although parents and caregivers are considered to be the key sources of social influence on very young children (McIntyre & Dusek, 1995), the mass media plays an increasingly important environmental role among two- to six-year-olds due to widespread exposure (Kaiser Family Foundation, 2003b). A study of youth media use estimated that 20% of 2- to 7-year-olds, almost 50% of 8- to 12-year-olds, and about 60% of 13- to 17-year-olds have television sets in their bedrooms (Gentile & Walsh, 2002). Depending on the child's developmental level, media content, and degree of exposure, media portrayal of violence can negatively influence youth health-risk behavior (American Academy of Pediatrics, Committee on Public Education, 2001; Johnson, Cohen, Smailes, Kasen, & Brook, 2002), sexuality (Escobar-Chaves, Tortolero, Markham, & Low, 2004), food consumption (Crespo et al., 2001; Dietz & Gortmaker, 1985), tobacco and alcohol use (Connolly, Casswell, Zhang, & Silva, 1994; USDHHS, Centers for Disease Control and Prevention, National Center for Chronic Disease Prevention and Health Promotion, Office on Smoking and Health, 1994), and suicide (Gould & Shaffer, 1986).

Childhood: Ages 6 Through 10. These years encompass the transitional periods from mid- to late childhood and the beginning of formal schooling. Socioeconomic factors and early language skills can predict academic achievement (Walker, Greenwood, Hart, & Carta, 1994). Healthy children who enter the formal education system ready to learn have a better chance of succeeding in school (McKenzie & Richmond, 1998) and are more likely to become productive citizens than are those whose early development is compromised.

As a crucial aspect of the developmental trajectory, Erikson (1959, 1963, 1968) hypothesized a lifelong and central role for vocational development. He described, in concert with maturation of biological systems within a sociocultural context, adaptive capacities that individuals must acquire as they move through developmental stages from birth through adulthood before they can successfully meet life's challenges. During the third of eight psychosocial stages of development, at about age five, children begin to enjoy using tools and caring for younger children. From this time until they are about 10 years of age, most children identify with work roles of parents or other significant persons (Havighurst, 1964). Encompassing Erikson's fourth psychosocial developmental stage, this is the time when children internalize the principle of work as they begin to take on tasks such as school work and chores that help them to develop a sense of industry. During this period they must distinguish between behaviors and circumstances related to work and play (Havighurst, 1964). During puberty most adolescents develop a range of identities that include an occupational or vocational identity that may set the stage for future work-related attitudes, behaviors, and pursuits (Vondracek, 1992).

Younger school-age children continue to experience dramatic gains in physical, social, and cognitive development. Their increased attention span supports focused learning of all types, including the solving of concrete problems (Ginsburg & Opper, 1988; Piaget, 1952) and reading. Social relationships and play, especially with peers, become important as conceptual identity evolves (Perry, Pollard, Blakley, Baker, & Vigilante, 1995). As children approach puberty, rapid physical growth is often associated with increasing independence from parents and greater importance of peer relationships to social well-being (Morison & Masten, 1991).

Adolescence: Ages 11 Through 17. Adolescence is "a period of personal development during which a young person must establish a personal sense of individual identity and feelings of self-worth which include an alteration of his or her body image, adaptation to more mature intellectual abilities, adjustment to society's demands for behavioral maturity, internalizing a personal value system, and preparing for adult roles" (Ingersoll, 1989, p. 2). During early adolescence this preparation is influenced by the fit between the individual and the environment, characterizing personal relationships and the adoption of school, work, and possibly family roles (Eccles et al., 1993).

The term *adolescent* usually refers to young people under the age of 18 (Federal Interagency Forum on Child and Family Statistics, 2004). During this period most adolescents have experienced physiological and psychosocial changes related to puberty (Connolly, Paikoff, & Buchanan, 1996). Cognitive function continues to develop to include abstract and logical conceptualization from about age 11 through adulthood (Piaget, 1952). Multilevel influences from peers (Yancey, Siegel, &

McDaniel, 2002), parents (Cox & Harter, 2003), and the media (Escobar-Chaves et al., 2004; Kaiser Family Foundation, 2003a, 2004) may shape adolescent health-related behavior and well-being through periods of vulnerability associated with psychological distress (Ge, Conger, & Elder, 1996). These external or environmental influences (Fullerton & Ursano, 1994) may result in early adoption of unhealthy practices, such as tobacco smoking, that often continue into adulthood (Crockett & Petersen, 1993; Fischhoff, 1992; Flay, d'Avernas, Best, Kersell, & Ryan, 1983; Jessor, 1984; Jessor, Donovan, & Costa, 1991; Quadrel, Fischhoff, & Davis, 1993).

Adolescent short-term health outcomes are likely to be affected largely through behaviors that result in unintentional and intentional injury, alcohol and other drug use, and infections such as HIV/AIDS and sexually transmitted disease (STD) (Grunbaum et al., 2002; Institute of Medicine, Committee on Prevention and Control of STDs, 1997; NCHS, 2001; Resnick et al., 1997). Among 5- to 24 year olds, only four causes account for nearly three-quarters of total mortality and much of the morbidity and social dysfunction experienced in this age group: motor vehicle accidents (29% mortality, i.e., 40% of motor vehicle accidents are alcohol-related); homicide (20% mortality); suicide (12% mortality); and unintentional injuries from fires, falls, and drownings (11% mortality). In addition, nearly one quarter of all new HIV infections, one quarter of all new infections with other STDs, and 870,000 pregnancies occur among U.S. adolescents annually (Grunbaum et al., 2002; NCHS, 2001). Although the primary threats to adolescents' health are related to the health-risk behaviors they or their caregivers choose to adopt (Annie E. Casey Foundation, 2004; CDC, National Center for Chronic Disease Prevention and Health Promotion, 2004a, 2004b; Children's Defense Fund, 1998), early initiation of health-compromising behavior (tobacco use, dietary patterns, and physical inactivity) is also implicated in the total mortality associated with the long-term development of chronic health problems of cardiovascular disease (39.4%) and cancer (23.5%) in adulthood (Basen-Engquist, Edmundson, & Parcel, 1996; Grunbaum et al., 2004; NCHS, 2003b). McGinnis and Foege (1993) estimated that 50% of adult mortality in the United States is related to unhealthy lifestyle choices, for example, tobacco use, often initiated during adolescence.

Transition to Adulthood. As adolescents transition to young adulthood, they depend less directly on their membership in a family group, become increasingly self-reliant, and develop a more cohesive sense of identity in their new social role (Rutter, 1989). The two most important developmental tasks for older adolescents and young adults involve forming and maintaining interpersonal relationships and developing a capacity for productive activity such as work or raising a family (Havighurst, 1972). Throughout adulthood social support, clear personal values, economic stability, and meaningful pursuits provide a strong foundation for health and well-being (Antonucci, 1991). Although most individuals complete their formal education or vocational training in late adolescence or early adulthood, the capacity for learning continues through the life course (Rutter & Rutter, 1993; Tennant & Pogson, 1995). Social roles and behavior are influenced by many factors such as socioeconomic status, age, race or ethnicity, culture, gender, sexual orientation, religiosity, academic and job skills, and health status.

Young Adulthood: Ages 18 to 40. Most young people leave home during late adolescence and young adulthood, either to continue their education, enter the labor force, or form new intimate relationships and/or family groups. As well as the primary focus of employment (Karasek & Theorell, 1990), the activities of parenthood, child rearing, civic participation, and contribution to the larger society provide new and challenging roles for many young adults. This is particularly true for differently abled young people who are pursuing education (Margalit, 2003) and employment opportunities (Boardman, Grove, Perkins, & Shepherd, 2003).

During this phase of the life course, an individual's biological endowment, personality characteristics, knowledge and beliefs about parenting and child development, cultural models (Harkness, Super, & Keefer, 1992), and personal experience of childhood and adolescence are likely to affect choices he or she will make as a parent (Luster & Okagaki, 1993). Whether familial interactions were positive or negative, most parenting practice is thought to be shaped intergenerationally and seldom remains static (Harkness et al., 1992). Past experience of parent-child closeness and the quality of family life provide a contextual influence on child rearing (Kolar, 1999). Although reproduction and child rearing may enhance an individual's psychosocial well-being, parenting may also involve significant economic, educational, and supervisory responsibilities that the individual must meet for the better part of two decades or more.

Middle Adulthood: Ages 41 to 65. As individuals and families mature, the balance between self and society may alter, particularly as preparation for change begins in work and caregiver roles. Parenting adult children; grand-parenting; and coping with chronic illness, loss, and lifestyle change may emerge as new challenges in midlife. Many people leave the workforce at or before age 65, particularly if they experience health problems (Dwyer & Mitchell, 1999); and they may face related economic, social, or individual role-related stress.

Late Adulthood: Ages 66 and Older. Although individuals vary greatly, physical and mental functions often decline after the sixth decade of life unless individuals maintain healthy levels of physical activity and adequate nutrition (Birren & Schaie,

2001; Mattson, Duan, Wan, & Guo, 2004). Although health, quality of life, and socioeconomic status may be less stable than during early adulthood, social support and maintenance of healthy lifestyle may promote continued well-being (Baltes & Baltes, 1990; Bossé, Levenson, Spiro, Aldwin, & Mroczek, 1992; Deeg, Kardaun, & Fozard, 1996; Wortman & Silver, 1990). Relationships with adult children may change as caregiver roles reverse during senescence (Stone, Cafferata, & Sangl, 1987).

Dynamics of Life-Course Development

Human development is a dynamic process that involves the interplay between exposure to various risks along experiential trajectories that are shaped by timing, context, and degree of individual resilience and adaptation to potentially harmful experience.

Risk. The term *risk* refers to specific conditions that make an individual susceptible to disease, reduced quality of life, or developmental disorders. According to Simeonsson (1994, p. 5),

> At risk status is not simply a concept that applies to problems of infancy and early childhood. It encompasses all developmental phases from the fetal period (drug exposure) and early childhood (learning problems) to the problems of delinquency, teen pregnancy, and school failure in adolescence.

Exposure to a variety of developmental risks during early childhood may influence mental health (Sameroff & Fiese, 2000), including family function (Raphael & Sprague, 1996).

Health-risk behavior encompasses voluntary activity characterized by violence, suicidality (ideation and behavior), use of tobacco, alcohol, and other drugs, early and unprotected sexual activity, as well as poor nutrition and inadequate physical activity. Although good parenting can act as a buffer to protect children from risk, transmission of unhealthy behavior can also occur intergenerationally (Wickrama, Conger, Wallace, & Elder, 1999).

Until recently, research on health determinants focused largely on measures of disease (NCHS, 2000) rather than on assets and resources. A growing literature examines the interplay between risk and protection, contributing in a dynamic fashion across time to poor health or well-being through the life course.

Life Exposures to Risk. Inequalities in human health and development exist from conception to adulthood and are similar to social and economic class gradients in their expression (Hertzman, 1998). Children living in low-income families are on average more likely to be vulnerable to poorer health and quality of life through their life course than are their peers from higher-income families (Duncan & Brooks-Gunn, 1997; McCain & Mustard, 1999). Health and developmental gradients emerge in early childhood relative to infant mortality and low birth weight; during school-age years in relation to behavioral and cognitive development; and throughout adulthood in terms of obesity, mental health, and long-term or recurring illness, as well as later experience of chronic disease and dementia (Keating & Hertzman, 1999).

Trajectories of Life Exposures to Risk. A *trajectory* is "a long term view of one dimension of an individual's life over time. These may be social states (such as work, marriage, socioeconomic position), psychological states (such as depression) or physiological states (such as lung function)" (Kuh et al., 2003, p. 781). Across the life course, an individual's unique life-exposure trajectory reflects differential exposure to a range of health-promoting and harmful events that are ultimately expressed as health and well-being (Hertzman et al., 2001). As a result of these fundamental life-course exposures, long-term health and social gradients will also emerge at group or population levels (Hertzman, 1990; Starfield, Riley, Witt, & Robertson, 2002). Many studies have regressed measures of behavior, cognition, and health against socioeconomic position (SEP), whether defined by income, occupation, or education (Ala-Mursula, Vahtera, Pentti, & Kivimaki, 2004; Avendaño et al., 2004; Case, Griffin, & Kelly, 1999; Claussen, Davey, & Thelle, 2003; Everson-Rose, Mendes de Leon, Bienias, Wilson, & Evans, 2003; Hertzman, 1999; Jackson, Wright, Kubzansky, & Weiss, 2004; Kunst, Geurts, & van den Berg, 1995; Macintyre, 1994; Marmot, Feeney, Shipley, North, & Syme, 1995; Power & Hertzman, 1997; Vescio, Smith, Giampaoli, & MATISS Research Group, 2003; Willms, 1999).

The data demonstrate a graded relationship, or gradient, with lowest levels of SEP having lowest health outcomes and at every level of the social hierarchical scale, those with higher levels of SEP on average having better health outcomes (Lawlor, Ebrahim, & Davey, 2004; Mustard, 2000). To illustrate, Figure 4.4 depicts cumulative death rates among 4,271 British adults age 26 to 54 by their socioeconomic position during childhood—those whose fathers were manual workers (i.e., indicator of poorer socioeconomic conditions) were twice as likely to die at age 54 compared to those whose fathers were not manual workers (6% vs. 3%, respectively) (Kuh, Hardy, Langenberg, Richards, & Wadsworth, 2002).

Using terminology from the field of life-course epidemiology, Hertzman and colleagues (2001) described three generic patterns through which these outcomes might be expressed, categorized as latency, cumulative, and pathway effects. During early development, individuals may experience life events that exert more than one type of effect, ultimately influencing their competence or well-being.

FIGURE 4.4. ADULT MORTALITY RELATED TO SOCIOECONOMIC CONDITIONS DURING CHILDHOOD.

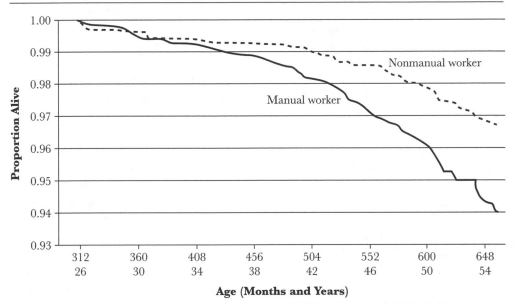

Cumulative Death Rates Age 26 to 54 Years by Father's Social Class in 4,271 (201 Deaths) Men and Women Born in March 1946

Note. Adapted from "Mortality in Adults Aged 26–54 Years Related to Socioeconomic Conditions in Childhood and Adulthood: Post War Birth Cohort Study," by D. Kuh, R. Hardy, C. Langenberg, M. Richards, & M. E. Wadsworth, 2002, *British Medical Journal, 325,* p. 1078, fig. 1. Used with permission of the BMJ Publishing Group.

Latent effects arise when, regardless of intervening experience, exposure to developmental or biological factors at a specific point in the trajectory does not affect health status until many years later (Keating & Hertzman, 1999). For example, full-term infants who are small for gestational age may be at increased risk for high blood pressure, heart disease, and adult-onset diabetes several decades later (Marmot & Wadsworth, 1997). Other evidence from fetal and infant exposure resulting in adult disease supports this long-term exposure–effect pattern through a direct association between early life events and adult coronary heart disease and hypertension (Barker, 1997; Barker, Osmond, Simmonds, & Wield, 1993). During the first seven years of life, British children who grew relatively rapidly, who were consistently read to during the preschool years, and who coped well with their transition into school were only one-fifth as likely to report fair or poor health status at age 33 than their peers who experienced slow growth, inconsistent stimulation by reading, and problematic school adjustment (Jefferis, Power, & Hertzman, 2002; Power, Li, & Manor, 2000). Similarly, cognitive-intellectual and social-emotional-behavioral development is influenced early in life but may exhibit distal health or social outcomes (Repetti, Taylor, & Seeman, 2002). An infant's nurturing experience with consistent, trusted, and affectionate caregivers positively influences development of neurobiological functioning as well as secure relational attachments later in childhood, adolescence, and adulthood (Bates, Maslin, & Frankel, 1985; Eisenberg, 1990; Francis & Meaney, 1999; Suomi, 1999).

Cumulative effects result from exposure to protective and risk factors that accumulate over the life course, depending on their duration, frequency, and intensity (Hertzman et al., 2001; Keating & Hertzman, 1999). Evidence of this pattern arising from multiple exposures to socioeconomic risk is provided by the stronger influence of low parental occupational class on poor adult health throughout childhood than at any single point in time (Power, Manor, & Matthews, 1999). A four-year study of the effects of welfare services on U.S. children living in poverty found that maternal factors such as education level and marital status, as well as early childhood experiences, predicted school performance and behavior problems at ages 10 and 11, but family economic stability emerged as a primary determinant (Moore, Glei, Driscoll, Zaslow, & Redd, 2002). A British longitudinal study of the effects of multiple exposures showed that adverse factors in early life (physical height and socioeconomic disadvantage during childhood), adolescence (behavioral adjustment), and adulthood (underweight or overweight and injury) predicted chronic illness and disability at age 33 (Jefferis et al., 2002; Power et al., 2000).

Social disadvantage may influence individual health trajectories cumulatively from birth onward, but researchers have also noted a strong association between the size of the social differences among members of a society and the overall health of that population. This *gradient effect* (Acheson, 1998; Keating & Hertzman, 1999), evident whether investigators consider current socioeconomic status or that of an individual's family of origin, appears steepest in populations with marked differences in individual social position. These cumulative effects appear to persist across the life course into old age (Power & Hertzman, 1997).

Pathway effects originate in early life when certain trajectories lead to social and behavioral experiences that, in a cascading fashion, eventually affect health, well-being, and competence. A good example of these cascading effects can be found in the influence of socioeconomic context of early childhood on readiness for learning (Duncan & Brooks-Gunn, 1997; Kohen & Hertzman, 1998). Differential status at birth is associated with varying levels of security, stability, and stimulation during early childhood that later influence the child's readiness to learn in school; this in turn puts children at risk for academic, social, and behavioral problems including mental illness, school dropout, violence, criminality, teenage pregnancy, tobacco smoking, and substance use (Hertzman & Wiens, 1996; Keating & Hertzman, 1999; Power, Manor, & Fox, 1991; Tremblay, 1999).

Moderators of Trajectories of Life Exposures to Risk. Individual experience of exposure to risk and its effects may be moderated throughout the life course, depending on the timing and context of exposure as well as on the person's adaptive ability, for example, resilience.

Timing and Context of Healthy Development. This section defines several important developmental terms: The *critical period* of development (Colombo, 1982) is "a limited time window in which an exposure can have adverse or protective effects on development and subsequent disease outcome" (Kuh et al., 2003, p. 780); *sensitive periods of development* occur when an exposure has a stronger effect on development and disease risk than it would at other times (Ben-Shlomo & Kuh, 2002, p. 288); and the *context* is the

> location of an individual by time and place, including group membership, class, ethnicity, residence, and gender relating to social and economic structure of society. Application of a life course perspective to contextual as well as individual effects on health implies understanding the effects of changing contexts over time on the life course of individuals (Kuh et al., 2003, p. 780).

According to the conceptual model posited by Hertzman and colleagues (2001), health status across an individual's life course is influenced by the interaction between daily experiences and latent, cumulative, and pathway effects. At each stage of development, particularly during critical and sensitive periods such as the first three years of life, physiological growth and eventual maturation directly affect health status (Cameron & Demerath, 2002). Over time health is concurrently influenced by interactions within the environmental context of individual, societal, and broader socioeconomic factors. These influences must be considered in an integrated fashion to better relate policy to human development and health (Hertzman et al., 2001).

> Health development is shaped by the dynamic and continuous interaction between biology and experiences and is framed by the constantly changing developmental contexts over the lifetime. These nested contexts include child rearing, access to resources, employment and health care, and the psychological environment that mediates behavior and stress responses to the trials and tribulations of daily life. The dynamic interaction between biology and experience

also is shaped by biobehavioral pathways that are genetically programmed and adaptively influenced by individuals, families, and social experiences and environments. Differences in the health development trajectories of individuals and populations reflect the cumulative and programmed effects of risk and protective factors on health development (Halfon & Hochstein, 2002, p. 10).

Transition Periods. During major transitions between developmental levels (Shonkoff & Marshall, 2000), humans may be especially vulnerable to external influences such as the physical, social, and cultural environments. Depending on their context, such transition-linked turning points represent developmental events that can potentially influence long-term behavior, cognition, or affect (Graber & Brooks-Gunn, 1996; Pickles & Rutter, 1991; Rutter, 1994). Although currently limited, research that examines how children and adolescents manage these transitions due to certain environmental or contextual factors (Brooks-Gunn & Duncan, 1997; Maggi, Hertzman, Kohen, & D'Angiulli, 2004; Willms, 2002; Yoshikawa, 1994) or to psychological or biological characteristics will contribute to our understanding of the developmental influences of risk and resilience throughout the life course (Graber & Brooks-Gunn, 1996).

> Developmental plasticity and vulnerability are complementary expressions of the same idea, with episodes of rapid change creating periods of enhanced vulnerability. This relationship implies that developmental trajectories can be altered more readily during sensitive periods of rapid developmental change than during other periods. Each transition represents an important point in development during which adverse and beneficial inputs can have a relatively greater effect on future health. Life transitions, such as starting nursery school, entering middle school, or entering or leaving the workforce, impose stress on adaptive and regulatory systems, requiring the developing individual to adapt to new routines and to adopt new response patterns (Halfon & Hochstein, 2002, p. 8).

Resilience to Risks and Related Assets. According to Hertzman (1998, p. 14), "the complex relationship between life course and social/economic-psychosocial conditions in a given society has a powerful determining effect on human health." Yet despite exposure to multiple risk factors during infancy and early childhood, many individuals develop into healthy, productive, and stable adolescents and adults. From an early developmental perspective, the term *resilience* refers to characteristics and resources that children and adolescents can rely on to effectively deal with stress and to remain on track developmentally through the transition into adulthood (Luthar & Zigler, 1991; Rutter, 1987) or to a dynamic process involving "maintenance of positive adaptation by individuals despite experiences of significant adversity" (Luthar, Cicchetti, & Becker, 2000, p. 543). Psychosocial resilience and protective mechanisms incorporate individual and socioenvironmental beliefs, attitudes, and behaviors that promote health. Garmezy (1982, p. xiii) described the resilient youth as "the healthy child in an unhealthy setting," referring to competence under potentially harmful conditions.

The key findings of several researchers, for example, Hertzman and Wiens (1996) in their review of child development and long-term health outcomes from a population perspective, as well as evidence from intervention studies (e.g., quality child care, family support, and early education), provide guidance for creating policies related to promoting healthy early childhood and adolescent development. A primary focus of research on child and adolescent health centers on the intrinsic and extrinsic factors associated with educational, emotional, and behavioral resilience early in the life course (Masten, 2001; Masten, Best, & Garmezy, 1990; Rutter, 1989), their developmental trajectories from childhood through adulthood (Kohen, Hertzman, & Brooks-Gunn, 1999; Roisman, Masten, Coatsworth, & Tellegen, 2004; Smith & Kuh, 2001; Suomi, 1999), and policies that support or inhibit resilience and healthy development (Weissberg, Caplan, & Harwood, 1991).

The Kauai Longitudinal Study (Werner, 1993; Werner & Smith, 1982) provided strong evidence that resilience involves a dynamic developmental process (Werner & Smith, 1992). Among a diverse birth cohort, about one-third of the 15% of children at risk for serious academic or conduct problems who experienced four or more early risk factors (e.g., perinatal stress, poverty, low parental education, and family conflict) still coped academically, got along with parents and peers, kept out of serious trouble, and grew up to be healthy adults. Beginning in early childhood, these resilient youngsters experienced fewer adverse events such as separations from caregivers and rapid arrival of younger siblings. Besides protective factors such as better physical health and appealing temperament as infants, they had more social resources such as nurturing parenting and strong bonds with prosocial adults, for example, those whose voluntary behavior is intended to benefit others. This group also possessed traits such as intellectual capability, responsibility, self-confidence, and achievement motivation that helped the individuals to capitalize on educational and occupational opportunities.

As noted in Chapter Two, population health monitoring should focus on positive developmental assets and resources rather than solely on the traditional outcomes of mortality and morbidity (Andrews & Ben-Arieh, 1999; Breslow, 1999; Lerner & Benson, 2003; Young, 2005). Healthy child and adolescent development is supported and strengthened by protective factors or assets within the context of the individual's needs. This is particularly true for those considered at risk of unhealthy development due to poverty, family dysfunction, school failure, exposure to harm, or adoption of health-risk behavior (Benson, Leffert, Scales, & Blyth, 1998). From a developmental perspective, healthy youth are considered to benefit from emotional attachment and commitment (bonding) to parents, family, peers, educators, and community members within the individual's culture. Lack of sufficient assets or resources may predispose vulnerable youth to problem behaviors such as substance use (Kumpfer & Turner, 1990).

Other assets that may shield or buffer youth from harm (Tolan, Guerra, & Kendall, 1995) are those that foster resilience, self-determination, self-efficacy, well-defined and positive identity, future aspirations, and prosocial norms. In an evaluation of 25 positive youth-development interventions with community, school, and/or family components, Catalano, Berglund, Ryan, Lonczak, and Hawkins (1998) found that the most effective programs improved positive youth-adult bonds, increased youth participation in positive social activities, and provided recognition for positive behaviors such as educational engagement, for example, the degree to which the youth made an effort to perform well in school.

While young people are developing decision-making skills, they are greatly influenced by peers (Fullerton & Ursano, 1994; Hymel, Comfort, Schonert-Reichl, & McDougall, 1996), parents (Darling & Steinberg, 1993), school personnel (Kumpfer & Turner, 1990), and the media (Escobar-Chaves et al., 2004; Singer, Slovak, Frierson, & York, 1998; Smith & Donnerstein, 1998). These and other environmental factors may shape their future educational attainment and health behavior (Hartup & Moore, 1990; Keefe, 1994; McBroom, 1994).

Rather than focus solely on surveillance of health-risk behavior through measures such as the Youth Risk Behavior Survey (Kolbe, 1990), some researchers also measure youth assets involving adult support, interaction with parents, and empathetic relationships in order to better understand their relationship to health (Leffert et al., 1998; Reininger et al., 2003; Scales & Leffert, 2004; Tolan et al., 1995). Half of the 40 assets that the Developmental Assets Framework (Leffert et al., 1998) measures are characterized as intrapersonal factors within the domains of education, community, values, social competency, and positive identity. Another 20 environmental factors are measured within the domains of support, empowerment, boundaries and expectations, and time. Using this framework, Scales and Leffert (2004) describe an additive protective effect so that the more assets young people have, the greater their likelihood of avoiding health-risk behaviors such as substance use or delinquency and negative outcomes such as teen pregnancy. While evaluating the Adolescent Health Attitude and Behavior Survey to measure risk behaviors, attitudes, and youth assets among almost 4,400 public high school students, Reininger and colleagues (2003) reported findings that suggested similar additive protective effects in relation to sexual activity. "Youth with more assets and more protective attitudes about sex engage in fewer risk behaviors" (p. 474).

Assets at the collective level, termed *social capital,* subsume social trust and social networks (Coleman, 1990; Kawachi & Kennedy, 1997; Putnam, 1993), that is, "those features of social organization, such as the extent of interpersonal trust between citizens, norms of reciprocity, and density of civic associations, that facilitate cooperation for mutual benefit" (Kawachi, Kennedy, & Glass, 1999, p. 1187). At the community level, assets are linked to social capital through effective schools (Edmonds, 1986), neighborhood affiliation, and social connectedness or cohesion (Potapchuk, Crocker, & Schechter, 1997; Putnam, 1995; Woolcock & Narayan, 2000). Bell (2001) advocates proactive development of youth resiliency through promotion of community partnerships, physical health, family and school connectedness (Cox & Harter, 2003; Resnick, Harris, & Blum, 1993; Resnick et al., 1997), improved parenting and parental monitoring of children (Crouter, MacDermid, McHale, & Perry-Jenkins, 1990), youth social skills (Hawkins, Catalano, Kosterman, Abbott, & Hill, 1999), and prevention or amelioration of the effects of violence and trauma (Ellickson & McGuigan, 2000).

Impact of Human Capital Development on Health

Because the breadth of policy influences on human development is so great (Evans, 2002), this chapter focuses on human learning and education as potentially critical mediators of the relationship among political, economic, and social factors and health. The evidence for a relationship between education and health is extensive and persuasive. Healthy, competent, and literate residents of a community are more likely to contribute to their own as well as to a collective economy through gainful employment, regular tax payment, and civic participation such as voting, while minimizing the cost to society through imprisonment, long-term welfare support, or expenditure for serious medical care. Although designed to promote the growth of individual human capital, health and education policy must also promote development of social capital at the level of the local community, state, and nation. Chapter Six further discusses the role of social capital in community development.

Direct and Indirect Causal Pathways

Studies in several countries have shown a direct relationship between years of education completed and life expectancy, as well as objective and self-reported measures of health (Deaton & Paxton, 1999; Elo & Preston, 1996; Grossman & Kaestner, 1997; Kaplan & Keil, 1993; Ross & Mirowsky, 1999; Ross & Van Willigen, 1997).

Findings also show that low levels of education and literacy are associated with earlier mortality, poorer health, adoption of health-risk behaviors, lack of use of preventive health care, and generation of very high health care costs (Feldman, Makuc, Kleinman, & Cornoni-Huntley, 1989; Kunst et al., 1995; Pappas, Queen, Hadden, & Fisher, 1993; Weiss, 1999; Williams, Baker, Parker, & Nurss, 1998; Winkleby, Jatulis, Frank, & Fortmann, 1992).

Although scholars have well established the relationship of education to health, they do not yet completely understand the precise pathways through which education mediates health. Primary candidates include a direct, causal effect as well as indirect effects through work and income, self-efficacy, social supports, and influences on healthy lifestyles (Lynch et al., 1998; Ross & Wu, 1995). There are a number of possible explanations, and although we consider them separately here, we emphasize that they are not mutually exclusive; one pathway may predominate at one stage of the life course, whereas another is more important at a different stage. They may also interact with and influence each other.

Ross and colleagues (Ross & Mirowsky, 1999; Ross & Wu, 1995) argue that education exerts its positive effects on health through four broad channels: by influencing work and economic conditions; by enhancing social and psychological resources; by enabling lifestyle and health behaviors; and directly, with no known mediators. Researchers both in this country and elsewhere have paid a great deal of attention to the work and income pathway. As noted earlier, the relationship between personal or household income and life expectancy appears to be a very robust one (Lynch et al., 1998; Ross et al., 2000; Wolfson, Kaplan, Lynch, Ross, & Backlund, 1999). Well-educated people are more likely to work full-time, have higher incomes, and be in more satisfying jobs. Better-educated people are less likely to experience financial hardship or to be unemployed.

Marmot's now classic Whitehall study (Marmot et al., 1991) has shown a gradient in health status and mortality across job classifications in the British civil service, leading Evans (2002) to surmise that somehow, one's position in the workplace hierarchy becomes embedded in one's biology. Marmot (2002) emphasizes the importance to health of a personal sense of control over working conditions and job demands. While examining the relative contributions of education, work, and income to health, Winkleby and colleagues (1992) have shown that although income, education, and occupation all contribute to risk factors for cardiovascular disease, the relationship is strongest for education.

Good evidence supports Ross and colleagues' (Ross & Mirowsky, 1999; Ross & Wu, 1995) proposed second pathway between education and health mediated by social and psychological resources. The critical factors inherent in these resources are not yet identified, but there are a great many promising candidates. Readers must understand that education is not just for inculcation of marketable skills. It is also critical for acquiring those "spiritual resources" and capacities that Fogel (2000, p. 178) describes that are necessary for making moral choices, making informed judgments, increasing personal sense of control, enabling mastery, and facilitating self-direction. Scholars have defined many of these capacities and studied their origins. A large literature exists on character development, self-control, self-efficacy, and resilience. Factors such as supportive parental guidance and modeling (Cohen, Richardson, & LaBree, 1994; Duncan, Duncan, & Hops, 1996; Wickrama et al., 1999); stable social bond to a competent, caring adult (Egeland, Carlson, & Sroufe, 1993); positive and consistent experience with goal setting and achievement (Bandura, 1986b; Earley & Lituchy, 1991; Finn & Rock, 1997); monitoring and limit setting by parents (Chilcoat & Anthony, 1996; Dishion & McMahon, 1998); peer modeling and support (Bandura, 1986a; Fagan & Wilkinson, 1998; Schunk, 1987); reinforcement by significant others (Edmundson et al., 1996; Rosenfield, Folger, & Adelman, 1980); clear and positive community values (Flay, Allred, & Ordway, 2001; McAlister, Puska, Salonen, Tuomilehto, & Koskela, 1982); and committed, capable, experienced teachers who can inspire with positive expectations (Langer, 2000; Teven, 2001) all have important influences on children's development. Research has shown that many of these learned capacities also have a positive effect on health.

Better-educated people tend to have more numerous, supportive, and informative associations with family, friends, and others in their community (Marmot, Bosma, Hemingway, Brunner, & Stansfeld, 1997); and a large literature exists on the positive health effects of social support (Berkman & Syme, 1979; Eckenrode, 1983; Gore, 1978; House, Landis, & Umberson, 1988).

Research also supports Ross and colleagues' third proposed pathway (Ross & Mirowsky, 1999; Ross & Wu, 1995), the influence of education on health-promoting behavior. Well-educated people are more likely to engage in positive health behaviors such as exercising, not smoking, not drinking heavily, and using the health care system appropriately (Lantz et al., 1998; Ross & Mirowsky, 1999; Ross & Wu, 1995). This relationship appears very early in the educational stream, at least by the eighth grade (Low, 2001); and like education's effect on mortality, it is dose-dependent: The more years of education a person receives, the less likely that individual is to engage in negative health behaviors (Flay et al., 1994; Greenlund et al., 1996; Kandel & Wu, 1995).

Direct Effects of Education on Health. Based on the remaining unexplained variance in her data, Ross and her colleagues (Ross & Mirowsky, 1999; Ross & Wu, 1995) have concluded that education has a positive effect on health that is independent of the three pathways of influence; other authors have offered indirect evidence that education actually causes health. Based on a longitudinal cohort study constructed from census data from the decades before, during, and after different U.S. states enacted compulsory education laws, Lleras-Muney (2002) demonstrated a strong positive effect of education on life expectancy (mortality). She concluded that education does produce health, but because her data could not illuminate the pathways through which the effect is transmitted, they do not permit the determination of a direct effect of education on health.

Kennedy (2003) examined the hypothesis that education causes health, testing an econometric model that included technical efficiency, allocative efficiency, and time preference as possible pathways. His analysis found support for an effect of all three. We have already discussed time preference in preceding sections, but for those readers not familiar with the terms, *allocative* and *technical efficiency* together are very roughly equivalent to the processes of choosing and using the most appropriate resources for maintaining and enhancing health. Self-efficacy, self-control, and self-direction would play important roles in these processes, as would *health literacy* (AMA, 1999), defined as "the degree to which individuals have the capacity to obtain, process, and understand basic health information and services needed to make appropriate health decisions" (Ratzan & Parker, 2000, p. iv). The same definition of health literacy has provided the basis for national health communication objectives in the *Healthy People 2010* report (USDHHS, 2002). Researchers have found strong evidence to support the association between low literacy, poor health status, and premature mortality in the United States and overseas (Cleland & van Ginniken, 1988; Grosse & Auffrey, 1989; Weiss, Hart, McGee, & D'Estelle, 1992).

We would add one more line of evidence to support the concept that education and associated learning have direct effects on the brain. Recent research has demonstrated that even in older adults, learning new material and mental exercise are associated with increases in neuronal connectivity, measurable changes in the size of the hippocampus and other forebrain structures—thought to be responsible for permanent memory—and protection against cognitive decline (Albert, 1995; Yamada, Mizuno, & Nabeshima, 2002).

Alternative Explanations. Of course, both education and health may depend on some other factor that researchers have not yet identified. This section examines evidence pertaining to this possible third factor as well as to the hypothetical directionality of causation.

Third-Factor Hypothesis. There are at least two good candidates for a third factor: *endowment,* that cluster of genetically inherited factors that predispose to achievement and good health, and so-called *time preference* or delay of gratification (Fuchs,

1982). Genetic factors are rarely included for study per se in social determinants research, but evidence appears both for some heritability of general intelligence (Dickens & Flynn, 2001; Kaprio, Pulkkinen, & Rose, 2002; Miller, Mulvey, & Martin, 2001; Neiss & Rowe, 2000) and for a relationship between IQ, success in education, and health (Eaves, Vance, Mann, & Parkerbohannon, 1990; Hicks, Langham, & Takenaka, 1982; Jimerson, Egeland, Sroufe, & Carlson, 2000; Lassiter & Bardos, 1995; Lavin, 1996; Morris, 1999). Given the probable range of IQs included in cited studies of the correlation between years of education and mortality, and given the good evidence that environmental factors play a significant role in shaping IQ (Dickens & Flynn, 2001), it seems unlikely that inherited IQ alone accounts for the observed relationship between education and health. Of course, other inherited traits such as personality, stature, longevity, proneness to specific diseases, and so on may play a role in both health and education; but as yet there is no credible evidence of their effects on the health of populations. Research has good evidence that education plays a role in promoting health that is independent of such personal endowments, including genetics.

Low time preference, the ability and inclination to postpone gratification in the expectation of future benefit, is an important factor that some authors (Fuchs, 1982) believe may help explain some of the observed connection between education and health. According to this hypothesis, those who are able to put off earning income will stay in school longer than those who cannot, and the same traits will lead to avoiding the immediate gratifications of tobacco smoking and overeating in expectation of a longer and healthier life.

Fuchs (1982) and Kennedy (2003), among others, have demonstrated that time preference does play a role, albeit a relatively small one, in both education and health. The key question is whether time preference is innate or learned. The evidence from sociological research supports the view that time preference is significantly influenced by social and cultural factors (Lawrance, 1991).

Using a Danish cohort data set, Arendt (2001) also examined the hypothesis that education and health are related through some third variable. The two candidate variables he chose to examine were "endowment" or genetic factors and time preference. His work, like Kennedy's (2003), showed that education has positive effects on health that are independent of either endowment or time preference. Due to the complexity of the retrospective design involving comparison of individuals of disparate age over a relatively short follow-up period (five years) without being able to control for income, researchers must interpret the findings with caution, particularly in view of the potential for bias due to multicollinearity, for example, when two or more predictor variables in the regression model are highly correlated.

Possible Reverse Causation. Although education may promote or even cause health, another possible explanation of the correlation between them is the reverse: Better health may lead to more and better education. Although it is obvious in some cases that poor health may interfere with education, the relationship is very likely bidirectional over the life course; and the preponderance of the evidence supports the concept that the initial relationship is strongly in the direction from education to health and not the other way around (Koivusilta, Rimpela, & Rimpela, 1999; Ross & Wu, 1996; Shakotko, Edwards, & Grossman, 1980).

Evidence for the Impact of Education on Health. Educational attainment predicts occupational success as well as positive health outcomes: Individuals with less education report poorer health and are more likely to die prematurely (Feldman et al., 1989; Kunst et al., 1995; Pappas et al., 1993). If education does contribute as much to health as the literature clearly suggests, then a policy initiative aimed at broad improvements in education across the United States could produce a benefit to U.S. society in at least two areas of clearly demonstrated need—education and health. But the challenge of optimizing educational opportunity and outcomes should be approached from an effective starting point, and many national and state governments have concluded that providing publicly supported education beginning in kindergarten is too late.

Early Childhood. A substantial amount of evidence points to the fact that children do not reach kindergarten with the same capacities for learning and that rather than reducing these differences, the traditional K–12 education system in place in many school districts, particularly those in urban poor communities, perpetuates and even magnifies the differences. Two of the most important factors determining success in education are family resources and the course and quality of early childhood development (Lee & Burkham, 2002). Jimerson et al. (2000) have shown that a child's home environment and early care giving are powerful predictors of whether the child remained in a traditional program or dropped out of high school. Early care has an effect on the child's ability to capitalize on ensuing opportunities and environmental resources (Sroufe & Egeland, 1991). From this perspective "the context from which the child emerges when entering elementary school provides a critical foundation for subsequent academic success" (Jimerson et al., 2000, p. 544).

Fuchs and Reklis (1997) have reported a striking relationship between mathematics achievement in the eighth grade and readiness to learn, measured in part by behavior and language skills, as children entered kindergarten in each state in the United States. The relationship is essentially linear; math scores are higher in states where more children come to kindergarten ready to learn. Investigators reported similar findings in Canada, linking readiness to learn at ages four and five to mathematical performance, general academic achievement, and juvenile delinquency rates (McCain & Mustard, 1999, p. 9).

Academic failure or school dropout represents a much greater problem to society than just a loss of human capital. Early leavers will be more likely to engage in health-risk behaviors, be imprisoned for criminal activity, experience more illness, earn much less, participate in federal welfare programs, create more social problems, and live shorter lives than will their classmates who remain to graduate (Ary, Duncan, Duncan, & Hops, 1999; Boisjoly, Harris, & Duncan, 1998; NCHS, 2000; U.S. Department of Justice, Bureau of Justice Statistics, 2000). Furthermore, there is a close association between academic performance and current health status among low-income minority adolescent schoolchildren (Low, 2001). Some of the greatest threats to adolescent and subsequent adult health make their first appearance during the school years, the result of health-risk behaviors that are themselves influenced by education (Grunbaum et al., 2002; Kulbok & Cox, 2002).

Promotion of social and emotional competence among children may positively affect their academic performance (Hawkins, 1997; Hawkins et al., 1999; Simeonsson, 1994), beginning at birth (Landry, Smith, Miller-Loncar, & Swank, 1998). As a result, the promotion of academic success has been highlighted as a U.S. health goal due to empirical support for the association between academic achievement during childhood and social and emotional well-being. "By addressing high school dropout rates as part of the nation's health promotion and disease prevention agenda, it may be possible to reduce unwarranted risk of problem behavior and improve the health of our young people" (USDHHS, 1991, p. 254).

Adolescence. Associations among socioeconomic status, academic performance, and adolescent health and development are well supported (Brooks-Gunn & Duncan, 1997; Cairns, Cairns, & Neckerman, 1989; Dryfoos, 1997; Hauser, 1997; Haveman & Wolfe, 1995; Hibbett & Fogelman, 1990; Lempers & Clark-Lempers, 1990; Resnick et al., 1997; Riley et al., 1998; Seydlitz & Jenkins, 1998; Vingilis, Wade, & Adlaf, 1998; Walker, Grantham-McGregor, Himes, Williams, & Duff, 1998).

In addition to the models of Hertzman et al. (2001) and Evans and Stoddart (1990, 2003) described in Chapter Two, and that of Halfon and Hochstein (2002) earlier in this chapter, child ecological conceptual models provide a more complete picture of the potential impact that adolescent school dropout has on the social well-being of youth, their families, and the wider communities in which they live. Although peer influence is strong during adolescence (Lau, Quadrel, & Hartman, 1990), the literature suggests that promoting youth health and educational achievement requires support from three primary environmental influences: the family, the school, and the community (Hurley & Lustbader, 1997; Poole,

1997). Teens report a direct relationship between life satisfaction and perceived parental support (Young, Miller, Norton, & Hill, 1995).

Both academic achievement and adolescent health status are associated with health-risk behaviors that make up some of the leading causes of adolescent morbidity and mortality: tobacco smoking, violence, suicide, alcohol and substance use, and sexual activity (Chung & Pardeck, 1997; Ellickson & McGuigan, 2000; Ellickson, McGuigan, Adams, Bell, & Hays, 1996; Rosenberg, O'Carroll, & Powell, 1992; Tresidder, Macaskill, Bennett, & Nutbeam, 1997; Weller et al., 1999). Among adolescents, these health-risk behaviors are often related to problem behaviors such as truancy, antisocial behavior, academic failure, and school dropout (Dryfoos, 1990; Hawkins, Catalano, & Miller, 1992; Institute of Medicine, Committee on Prevention of Mental Disorders, 1994; Jessor & Jessor, 1977). "Out of school adolescents are more likely than those in school to smoke, to use alcohol, marijuana, or cocaine, to have been involved in a physical fight, and to have been sexually active" (NCHS, 2000, p. 32).

Evidence for the Impact of Work on Health. In a life-course perspective, after early childhood experience, family, and education, the next most important influences on human development are in the workplace: its organization, supports, and demands (Evans, 2002; Marmot, 2002). Chapter Five will consider work and income more fully as determinants of health; but we emphasize that learning, formal education, skills training, and vocation are interdependent. Young people who graduate from high school are more likely to find satisfying employment than are peers who drop out, because job opportunities that provide positive working conditions are greater for young people who have graduated and developed effective work-related skills.

Most adults spend the greater part of their day in a work environment at home or elsewhere. Workers are differentially exposed to physical, chemical, biological, and/or psychosocial stimuli that, depending on the individual's characteristics, competencies, and endowments, may influence health and well-being (Marmot, Siegrist, Theorell, & Feeney, 1999). This is particularly true if there is a lack of reciprocity between the effort expended and the perceived reward gained from work (effort-reward imbalance model, i.e., conceptual balance between effort and reward and between workplace demands and control) (Siegrist, 1996; Siegrist, Klein, & Voigt, 1997), especially among individuals with limited economic and psychosocial resources (Kristenson et al., 2004). Karasek and Theorell (1990) and others (Niedhammer et al., 2004; Schieman, McBrier, & Van Gundy, 2003) link positive psychosocial working conditions with well-being and cardiovascular health in adulthood.

Within the context of individual preferences, some employment conditions may elicit expectation of unpleasant outcomes, strong emotional and physiological responses, chronically stressful experience, and poor coping (Vahtera, Pentti, & Kivimaki, 2004), contributing over the short and long term to health inequalities (Siegrist & Marmot, 2004), cardiovascular disease (Kuh & Smith, 2004; Marmot et al., 1997), or poor self-reported health (Marmot et al., 1995; Niedhammer et al., 2004). Evans (2002) noted that data from the Whitehall study of the British civil service (Marmot, 2002) revealed a compelling gradient in health status and mortality across job classifications, suggesting that workplace position in that hierarchy may directly influence an individual's physiological functioning. Marmot and others emphasize the importance to health of a sense of control over one's working conditions and job demands (Bosma et al., 1997; Marmot, 2002; Siegrist et al., 2004). In the Whitehall II study of 10,314 British civil servants age 35 to 55, Marmot and colleagues (1991) found that workers with unpleasant jobs were more prone to disability and absenteeism, to premature death, and to a range of major causes of mortality than were peers employed in jobs they enjoyed, especially when they were socially isolated. Women may experience additional stress related to balancing work and home life due to family- and housework-related roles (Scandura & Lankau, 1997).

Although few dispute that factors related to the quality of experience in the workplace influence the health of adults, scholars do not think that occupational factors are primary factors in general population health outcomes. In their study examining the relative contributions of education, work, and income to health, Winkleby and colleagues (1992) have shown that although income, education, and occupation all contribute to risk factors for cardiovascular disease, the relationship is strongest for education.

Current Policies That Address Fundamental Determinants

No broad policies extant in the United States are specifically based on research on the fundamental determinants of health that deal directly with human development. During the Clinton administration, the Educational Excellence for All Children Act (1999), based on a 1965 initiative in the Lyndon Baines Johnson administration and later renamed the Academic Achievement for All Act, was introduced to establish higher national academic and health expectations among young people than had previously existed. The ensuing No Child Left Behind Act (2002), which President George W. Bush enacted in January 2002, focused on intervention for specific aspects of sociocognitive development in young children. Neither act received adequate funding to meet its objectives nor addressed well-researched, crucial social and emotional development issues inherent in promoting healthy developmental trajectories (National Research Council, 2000; Shonkoff,

2003, p. 4). Other legislation that addressed a wide spectrum of early developmental issues, such as the Leave No Child Behind Act (2003) or the Educational Excellence for All Learners Act (2003), were not enacted.

> The politics of resource allocation would be guided more constructively by empirical research if we moved beyond the basic question of *whether* early childhood interventions work and began to seriously address the more compelling challenge of *how* to achieve a maximum return on our early childhood investments (Shonkoff, 2003, p. 5).

Effective Education Policies in the United States

"Raising the academic achievement of all students while closing the gap in performance between majority and affluent students and minority and disadvantaged students is the fundamental challenge facing American education today" (Smrekar, Guthrie, Owens, & Sims, 2001, p. ii.).

Head Start and Early Head Start. The largest targeted early childhood intervention programs in the United States are Head Start, for children four and five years old, a program that the federal Department of Health and Human Services created in 1965; and Early Head Start, for pregnant mothers and for children up to three years of age, created in 1994. These needs-tested programs now serve just fewer than one million children, providing comprehensive child development, educational, health, nutritional, social, and family services. Services are offered either in centers or in the child's home, or both, depending on family need and preference. The trained Head Start service providers are locally based grantees of the USDHHS; they have a significant degree of discretion over program content but also are held accountable for meeting developmental standards that the national program directors set. Earlier published evaluations of the programs and their outcomes have shown mixed results (McGroder, 1990). A comprehensive, seven-year national examination of Early Head Start showed that this version of early, planned interventions for mothers-to-be and very young children had only modest but generally positive effects on learning, and depending on the age of the mother and the number of social risk factors involved, similar effects on the parenting that supports the child's learning through the first three years of life (Mathematica Policy Research, 2002).

From its inception Head Start has received two streams of funding: one for service provision and a second for development and testing of new approaches to care and development. While this second stream offers at least the possibility of continuous improvement in a social program that could have profound effects on the children and families that it serves (S. L. Kagan, personal communication, May 18, 2003), in one critical respect it has not worked well. A comprehensive evaluation of Head Start (USDHHS, Office of the Assistant Secretary for Planning and Evaluation, 2003b) concluded that children in Head Start are not getting what they need to succeed in school. Citing a serious lack of coordination of services and too little attention to development of cognitive skills, the department supports the proposals of the Bush administration to provide more skilled caregivers and a greater emphasis on letter and number recognition, prereading, and language skills. The proposed changes are consistent with an extensive literature on the observed lifetime benefits of early interventions; if fully implemented, they could significantly strengthen the program. At the time of writing, however, it appears that the administration's mandates for change will not receive full funding, and it remains to be seen what the programs can accomplish with less than optimal resources.

Department of Defense (DoD) Schools. The Department of Defense (DoD) schools, which serve approximately 112,000 children who are dependents of U.S. military personnel in the continental United States and around the globe, have adopted an effective education policy. Although fewer than 10% of students enrolled in DoD schools come from single-parent families (compared to the national rate of 27%), a large proportion are minorities (40%) and experience high rates of mobility due to parental transfers (35%), poverty (50% qualify for the free or reduced-cost school lunch program), and low level of parent education (75% have only high school) (Smrekar et al., 2001). Yet minority students in DoD schools perform significantly better than their non-DoD school peers, and their average scores on National Assessment of Academic Progress tests are among the highest in the nation. High levels of academic achievement and standardized test scores have consistently ranked all DoD school students among the best-performing when compared to individual state reports (DoD Education Activity, 2003; Smrekar et al., 2001).

According to Smrekar and colleagues (2001, p. i), DoD policy aimed at promotion of high academic standards is driven by the key determinants of achievement, including the following:

- Centralized direction setting with local decision making
- Policy coherence and regular data flow regarding instructional goals, assessments, accountability, and professional training and development
- Sufficient financial resources linked to instructionally relevant strategic goals
- Staff development that is job-embedded, intensive, sustained over time, relevant to school improvement goals, and linked to student performance
- Small school size, conducive to trust, communication, and sense of community

- Academic focus and high expectations for all students
- Continuity of care for children in high-quality preschool and after-school programs
- A "corporate commitment" to public education that is material and symbolic and that is visible and responsive to parents within the school community

The inclusion of quality care for preschool children, supervised after-school programs, staff support and development, and policy that is informed by student performance are factors that, in combination with parent involvement and social cohesion, support the development of human capital within DoD schools.

Economic Policies. Policy recommendations to assist low-income parents to provide for basic child needs such as preschool, child care, and health care include "a raise in the minimum wage, expansion of the federal Earned Income Tax Credit, a decreased payroll tax burden on low-wage workers, and health insurance for working parents" (Gershoff, 2003, p. 8). Job creation, although a positive step, has not been shown to be sufficient to close the gap between economically secure children and those living in poverty (Cauthen & Lu, 2003). Chapter Five further discusses the related economic policies.

Policies in Other Countries

Other developed countries have addressed these issues through public policies that explicitly link maternal and family health, infant and child care, play groups, preschool, kindergarten, and K–12 on a continuum focused on the goal of optimal human development (Children Families and Learning Network, 1999; Korpi, 2000). We will offer evidence that a single set of policies, coupled with greater public investments aimed at strengthening early child development and education, will accomplish five highly desirable outcomes: The policies can increase the stock of human capital, raise individual incomes, decrease income differentials, improve overall health status, and improve economic growth (Rehme, 2001). The benefits could be substantial.

Several European countries and Canada have long experience with human development policies focused on the family, child care, and education. France, Italy, and the Canadian province of Quebec have all moved to provide universal free or low-cost developmentally oriented child care. Sweden, England, and Scotland have transferred national responsibility for early childhood education and care from welfare to education departments. Changes in practice as a result of these policy initiatives differ across countries, but their policy rationales are based on the same evidence about the critical importance of a child's early years.

In Sweden legislation on child care is in the School Act, and the National Agency for Education now has supervisory responsibility. The agency has developed a national curriculum for children from ages one to five, making preschool the first step in lifelong learning and a "strong and equal part of the school system" (Korpi, 2000, p. 3). The Scottish Council Foundation has examined the issues surrounding the integration of child care and education and has concluded that an integrated system of early childhood services should be accessible to every child (Children Families and Learning Network, 1999). This would include a guaranteed place in preschool when children reach age three to five that links from earlier quality child care, emphasizing coherence and continuity to avoid transitional disruption between day care, play settings, nursery or preschool, and kindergarten. Implementation of these principles in practice began in 1998 in a pilot program, the New Community Schools Initiative, which is now being extended to all schools in Scotland. The aim is an integrated and child-centered approach to education, health, and family support.

England provides government funding for children's centers to bring care, education, and other child and family services together; but so far these have been created only in economically deprived areas, somewhat like Head Start centers in the United States. Perhaps most importantly, England has consolidated all authority for educational and children's services under one national inspectorate (United Nations Educational, Scientific, and Cultural Organization, Early Childhood and Family Education Section, 2003).

Among all Western countries, France has what most regard as the most comprehensive set of policies in the relevant domains, and we believe its approach can serve as a model of what would be desirable in the United States (Kamerman, 2002a; Kamerman et al., 2003). France has an explicit family policy that has evolved over several decades and now involves a rich array of child-related cash benefits and services. The cash benefits are very generous, and the child-related services are among the most extensive in the world. Five objectives guide French family policy: to compensate families for the economic costs of child rearing through solidarity; to encourage a higher birth rate by encouraging pronatalism, that is, attitudes or policies that promote childbearing; to redistribute income to low-income families with children in order to promote social justice; to protect the well-being of children; and to protect parental choice among family types regardless of whether parents choose to work outside the home or to remain at home to rear children. The emphasis on the five objectives fluctuates over time, especially between pronatalism and social justice, depending on the predominant values of the government of the day; but whether left-leaning or conservative, in difficult economic times or in times of plenty, all modern French governments have reaffirmed a commitment to support for families and children.

A central feature of child services in France is a universal, voluntary, and free preschool system (*maternelles*) that covers all children ages three to six and nearly half of all children from the ages of three months to two years (*crèches*). Care, socialization, development, and school readiness are recurrent themes; and all teachers and teacher assistants from the *maternelle* level onward must receive federally prescribed training and certification. France has extensive provisions for family leaves for both parents, subsidizes infant and toddler care, and has an exemplary maternal and child health care system that covers every mother and child. Ninety-six percent of all infants in France are born to mothers who received early prenatal care; and by age two, 90% of children have received all recommended vaccinations.

Although cultural factors and attitudes toward individual and collective responsibility vary widely across the countries whose policies we have reviewed here, along with the United States, they all share a commitment to publicly supported education as a critical factor in developing human capital.

Strengths and Limitations of Current Policies

The current U.S. policies that address education have inherent strengths and weaknesses. The greatest strengths lie in the near-universal commitment to publicly supported basic education from age 5 or 6 through age 16 and in the strong policy support for access to postsecondary education, resulting in one of the highest university or postsecondary participation rates in the world.

The limitations are in part conceptual, evidenced by the incomplete understanding of the foundational importance of early childhood factors both to success in the educational system and in life, and they are in part political-economic. Education and child care are the responsibility of each state, and in most states, responsibility devolves further to municipalities. Funding of early child care is largely from private sources (except for certain needy families, as we will note), whereas local ad valorem taxes, with or without state tax–funded supplements, support K–12 schooling. Parents can send their children to private schools, whether parochial, sectarian, or secular, but this is a major expense for any family; and the choice is generally available only to families that are relatively well-off. The Bush administration and some states support the practice of giving vouchers to all parents who want their children to attend private schools, but because the money that such vouchers represent is taken from the available funds for public schools, and in most cases is not enough to cover the high tuition costs in good private schools, the effects of the policy are mixed, at best.

A few states have curricular and staffing standards for K–12 education and for child-care centers and prekindergarten programs; but where they exist, standards related to the earliest and arguably the most important period of human development and education tend to be minimal and to vary widely across the country. Similarly, funding levels for publicly supported early care and K–12 education vary widely from region to region even within the same state, resulting in significant disparities in both opportunity and outcomes across the nation (a topic we will discuss further). Attempts by federal and even state policymakers to pass laws that might promote more equity and effectiveness in child care and education have encountered opposition rooted in the traditional values of choice and local control of education. Champions of personal choice can regard this as a strength. Others can see it as a limitation because it perpetuates significant variations in quality, performance, and outcomes.

To address early child development in its No Child Left Behind initiative, Bush administration policy emphasizes cognitive skill building to improve school performance (National Research Council, 2000); but it has not supported critical parts of the initiative related to teacher training, nor does it support social skill training for students' self-regulation and healthy interpersonal relationships. As Gershoff (2003, p. 4) has observed: "Whether children are able to control their impulses and to get along with other children in early childhood forecasts the success with which they manage the challenges of their later lives."

Equity, Effectiveness, and Efficiency Analyses of Policies

Any discussion of equity, efficiency, and effectiveness in relation to human development across an entire population immediately leads to the question: By what standards can development be measured, let alone judged? There are no universally accepted methods for accurately measuring human development. Traditionally, the standard has been an economic one, indexed by growth in national income; but more recently, the United Nations Development Programme (2002) has begun to use a human development index (HDI). The HDI for any country is calculated using a mix of indicators including that nation's life expectancy at birth; adult literacy rate; gross domestic product (GDP) per capita; an education index; the combined primary, secondary, and tertiary education enrollment ratio; and the GDP per capita rank among all countries, minus the HDI rank. The index therefore gives weight to life expectancy and participation in education, as well as to national income, and also takes into consideration the difference between potential (as indicated by income) and actual achievement (as indicated by the calculated HDI level).

Some, most frequently the more conservatively aligned economists like those at the Fraser Institute, have questioned the utility of the HDI in assessing progress in development. Though critics argue that the HDI does not give sufficient weight to income growth per se (Grubel, 1998), Philipson and Soares (2001) have shown that when compared to national full-income measures that incorporated life expectancy gains over the period 1962 to 1997, the HDI may accurately rank countries in an ordinal fashion because the nonincome aspects of human development that it includes are themselves highly correlated with a nation's wealth. The HDI ranks the United States sixth among all developed nations, behind Norway, Sweden, Canada, Belgium, and Australia. Although still very good in relation to most countries in the world, this relatively poor ranking in comparison to countries whose per capita national incomes (Norway excepted) are considerably lower than the United States is a function primarily of life expectancies that are among the lowest in the Organisation for Economic Co-operation and Development (OECD); and literacy rates for adults that also are lower than in many peer countries. The USDE NCES (2001b) estimates that 90 million U.S. adults have marginal or substandard literacy skills, and most of them are white and native-born. Furthermore, the group's statistics indicate that more than 60% of poor children in the fourth grade can't read and that only 31% of all fourth graders read at or above a basic standard (2001b).

Although the HDI does not include a factor for child poverty, which is itself a potent determinant of human development, the poverty rate in the United States is not only higher than in many peer countries, it is rising (U.S. Census Bureau, 2003b). Including a child poverty measure in calculating the index would drop the United States even further down the ranks. As measured by the HDI, therefore, we would argue that policies dealing with human development in the United States are not optimally effective. To the extent that healthy life expectancy, literacy rates, and poverty rates are both a reflection of and contributors to human development, the United States could do better.

In view of the central importance of education to human development, the evidence suggests that existing U.S. educational policies are effective for some but quite ineffective for others. Although educational attainment varies widely across student populations within individual schools, school districts, and states, the education gradient is most dramatically illustrated in the differences in student standardized test scores from northern to southern states. On average, children in many northern states do as well as their age peers anywhere in the world in reading and math; Maine, North Dakota, Minnesota, and Iowa are consistently among the best. Children in the South do much more poorly; in some states, such as Mississippi and Arkansas, students' math and reading scores are consistently on a par with the worst-performing countries in the OECD (USDE NCES, 1997). Children growing up in states closer to the Mason-Dixon Line generally achieve scores in the mid range compared to their peers in the northern and southern states. Interesting exceptions to the otherwise neatly aligned gradient are Texas and North

Carolina, where both states' K–12 educational institutions have adopted standardized curricula (Figure 4.5).

Grossman (1972) theorized a central role for education as a means for greater efficiency in health production in part because better-educated individuals are more likely to understand technology and information as well as to more efficiently use their time to access medical and other health-enhancing market inputs. A look at the wide array of early childhood care and education arrangements across the country shows the grossly uneven outcomes in terms of readiness to learn on entry to kindergarten and the high loss ratio (dropouts) in middle and high schools; the present arrangements in the United States are far from optimally effective and,

FIGURE 4.5.   FOURTH-GRADE STANDARDIZED NATIONAL ASSESSMENT OF EDUCATIONAL PROGRESS MATH SCORES BY PERCENT OF U.S. STUDENTS ELIGIBLE FOR NATIONAL FREE OR REDUCED-COST LUNCH PROGRAM, 2000, BY STATE AND DISTRICT OF COLUMBIA.

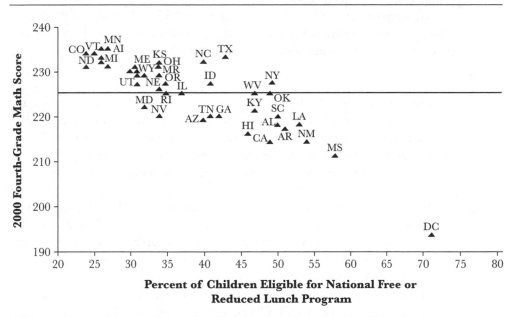

Note. From *Which American Children Will Succeed? Personal and Social Determinants of Educational Attainment and Health,* by M. D. Low, B. J. Low, E. Baumler, P. Huynh, and P. Cronin (paper presented at the June 2002 Annual International Conference on Social Sciences, Honolulu, HI), p. 5, fig. 1.3; and *Student Academic Success and Health Outcomes: Policy Implications,* by B. J. Low, E. Baumler, K. M. Cardarelli, J. M. Sterner, and M. D. Low (paper presented at the November 2003 annual conference of the American Public Health Association, Washington, DC), slide 18. Used with permission.

given the (avoidable) human capital losses from the process, relatively inefficient as well.

As this chapter has indicated so far, the efficiency question is very difficult to address in relation to the broad scope of human development. U.S. ideals and enshrined ethical principles preclude a range of alternative approaches to the production of human capital that may well be more efficient, from a strictly economic viewpoint, than the ones we currently employ. For example, eugenics, forced sterilization, and selective abortion occupy one end of a spectrum of possibilities that no ethical person would advocate. Further toward the bounds of acceptability, the directed streaming of children into trade school, university, or professional schools based on institutional assessments of ability and aptitude may well be a more efficient way of creating the human capital needed for the nation's development than the current practice of holding university graduation as the expectation for everyone, regardless of individual endowments. Such streaming practices are not only accepted but normative in Europe and Asia, but we are not aware of any evidence of their efficiency vis à vis the more one-standard-fits-all approach in Canada and the United States.

We propose that in view of the critical importance of human health and development to the individual and to society, standards of equity and effectiveness should take precedence in questions of policy. Nobel laureate Amartya Sen (2002, p. 659) said:

> health equity cannot but be a central feature of the justice of social arrangements in general. The reach of health equity is immense. . . . it must come to grips with the larger issue of fairness and justice in social arrangements, including economic allocations. Health equity is most certainly not just about the distribution of *health*, not to mention the even narrower focus on the distribution of *health care*.

Woodward and Kawachi (2000, p. 295) observe that, "Health is an exquisitely sensitive mirror of social circumstances." They define *health inequities* as differences in health status between groups of people, differences that are unfair and unjust because they are systematically related to some characteristic of the group, such as skin color, income, or place of residence, and because they are avoidable. Like Sen (2002) and others writing on the subject, Woodward and Kawachi (2000) argue not for equality of health status but for equality of opportunity to access the resources necessary for good health. Those resources include assets that are both material and nonmaterial or spiritual, according to Fogel (2000); in the context of contemporary U.S. life, individuals either gain them in the earliest stages of life through developmentally appropriate care and education or, lacking a fair start, are left at a significant (and inequitable) disadvantage.

Although there is a growing understanding in the United States of the foundational importance of early childhood to success later on in education and in life, that critical aspect of human development has not yet been effectively linked with the rest of the educational process, in the minds of either national-level policymakers or the general public (Carnegie Corporation of New York, 1994; Keating & Hertzman, 1999; Gershoff, 2003). As a result, policies dealing with this period in the life course, such as family leave and the availability and cost of child care, vary greatly from one region of the country to another and even from one employer to another within the same community.

In an environment that must deal with overall school dropout rates that, depending on measurement methods and study sample, range from 4.2% (NCHS, 2000) to 8.7% (U.S. Census Bureau, 2003a) to 11% (USDE NCES, 2003a, 2003b) to 16% (U.S. Census Bureau, 2003b) or even 23% (Annie E. Casey Foundation & Population Reference Bureau, 2003), more information is needed to help educators to better understand how to keep adolescents in school. Poor academic achievement may be associated with higher levels of health-risk behavior and lower levels of social competence and socioeconomic position (SEP), negatively mediating short- and long-term health outcomes (Durlak, 1995; Jordan, Lara, & McPartland, 1996; Mortimore, 1995; Willis, 1987). Effective, innovative programs and policies that promote child and youth resilience and graduation from high school may positively affect short- and long-term health (Hauser, 1997). These data, confirmed by other studies (Dearing, McCartney, & Taylor, 2001) and reviews of evidence (Aber, Bennett, Conley, & Li, 1997; Brooks-Gunn & Duncan, 1997; Children's Defense Fund, 1997; Huston, 1991; McLoyd, 1998; Seccombe, 2000), provide serious implications for U.S. policy.

We recommend further federal, state, and local policy change to promote equity in child access to school resources. The USDE NCES (2000) reported that schools with disproportionately high enrollment of children from low-income families have fewer resources such as experienced teachers, access to computers and the Internet, and smaller class size. Further inequity is highlighted by the disproportion of minority children in lower-quality schools (National Education Association, 2001).

Anderson, Scrimshaw, Fullilove, and Fielding (2003) have extensively reviewed and summarized the effectiveness of U.S. early childhood development programs. With a multidisciplinary team that included the Task Force on Community Preventive Services, Anderson and colleagues examined the impact of community-based interventions to improve population health in three broad categories: "*social institutions,* including cultural and religious institutions, economic systems, and political structures; *surroundings,* including neighborhoods, workplaces, towns, cities, and built environments; and *social relationships,* including position in social hierarchy, differential treatment of social groups, and social networks" (p. 12). Addressing these issues requires a broad public policy approach.

Recommendations

We would argue that one of the best ways for the United States to improve the health of the whole population is to focus policies on optimizing both early childhood development and education. In this chapter we have tried to show that in one critical sense, they are the same thing: Adequate social and cognitive development in childhood is a necessary foundation for success in education, which in turn is necessary for health and success in life. The discussion that follows provides a series of specific policy recommendations to enhance the availability and integration of early childhood development and education.

Expand the Availability of Comprehensive Preschool Education Programs

According to Gershoff (2003, p. 7) at the National Center for Children in Poverty, compelling evidence of the importance of early success in education as a contributor to health supports

> a broad perspective on factors that promote school readiness and early school success. They are particularly relevant to a current policy debate about the emphasis primarily on interventions that develop academic skills versus those that include attention to both health issues (with necessary attention to obesity) and social and emotional competence.

Efforts to improve poor children's access to high-quality, well-regulated child care and preschools are still inadequate despite increases in the de facto number and availability and related funding of such programs since the initiation of welfare reform. To address the achievement gap between low-income children and their more economically secure peers, the nation needs more preschools, especially those similar to Head Start that provide comprehensive services such as immunizations and parent education (Center for Law and Social Policy, 2004).

Expand the Availability of Parenting Education Programs

Because learning starts at birth or before and because education is so important to health, policymakers in the United States should think of our collective responsibilities for universal education as starting at least when a child is born, not just when she enters kindergarten. Because no one is born knowing how to be a good parent, the policy should include parental education (Pfannenstiel, Lambson, and Yarnell, 1996).

Link Formal Child-Care and K–12 Education Programs

The suggested new kind of public policy would explicitly link child care with what people in the United States have traditionally thought of as formal education. This will require a different approach from the usual compartmentalized thinking that characterizes most governmental policymaking. All agencies, from education to health to finance to social welfare, will have to agree on common objectives and create integrated policies to promote and support the new programs. All must understand that promoting good health is not the sole purview of the health care system.

The nation can also draw on several models of integrated policymaking. As the previous section described, although France, Scotland, Sweden, and England are far ahead of the United States on the national level, some U.S. states have made remarkable strides in this direction in recent years. Georgia's Bright From the Start program, which links child care, family support, and education, stands out as an excellent example of what can be accomplished with enlightened and determined leadership from the top (Georgia Department of Early Care and Learning, n.d.).

The authors would recommend policies that, like Georgia's Bright From the Start program, anticipate linkages to models of improved K–12 education such as the DoD has achieved over many years. There is strong evidence that no prescription for remedy of K–12 education in the United States will have the hoped-for benefits until it levels the prekindergarten playing field. The early years of life are clearly critical to a child's chances both in the public education system and in the broader society, and our nation should act on that knowledge to ensure that this public good is all that it can be, for the future of our children and our country.

Develop and Apply Quality Standards
for Integrated Child-Care and Education Programs

The Head Start and Early Head Start programs, a consortium of educators and child development experts led by the National Center for Children and Families at Columbia University and by the Canadian Centre for Studies of Children at Risk at McMaster University, among others, have all developed standards and model curricula that are adaptable to any community, including ones in developing countries (Center for the Study of Social Policy, 2003; Consultative Group on Early Childhood Care and Development, 1999; Offord Centre for Child Studies, 2004).

The essential elements of a U.S. human development–oriented health policy would include at a minimum appropriate prenatal care, provision for parent training and financial support where necessary, quality child care delivered by well-qualified child development specialists, progressive introduction of elemental education beginning at a few months of age, and regular assessment to ensure that children are meeting developmental and cognitive milestones prior to entering kindergarten. Early Head Start already offers many of these things to some needy families and children, with some benefit. However, far too few children qualify; program quality is uneven; and by the USDHHS's (2003b) own assessment, the program does too little for the child's cognitive development. The authors would recommend that, like public education, versions of these programs should be universally available to all children and families who choose to take part (McCain & Mustard, 1999).

Funding sources, standard setting, and jurisdiction are subjects for debate, but we would argue for substantial federal oversight and support in all these areas. The available evidence indicates that in childhood development and education programs, quality counts. Although approximately one-third of all elementary schools in the nation have already started prekindergarten education programs, with very few exceptions (e.g., the state of Georgia), coordination with other child-related services, age at entry, access, and quality vary greatly across districts; and many of these programs are in jeopardy because of inadequate or uncertain funding (Olson, 2002; Windham, 1999). If this nation is going to come close to eliminating educational and health disparities, we cannot leave the task entirely to regions of the country that are already suffering economic and social privation, with little prospect for change.

Although quality early childhood care and development programs have been created, tested, and validated so that existing models could be adapted and implemented anywhere, commitment to local control and funding of education in this country makes standardization of any aspect of education a challenge. The evidence from studies of education policies and outcomes in other countries, from comparisons of achievement scores in states with statewide standardized curricula and those without, and from the successes of the DoD school system (Institute for Defense Analyses, 2000; Smrekar et al., 2001) indicates that we already know a great deal about how to promote excellent outcomes in schools. Family resources and involvement; appropriate curricular and assessment standards; significant school-level autonomy over pedagogical methods; and well-qualified, experienced teachers are some of the critical elements in the mix.

Create New Models for Funding Integrated Child-Care and Development Programs

In the United States, the principle of universal access to education is largely accepted, and taxation provides the funding. If this nation takes the next step and agrees that collective responsibility really should begin at birth rather than on entrance to kindergarten, we will have to face the question of who pays for the necessary care and development support. One obvious possibility would be to give school districts that responsibility and the necessary taxing authority, as some European centers have done. The existing and planned policies for linking care and education in Europe are all at least subsidized by substantial cash contributions from the federal government.

On the other hand, given that 70% of all child care in the United States is currently paid for by individuals and provided in the private sector, it would not be wise to attempt to move child-care and development programs entirely under the public schools' jurisdiction and pay all of the costs through taxes. Rather, the United States could develop a made-in-the-USA model that incorporates intersectoral, collaborative standard setting and curricular design, with multiple funding streams from federal, state, local, and private sources. A good starting point would be for state and local child-care providers and payers to work under federal oversight to agree on consistent care and development objectives and a common set of measurement standards for assessing a child's developmental progress. Without them, further investments can't be targeted effectively, and disparities will persist.

Recognize the Benefits of a New Policy That Education Starts at Birth

We believe that the right education policy would result in significant improvement in the health of the U.S. population and would help to reduce both the health disparities that afflict so many and the income inequalities that breed social problems in all regions of the country. Evidence supports this expectation beyond what we have offered so far in this chapter. In his study of redistribution of personal incomes, education, and economic performance in OECD countries, Rehme (2001) has shown the negative relationship between income inequality and economic growth—less inequality, more growth—and indicated that, in relatively wealthy countries, spending more on education would both enhance growth and decrease pre- and posttax inequality. In the context of our thesis, then, Rheme's work points to the possibility of combining and achieving four highly desirable objectives. The right education policy would not only strengthen educational attainment and the stock of human capital, it would improve overall health status, reduce income inequality, and promote economic growth.

We would stress once more that human learning is continuous from birth and that changes in the quality of K–12 education alone, as important as such changes may be, can't and won't be a panacea. Education, without appropriate early interventions aimed at improvements in children's social and cognitive development, may have little protective effect for children and adolescents in households with incomes well below the poverty level (Krieger & Fee, 1994). Our suggested approach would link early child care, family support, and developmental enrichment with the subsequent processes of K–12 education in a seamless continuum, thereby minimizing educational and health risks for all children, including those who are even now being left behind.

This chapter has documented the important role that early childhood development and education play in the prospects for economic well-being and health. Chapter Five probes the direct impact of economic factors and policies in enhancing human health and development.

References

Aber, J. L., Bennett, N. G., Conley, D. C., & Li, J. L. (1997). The effects of poverty on child health and development. *Annual Review of Public Health, 18,* 463–483.

Acheson, D. (1998). *Independent inquiry into inequalities in health report.* London: Stationery Office.

Ala-Mursula, L., Vahtera, J., Pentti, J., & Kivimaki, M. (2004). Effect of employee worktime control on health: A prospective cohort study. *Occupational and Environmental Medicine, 61,* 254–261.

Albert, M. S. (1995). How does education affect cognitive function? *Annals of Epidemiology, 5,* 76–78.

American Academy of Pediatrics, Committee on Public Education. (2001). Media violence. *Pediatrics, 108,* 1222–1226.

American Medical Association, Ad Hoc Committee on Health Literacy for the Council on Scientific Affairs. (1999). Health literacy: Report of the Council on Scientific Affairs. *Journal of the American Medical Association, 281,* 552–557.

Anderson, L. M., Scrimshaw, S. C., Fullilove, M. T., & Fielding, J. E. (2003). The Community Guide's model for linking the social environment to health. *American Journal of Preventive Medicine, 24*(Suppl. 3), 12–20.

Andrews, A. B., & Ben-Arieh, A. (1999). Measuring and monitoring children's well-being across the world. *Social Work, 44,* 105–115.

Annie E. Casey Foundation. (2004). *Kids count data book: State profiles of child well-being: Moving youth from risk to opportunity.* Baltimore: Author.

Annie E. Casey Foundation & Population Reference Bureau. (2003). *The growing number of kids in severely distressed neighborhoods: Evidence from the 2000 census.* Baltimore, MD; Washington, DC: Annie E. Casey Foundation.

Antonucci, T. C. (1991). Attachment, social support, and coping with negative life events in mature adulthood. In E. M. Cummings, A. L. Greene, & K. H. Karraker (Eds.), *Life-span developmental psychology: Perspectives on stress and coping* (pp. 261–276). Hillsdale, N.J.: Erlbaum.

Arendt, J. N. (2001). *Education effects on health: Causal or from unobserved components? A panel analysis with endogenous education.* Retrieved October 26, 2004, from http://www.econ.ku.dk/okojn/public/research/jarendt.pdf

Ary, D. V., Duncan, T. E., Duncan, S. C., & Hops, H. (1999). Adolescent problem behavior: The influence of parents and peers. *Behaviour Research and Therapy, 37,* 217–230.

Australian Institute of Family Studies. (2002). *Introducing the Longitudinal Study of Australian Children* (LSAC Discussion Paper No. 1). Melbourne: Author.

Avendaño, M., Kunst, A. E., Huisman, M., van Lenthe, F., Bopp, M., Borrell, C., et al. (2004). Educational level and stroke mortality: A comparison of 10 European populations during the 1990s. *Stroke, 35,* 432–437.

Baltes, P. B., & Baltes, M. M. (1990). Psychological perspectives on successful aging: The model of selective optimization with compensation. In P. B. Baltes & M. M. Baltes (Eds.), *Successful aging: Perspectives from the behavioral sciences* (pp. 1–34). New York: Cambridge University Press.

Bandura, A. (1986a). The explanatory and predictive scope of self-efficacy theory. *Journal of Social and Clinical Psychology, 4,* 359–373.

Bandura, A. (1986b). *Social foundations of thought and action: A social cognitive theory.* Englewood Cliffs, NJ: Prentice Hall.

Baranowski, T., & Nader, P. R. (1985). Family health behavior. In D. C. Turk & R. D. Kerns (Eds.), *Health, illness, and families: A life-span perspective* (pp. 51–80). New York: Wiley.

Barker, D.J.P. (1997). Fetal nutrition and cardiovascular disease in later life. *British Medical Bulletin, 53,* 96–108.

Barker, D.J.P., Osmond, C., Simmonds, S. J., & Wield, G. A. (1993). The relation of small head circumference and thinness at birth to death from cardiovascular disease in adult life. *British Medical Journal, 306,* 422–426.

Basen-Engquist, K., Edmundson, E. W., & Parcel, G. S. (1996). Structure of health risk behavior among high school students. *Journal of Consulting and Clinical Psychology, 64,* 764–775.

Bates, J. E., Maslin, C. A., & Frankel, K. A. (1985). Attachment security, mother-child interaction, and temperament as predictors of behavior-problem ratings at age three years. *Monographs of the Society for Research in Child Development, 50,* 167–193.

Becker, G. S. (1964). *Human capital* (National Bureau of Economic Research: General Series No. 80). New York: National Bureau of Economic Research.

Becker, G. S. (1991). *A treatise on the family* (Enl. ed.). Cambridge, MA: Harvard University Press.

Bell, C. C. (2001). Cultivating resiliency in youth. *Journal of Adolescent Health, 29,* 375–381.

Ben-Shlomo, Y., & Kuh, D. (2002). A life course approach to chronic disease epidemiology: Conceptual models, empirical challenges and interdisciplinary perspectives. *International Journal of Epidemiology, 31,* 285–293.

Benson, P. L., Leffert, N., Scales, P. C., & Blyth, D. (1998). Beyond the "village" rhetoric: Creating healthy communities for children and adolescents. *Applied Developmental Science, 2,* 138–159.

Bergen, D. (2002, Spring). The role of pretend play in children's cognitive development. *Early Childhood Research and Practice, 4*(1). Retrieved November 16, 2004, from http://ecrp.uiuc.edu/v4n1/bergen.html

Berkman, L. F., & Syme, S. L. (1979). Social networks, host resistance, and mortality: A nine-year follow-up study of Alameda County residents. *American Journal of Epidemiology, 109,* 186–204.

Birren, J. E., & Schaie, K. W. (Eds.). (2001). *Handbook of the psychology of aging* (5th ed.). San Diego, CA: Academic Press.

Boardman, J., Grove, B., Perkins, R., & Shepherd, G. (2003). Work and employment for people with psychiatric disabilities. *British Journal of Psychiatry, 182,* 467–468.

Boisjoly, J., Harris, K. M., & Duncan, G. J. (1998). Trends, events, and duration of initial welfare spells. *Social Service Review, 72,* 466–492.

Bosma, H., Marmot, M. G., Hemingway, H., Nicholson, A. C., Brunner, E., & Stansfeld, S. A. (1997). Low job control and risk of coronary heart disease in Whitehall II (prospective cohort) study. *British Medical Journal, 314,* 558–565.

Bossé, R., Levenson, M. R., Spiro, A., III, Aldwin, C. M., & Mroczek, D. K. (1992). For whom is retirement stressful? Findings from the Normative Aging Study. In B. Vellas & J. L. Albarède (Eds.), *Facts and research in gerontology 1992* (pp. 223–240). New York: Springer.

Brandtjen, H., & Verny, T. (2001). Short and long term effects on infants and toddlers in full time daycare centers. *Journal of Prenatal and Perinatal Psychology and Health, 15,* 239–286.

Breslow, L. (1999). From disease prevention to health promotion. *Journal of the American Medical Association, 281,* 1030–1033.

Bronfenbrenner, U. (1979). *The ecology of human development: Experiments by nature and design.* Cambridge, MA: Harvard University Press.

Brooks-Gunn, J., & Duncan, G. J. (1997). The effects of poverty on children. *Future of Children, 7,* 55–71.

Brown, B. V. (1997). Indicators of children's well-being: A review of current indicators based on data from the federal statistical system. In R. M. Hauser, B. V. Brown, & W. R. Prosser (Eds.), *Indicators of children's well-being* (pp. 3–35). New York: Russell Sage Foundation.

Bruer, J. T. (1998). Brain science, brain fiction. *Educational Leadership, 56,* 14–18.

Bruner, J. S., Jolly, A., & Sylva, K. (Eds.). (1976). *Play: Its role in development and evolution.* New York: Basic Books.

Cairns, R. B., Cairns, B. D., & Neckerman, H. J. (1989). Early school dropout: Configurations and determinants. *Child Development, 60,* 1437–1452.

Cameron, N., & Demerath, E. W. (2002). Critical periods in human growth and their relationship to diseases of aging. *American Journal of Physical Anthropology, 119*(Suppl. 35), 159–184.

Campbell, T. L. (1986). Family's impact on health: A critical review. *Family Systems Medicine, 4,* 135–328.

Carnegie Corporation of New York. (1994). *Starting points: Meeting the needs of our youngest children: The report of the Carnegie Task Force on Meeting the Needs of Young Children.* New York: Author.

Case, R., Griffin, S., & Kelly, W. M. (1999). Socioeconomic gradients in mathematical ability and their responsiveness to intervention during early childhood. In D. P. Keating & C. Hertzman (Eds.), *Developmental health and the wealth of nations: Social, biological, and educational dynamics* (pp. 125–150). New York: Guilford Press.

Catalano, R. F., Berglund, M. L., Ryan, J.A.M., Lonczak, H. S., & Hawkins, J. D. (1998). *Positive youth development in the United States: Research findings on evaluations of positive youth development programs.* Seattle: University of Washington, School of Social Work, Social Development Research Group.

Cauthen, N. K., & Lu, H.-H. (2003). *Employment alone is not enough for America's low-income children and families* (Living at the Edge Research Brief No. 1). New York: National Center for Children Living in Poverty.

Center for Law and Social Policy. (2004, January). *Head Start comprehensive services: A key support for early learning for poor children* (CLASP Policy Brief Head Start Series Publication No. 04-03). Washington, DC: Author.

Center for the Study of Social Policy. (2003). *"Policy counts": Setting and measuring benchmarks for state policies: A concept paper.* Washington, DC: Author.

Centers for Disease Control and Prevention, National Center for Chronic Disease Prevention and Health Promotion. (2004a). *Healthy schools healthy youth! home page.* Retrieved February 9, 2005, from http://www.cdc.gov/HealthyYouth/index.htm

Centers for Disease Control and Prevention, National Center for Chronic Disease Prevention and Health Promotion. (2004b). *Healthy youth! YRBSS data files and documentation 1991 to 2003.* Retrieved February 9, 2005, from http://www.cdc.gov/HealthyYouth/yrbs/data/index.htm

Chandola, T., Kuper, H., Singh-Manoux, A., Bartley, M., & Marmot, M. (2004). The effect of control at home on CHD events in the Whitehall II study: Gender differences in psychosocial domestic pathways to social inequalities in CHD. *Social Science and Medicine, 58,* 1501–1509.

Chechik, G., Meilijson, I., & Ruppin, E. (1999). Neuronal regulation: A mechanism for synaptic pruning during brain maturation. *Neural Computation, 11,* 2061–2080.

Chilcoat, H. D., & Anthony, J. C. (1996). Impact of parent monitoring on initiation of drug use through late childhood. *Journal of the American Academy of Child and Adolescent Psychiatry, 35,* 91–100.

Children Families and Learning Network. (1999). *Children, families and learning: A new agenda for education* (Paper No. 10). Edinburgh: Scottish Council Foundation.

Children's Defense Fund. (1997). *Poverty matters: The cost of child poverty in America.* Washington, DC: Author.

Children's Defense Fund. (1998). *The state of America's children yearbook 1998.* Washington, DC: Author.

Chung, W. S., & Pardeck, J. T. (1997). Explorations in a proposed national policy for children and families. *Adolescence, 32,* 429–436.

Claussen, B., Davey, S. G., & Thelle, D. (2003). Impact of childhood and adulthood socio-economic position on cause specific mortality: The Oslo Mortality Study. *Journal of Epidemiology and Community Health, 57,* 40–45.

Cleland, J. G., & van Ginneken, J. K. (1988). Maternal education and child survival in developing countries: The search for pathways of influence. *Social Science and Medicine, 27,* 1357–1368.

Cohen, D. A., Richardson, J., & LaBree, L. (1994). Parenting behaviors and the onset of smoking and alcohol use: A longitudinal study. *Pediatrics, 94,* 368–375.

Coleman, J. S. (1988). Social capital in the creation of human capital. *American Journal of Sociology, 94*(Suppl.), 95–120.

Coleman, J. S. (1990). Social capital. In J. S. Coleman (Ed.), *Foundations of social theory* (pp. 300–324). Cambridge, MA: Harvard University Press.

Colombo, J. (1982). The critical period concept: Research, methodology, and theoretical issues. *Psychological Bulletin, 91,* 260–275.

Connolly, G. M., Casswell, S., Zhang, J. F., & Silva, P. A. (1994). Alcohol in the mass media and drinking by adolescents: A longitudinal study. *Addiction, 89,* 1255–1263.

Connolly, S. D., Paikoff, R. L., & Buchanan, C. M. (1996). Puberty: The interplay of biological and psychosocial processes in adolescence. In G. R. Adams, R. Montemayor, & T. P. Gullotta (Eds.), *Psychosocial development during adolescence: Progress in developmental contextualism* (pp. 259–299). Thousand Oaks, CA: Sage.

Consultative Group on Early Childhood Care and Development. (1999). *The costs and affordability of early childhood care and development programs.* Washington, DC: World Bank.

Cox, M. J., & Harter, K.S.M. (2003). Parent-child relationships. In M. H. Bornstein, L. Davidson, C.L.M. Keyes, & K. Moore (Eds.), *Well-being: Positive development across the life course* (pp. 191–204). Mahwah, NJ: Erlbaum.

Crespo, C. J., Smit, E., Troiano, R. P., Bartlett, S. J., Macera, C. A., & Andersen, R. E. (2001). Television watching, energy intake, and obesity in U.S. children: Results from the third National Health and Nutrition Examination Survey, 1988–1994. *Archives of Pediatrics and Adolescent Medicine, 155,* 360–365.

Crockett, L. J., & Petersen, A. C. (1993). Adolescent development: Health risks and opportunities. In S. G. Millstein, A. C. Petersen, & E. O. Nightingale (Eds.), *Promoting the health of adolescents: New directions for the twenty-first century* (pp. 13–37). New York: Oxford University Press.

Crouter, A. C., MacDermid, S. M., McHale, S. M., & Perry-Jenkins, M. (1990). Parental monitoring and perceptions of children's school performance and conduct in dual-earner and single-earner families. *Developmental Psychology, 26,* 649–657.

Darling, N., & Steinberg, L. (1993). Parenting style as context: An integrative model. *Psychological Bulletin, 113,* 487–496.

Daw, N. W. (1995). *Visual development.* New York: Plenum Press.

Dawson, G. (1994). Development of emotional expression and emotion regulation in infancy: Contributions of the frontal lobe. In G. Dawson & K. W. Fischer (Eds.), *Human behavior and the developing brain* (pp. 346–378). New York: Guilford Press.

Dearing, E., McCartney, K., & Taylor, B. A. (2001). Change in family income-to-needs matters more for children with less. *Child Development, 72,* 1779–1793.

Deaton, A. (2002). Policy implications of the gradient of health and wealth: An economist asks, would redistributing income improve population health? *Health Affairs, 21*(2), 13–30.

Deaton, A., & Paxton, C. (1999). *Mortality, education, income, and inequality among American cohorts* (NBER Working Paper No. w7140). Cambridge, MA: National Bureau of Economic Research.

DeCasper, A. J., Lecanuet, J. P., Busnel, M. C., Granier-Deferre, C., & Maugeais, R. (1994). Fetal reactions to recurrent maternal speech. *Infant Behavior and Development, 17,* 159–164.

Deeg, D.J.H., Kardaun, J.W.P.F., & Fozard, J. L. (1996). Health, behavior, and aging. In J. E. Birren & K. W. Schaie (Eds.), *Handbook of the psychology of aging* (pp. 129–149). San Diego, CA: Academic Press.

Department of Defense Education Activity. (2003, November 13). *DoD school students continue to improve in mathematics: Overseas eighth graders move to third in nation: Measurable improvements by all groups tested* [News release]. Retrieved November 3, 2004, from http://www.odedodea.edu/communications/news/releases/111303_math.htm

DeWitt, S. J., Sparks, J. W., Swank, P. R., Smith, K., Denson, S. E., & Landry, S. H. (1997). Physical growth of low birthweight infants in the first year of life: Impact of maternal behaviors. *Early Human Development, 47,* 19–34.

Dickens, W. T., & Flynn, J. R. (2001). Heritability estimates versus large environmental effects: The IQ paradox resolved. *Psychological Review, 108,* 346–369.

Dietz, W. H., Jr., & Gortmaker, S. L. (1985). Do we fatten our children at the television set? Obesity and television viewing in children and adolescents. *Pediatrics, 75,* 807–812.

Dishion, T. J., & McMahon, R. J. (1998). Parental monitoring and the prevention of child and adolescent problem behavior: A conceptual and empirical formulation. *Clinical Child and Family Psychology Review, 1,* 61–75.

Doherty, G. (1997). *Zero to six: The basis for school readiness.* Hull, Quebec: Human Resources Development Canada.

Dowling, J. E. (1998). *Creating mind: How the brain works.* New York: Norton.

Dryfoos, J. G. (1990). *Adolescents at risk: Prevalence and prevention.* New York: Oxford University Press.

Dryfoos, J. G. (1997). New approaches to the organization of health and social services in schools. In Institute of Medicine, Committee on Comprehensive School Health Programs in Grades K-12, *Schools and health: Our nation's investment* (pp. 365–415). Washington, DC: National Academies Press.

Duncan, G. J., & Brooks-Gunn, J. (Eds.). (1997). *Consequences of growing up poor.* New York: Russell Sage Foundation.

Duncan, T. E., Duncan, S. C., & Hops, H. (1996). The role of parents and older siblings in predicting adolescent substance use: Modeling development via structural equation latent growth methodology. *Journal of Family Psychology, 10,* 158–172.

Durlak, J. A. (1995). Prevention of academic problems. In J. A. Durlak (Ed.), *School-based prevention programs for children and adolescents* (pp. 43–58). Thousand Oaks, CA: Sage.

Dwyer, D. S., & Mitchell, O. S. (1999). Health problems as determinants of retirement: Are self-rated measures endogenous? *Journal of Health Economics, 18,* 173–193.

Earley, P. C., & Lituchy, T. R. (1991). Delineating goal and efficacy effects: A test of three models. *Journal of Applied Psychology, 76,* 81–98.

Eaves, R. C., Vance, R. H., Mann, L., & Parkerbohannon, A. (1990). Cognition and academic achievement: The relationship of the Cognitive Levels Test, the Keymath Revised, and the Woodcock Reading Mastery Tests Revised. *Psychology in the Schools, 27,* 311–318.

Eccles, J. S., Midgley, C., Wigfield, A., Buchanan, C. M., Reuman, D., Flanagan, C., et al. (1993). Development during adolescence: The impact of stage-environment fit on young adolescents' experiences in schools and in families. *American Psychologist, 48,* 90–101.

Eckenrode, J. (1983). The mobilization of social supports: Some individual constraints. *American Journal of Community Psychology, 11,* 509–528.

Edmonds, R. (1986). Characteristics of effective schools. In U. Neisser (Ed.), *The school achievement of minority children: New perspectives* (pp. 93–104). Hillsdale, NJ: Erlbaum.

Edmundson, E., Parcel, G. S., Feldman, H. A., Elder, J., Perry, C. L., Johnson, C. C., et al. (1996). The effects of the Child and Adolescent Trial for Cardiovascular Health upon psychosocial determinants of diet and physical activity behavior. *Preventive Medicine, 25,* 442–454.

Educational Excellence for All Children Act. H.R. 2300, 106th Cong. (1999).

Educational Excellence for All Learners Act. S8, 108th Congress. (2003).

Edudata Canada. (n.d.). *Early Development Instrument (EDI).* Retrieved November 12, 2004, from http://www.edudata.educ.ubc.ca/Data_Pages/EDIsplash.htm

Egeland, B., Carlson, E., & Sroufe, L. A. (1993). Resilience as process. *Development and Psychopathology, 5,* 517–528.

Ehrenberg, H. M., Dierker, L., Milluzzi, C., & Mercer, B. M. (2003). Low maternal weight, failure to thrive in pregnancy, and adverse pregnancy outcomes. *American Journal of Obstetrics and Gynecology, 189,* 1726–1730.

Eisenberg, L. (1990). The biosocial context of parenting in human families. In N. A. Krasnegor & R. S. Bridges (Eds.), *Mammalian parenting: Biochemical, neurobiological, and behavioral determinants* (pp. 9–24). New York: Oxford University Press.

Elder, G. H., Jr. (1998). The life course as developmental theory. *Child Development, 69,* 1–12.

Ellickson, P. L., & McGuigan, K. A. (2000). Early predictors of adolescent violence. *American Journal of Public Health, 90,* 566–572.

Ellickson, P. L., McGuigan, K. A., Adams, V., Bell, R. M., & Hays, R. D. (1996). Teenagers and alcohol misuse in the United States: By any definition, it's a big problem. *Addiction, 91,* 1489–1503.

Elo, I. T., & Preston, S. H. (1996). Educational differentials in mortality: United States, 1979–85. *Social Science and Medicine, 42,* 47–57.

Erikson, E. H. (1959). Identity and the life cycle: Selected papers. *Psychological Issues, 1,* 1–171.

Erikson, E. H. (1963). *Childhood and society* (2nd, rev., and enl. ed.). New York: Norton.

Erikson, E. H. (1968). *Identity, youth, and crisis.* New York: Norton.

Escobar-Chaves, S. L., Tortolero, S., Markham, C., & Low, B. J. (2004). *Impact of the media on adolescent sexual attitudes and behaviors.* Austin, TX: Medical Institute.

Evans, R. G. (2002). *Interpreting and addressing inequalities in health: From Black to Acheson to Blair to . . . ?: Seventh annual lecture.* London: Office of Health Economics.

Evans, R. G., Barer, M. L., & Marmor, T. R. (Eds.). (1994). *Why are some people healthy and others not? The determinants of health of populations.* New York: Aldine de Gruyter.

Evans, R. G., & Stoddart, G. L. (1990). Producing health, consuming health care. *Social Science and Medicine, 31,* 1347–1363.

Evans, R. G., & Stoddart, G. L. (2003). Consuming research, producing policy? *American Journal of Public Health, 93,* 371–379.

Everson-Rose, S. A., Mendes de Leon, C. F., Bienias, J. L., Wilson, R. S., & Evans, D. A. (2003). Early life conditions and cognitive functioning in later life. *American Journal of Epidemiology, 158,* 1083–1089.

Fagan, J., & Wilkinson, D. L. (1998). Social contexts and functions of adolescent violence. In D. S. Elliott, B. A. Hamburg, & K. R. Williams (Eds.), *Violence in American schools: A new perspective* (pp. 55–93). New York: Cambridge University Press.

Federal Interagency Forum on Child and Family Statistics. (2004). *America's children in brief: Key national indicators of well-being, 2004.* Washington, DC: Author.

Feldman, J. J., Makuc, D. M., Kleinman, J. C., & Cornoni-Huntley, J. (1989). National trends in educational differentials in mortality. *American Journal of Epidemiology, 129,* 919–933.

Felitti, V. J., Anda, R. F., Nordenberg, D., Williamson, D. F., Spitz, A. M., Edwards, V., et al. (1998). Relationship of childhood abuse and household dysfunction to many of the leading causes of death in adults: The Adverse Childhood Experiences (ACE) Study. *American Journal of Preventive Medicine, 14,* 245–258.

Finn, J. D., & Rock, D. A. (1997). Academic success among students at risk for school failure. *Journal of Applied Psychology, 82,* 221–234.

Fischhoff, B. (1992). Risk taking: A developmental perspective. In J. F. Yates (Ed.), *Risk-taking behavior* (pp. 133–162). New York: Wiley.

Flay, B. R., Allred, C. G., & Ordway, N. (2001). Effects of the Positive Action Program on achievement and discipline: Two matched-control comparisons. *Prevention Science, 2,* 71–89.

Flay, B. R., d'Avernas, J. R., Best, J. A., Kersell, M. W., & Ryan, K. B. (1983). Cigarette smoking: Why young people do it and ways of preventing it. In P. J. McGrath & P. Firestone (Eds.), *Pediatric and adolescent behavioral medicine: Issues in treatment* (pp. 132–183). New York: Springer.

Flay, B. R., Hu, F. B., Siddiqui, O., Day, L. E., Hedeker, D., Petraitis, J., et al. (1994). Differential influence of parental smoking and friends' smoking on adolescent initiation and escalation of smoking. *Journal of Health and Social Behavior, 35,* 248–265.

Flint, B. M., & Kilgour, M. (1966). *The child and the institution: A study of deprivation and recovery.* Toronto, Ontario, Canada: University of Toronto Press.

Fogel, R. W. (2000). *The fourth great awakening and the future of egalitarianism.* Chicago: University of Chicago Press.

Foundation for Child Development Index of Child Well-Being Project. (2004). *The Child Well-Being Index (CWI) 1975–2002, with projections for 2003: An index of the social well-being of our nation's children.* Durham, NC: Duke University.

Founder's Network. (2004). *The early years: Early Development Instrument.* Retrieved November 12, 2004, from http://www.founders.net/ey/communities.nsf/0/7b7ecca25d919a3 c85256603007957da?

Francis, D. D., & Meaney, M. J. (1999). Maternal care and the development of stress responses. *Current Opinion in Neurobiology, 9,* 128–134.

Fuchs, V. R. (1982). Time preference and health: An exploratory study. In V. R. Fuchs (Ed.), *Economic aspects of health* (pp. 93–120). Chicago: University of Chicago Press.

Fuchs, V. R., & Reklis, D. M. (1997, Summer). Adding up the evidence on readiness to learn. *Jobs and Capital,* pp. 26–29.

Fullerton, C. S., & Ursano, R. J. (1994). Preadolescent peer friendships: A critical contribution to adult social relatedness. *Journal of Youth and Adolescence, 23,* 43–63.

Garbarino, J., & Ganzel, B. (2000). The human ecology of early risk. In J. P. Shonkoff & S. J. Meisels (Eds.), *Handbook of early childhood intervention* (2nd ed., pp. 76–93). New York: Cambridge University Press.

Garmezy, N. (1982). Foreword. In E. E. Werner & R. S. Smith (Eds.), *Vulnerable, but invincible: A longitudinal study of resilient children and youth* (pp. xiii–xix). New York: McGraw-Hill.

Gazzaniga, M. S., Volpe, B. T., Smylie, C. S., Wilson, D. H., & LeDoux, J. E. (1979). Plasticity in speech organization following commissurotomy. *Brain, 102,* 805–815.

Ge, X., Conger, R. D., & Elder, G. H., Jr. (1996). Coming of age too early: Pubertal influences on girls' vulnerability to psychological distress. *Child Development, 67,* 3386–3400.

Gentile, D. A., & Walsh, D. A. (2002). A normative study of family media habits. *Journal of Applied Developmental Psychology, 23,* 157–178.

Georgia Department of Early Care and Learning. (n.d.). *About Bright from the Start.* Retrieved July 12, 2005, from http://www.decal.state.ga.us/about_Decal.html

Gershoff, E. (2003). *Low income and the development of America's kindergartners* (Living at the Edge Research Brief No. 4). New York: National Center for Children Living in Poverty.

Ginsburg, H. P., & Opper, S. (1988). *Piaget's theory of intellectual development* (3rd ed.). Englewood Cliffs, NJ: Prentice-Hall.

Goals 2000: Educate America Act. Pub. L. No. 103-227, 104 Stat. 125 (1994).

Godfrey, K. M., & Barker, D. J. (2001). Fetal programming and adult health. *Public Health Nutrition, 4,* 611–624.

Gore, S. (1978). The effect of social support in moderating the health consequences of unemployment. *Journal of Health and Social Behavior, 19,* 157–165.

Gould, M. S., & Shaffer, D. (1986). The impact of suicide in television movies: Evidence of imitation. *New England Journal of Medicine, 315,* 690–694.

Graber, J. A., & Brooks-Gunn, J. (1996). *Transitions and turning points: Navigating the passage from childhood through adolescence* (CIAR Document Code HD-R7). Toronto, Ontario, Canada: Canadian Institute for Advanced Research.

Graham, H. (2004). Tackling inequalities in health in England: Remedying health disadvantages, narrowing health gaps or reducing health gradients? *Journal of Social Policy, 33,* 115–131.

Greenlund, K. J., Liu, K., Dyer, A. R., Kiefe, C. I., Burke, G. L., & Yunis, C. (1996). Body mass index in young adults: Associations with parental body size and education in the CARDIA Study. *American Journal of Public Health, 86,* 480–485.

Greenough, W. T. (1997). We can't focus just on ages zero to three. *APA Monitor, 28,* 19.

Greenough, W. T., Withers, G. S., & Anderson, B. J. (1992). Experience-dependent synaptogenesis as a plausible memory mechanism. In I. Gormezano & E. A. Wasserman (Eds.), *Learning and memory: The behavioral and biological substrates* (pp. 209–229). Hillsdale, NJ: Erlbaum.

Grosse, R. N., & Auffrey, C. (1989). Literacy and health status in developing countries. *Annual Review of Public Health, 10,* 281–297.

Grossman, M. (1972). On the concept of health capital and the demand for health. *Journal of Political Economy, 80,* 223–255.

Grossman, M., & Kaestner, R. (1997). Effects of education on health. In J. R. Behrman & N. Stacey (Eds.), *The social benefits of education* (pp. 69–123). Ann Arbor: University of Michigan Press.

Grubel, H. G. (1998). Economic freedom and human welfare: Some empirical findings. *Cato Journal, 18,* 287–304.

Grunbaum, J. A., Kann, L., Kinchen, S. A., Williams, B., Ross, J. G., Lowry, R., et al. (2002). Youth risk behavior surveillance: United States, 2001. *Morbidity and Mortality Weekly Report—Surveillance Summaries, 51*(Suppl. 4), 1–62.

Grunbaum, J. A., Kann, L., Kinchen, S. A., Ross, J. G., Hawkins, J., Lowry, R., et al. (2004). Youth risk behavior surveillance: United States, 2003. *Morbidity and Mortality Weekly Report—Surveillance Summaries, 53*(Suppl. 2), 1–96.

Grunfeld, N. (1995). *Pregnancy week by week* (New ed.). New York: Smithmark.

Grzywacz, J. G., & Fuqua, J. (2000). The social ecology of health: Leverage points and linkages. *Behavioral Medicine, 26,* 101–115.

Halfon, N., & Hochstein, M. (2002). Life course health development: An integrated framework for developing health, policy, and research. *Milbank Quarterly, 80,* 433–479.

Hall, A. J., Yee, L. J., & Thomas, S. L. (2002). Life course epidemiology and infectious diseases. *International Journal of Epidemiology, 31,* 300–301.

Harkness, S., Super, C. M., & Keefer, C. H. (1992). Learning to be an American parent: How cultural models gain directive force. In R. G. D'Andrade & C. Strauss (Eds.), *Human motives and cultural models* (pp. 163–178). New York: Cambridge University Press.

Hart, B., & Risley, T. R. (1995). *Meaningful differences in the everyday experience of young American children.* Baltimore: Brookes.

Hartup, W. W., & Moore, S. G. (1990). Early peer relations: Developmental significance and prognostic implications. *Early Childhood Research Quarterly, 5,* 1–17.

Hauser, R. M. (1997). Indicators of high school completion and dropout. In R. M. Hauser, B. V. Brown, & W. R. Prosser (Eds.), *Indicators of children's well-being* (pp. 152–184). New York: Russell Sage Foundation.

Haveman, R., & Wolfe, B. (1995). The determinants of children's attainments: A review of methods and findings. *Journal of Economic Literature, 33,* 1829–1878.

Havighurst, R. J. (1964). Youth in exploration and man emergent. In H. Borow (Ed.), *Man in a world at work* (pp. 215–236). Boston: Houghton Mifflin.

Havighurst, R. J. (1972). *Developmental tasks and education* (3rd ed.). New York: David McKay.

Hawkins, J. D. (1997). Academic performance and school success: Sources and consequences. In R. P. Weissberg, T. P. Gullotta, R.I.L. Hampton, B. A. Ryan, & G. R. Adams (Eds.), *Enhancing children's wellness* (pp. 278–305). Thousand Oaks, CA: Sage.

Hawkins, J. D., Catalano, R. F., Kosterman, R., Abbott, R., & Hill, K. G. (1999). Preventing adolescent health-risk behaviors by strengthening protection during childhood. *Archives of Pediatrics and Adolescent Medicine, 153,* 226–234.

Hawkins, J. D., Catalano, R. F., & Miller, J. Y. (1992). Risk and protective factors for alcohol and other drug problems in adolescence and early adulthood: Implications for substance-abuse prevention. *Psychological Bulletin, 112,* 64–105.

Healy, T., Côté, S., Helliwell, J. F., Field, S., Centre for Educational Research and Innovation, & Organisation for Economic Co-operation and Development. (2001). *The well-being of nations: The role of human and social capital.* Paris: Organisation for Economic Co-operation and Development.

Hertzman, C. (1990). *Where are the differences which make a difference? Thinking about the determinants of health* (CIAR Document Code PHWP-8). Toronto, Ontario, Canada: Canadian Institute for Advanced Research.

Hertzman, C. (1998). The case for child development as a determinant of health. *Canadian Journal of Public Health—Revue Canadienne de Santé Publique, 89*(Suppl. 1), 14–19.

Hertzman, C. (1999). Population health and human development. In D. P. Keating & C. Hertzman (Eds.), *Developmental health and the wealth of nations: Social, biological, and educational dynamics* (pp. 21–40). New York: Guilford Press.

Hertzman, C., McLean, S. A., Kohen, D. E., Dunn, J., & Evans, T. (2002). *Early development in Vancouver: Report of the Community Asset Mapping Project (CAMP).* Ottawa, Ontario, Canada: Canadian Population Health Initiative.

Hertzman, C., Power, C., Matthews, S., & Manor, O. (2001). Using an interactive framework of society and lifecourse to explain self-rated health in early adulthood. *Social Science and Medicine, 53,* 1575–1585.

Hertzman, C., & Wiens, M. (1995). *Child development and long-term outcomes: A population health perspective and summary of successful interventions* (CIAR Document Code HDPH-1). Toronto, Ontario, Canada: Canadian Institute for Advanced Research.

Hertzman, C., & Wiens, M. (1996). Child development and long-term outcomes: A population health perspective and summary of successful interventions. *Social Science and Medicine, 43,* 1083–1095.

Hibbett, A., & Fogelman, K. (1990). Future lives of truants: Family formation and health-related behaviour. *British Journal of Educational Psychology, 60,* 171–179.

Hicks, L. E., Langham, R. A., & Takenaka, J. (1982). Cognitive and health measures following early nutritional supplementation: A sibling study. *American Journal of Public Health, 72,* 1110–1118.

Hockfield, S., & Lombroso, P. J. (1998). Development of the cerebral cortex: IX. Cortical development and experience: I. *Journal of the American Academy of Child and Adolescent Psychiatry, 37,* 992–993.

House, J. S., Landis, K. R., & Umberson, D. (1988). Social relationships and health. *Science, 241,* 540–545.

Hurley, L. P., & Lustbader, L. L. (1997). Project Support: Engaging children and families in the educational process. *Adolescence, 32,* 523–531.

Huston, A. C. (Ed.). (1991). *Children in poverty: Child development and public policy.* New York: Cambridge University Press.

Huttenlocher, P. R. (1984). Synapse elimination and plasticity in developing human cerebral cortex. *American Journal of Mental Deficiency, 88,* 488–496.

Hymel, S., Comfort, C., Schonert-Reichl, K., & McDougall, P. (1996). Academic failure and school dropout: The influence of peers. In J. Juvonen & K. R. Wentzel (Eds.), *Social motivation: Understanding children's school adjustment* (pp. 313–345). New York: Cambridge University Press.

Ingersoll, G. M. (1989). *Adolescents* (2nd ed.). Englewood Cliffs, NJ: Prentice-Hall.

Institute for Defense Analyses. (2000). *Review of Department of Defense education activity (DODEA) schools: Vol. 2. Quantitative analysis of educational quality* (IDA Paper P-3544). Alexandria, VA: Author.

Institute of Medicine, Committee on Prevention and Control of Sexually Transmitted Diseases. (1997). *The hidden epidemic: Confronting sexually transmitted diseases.* Washington, DC: National Academies Press.

Institute of Medicine, Committee on Prevention of Mental Disorders. (1994). *Reducing risks for mental disorders: Frontiers for preventive intervention research.* Washington, DC: National Academies Press.

Irwin, C. (1993). Adolescence and risk taking: How are they related? In N. J. Bell & R. W. Bell (Eds.), *Adolescent risk taking* (pp. 7–28). Newbury Park, CA: Sage.

Jackson, B., Wright, R. J., Kubzansky, L. D., & Weiss, S. T. (2004). Examining the influence of early life socioeconomic position on pulmonary function across the life span: Where do we go from here? *Thorax, 59,* 186–188.

Janus, M., & Offord, D. (2000). Readiness to learn at school. *ISUMA: Canadian Journal of Policy Research, 1,* 71–75.

Jefferis, B. J., Power, C., & Hertzman, C. (2002). Birth weight, childhood socioeconomic environment, and cognitive development in the 1958 British birth cohort study. *British Medical Journal, 325,* 305–310.

Jessor, R. (1984). Adolescent development and behavioral health. In J. D. Matarazzo, S. M. Weiss, J. A. Herd, & N. E. Miller (Eds.), *Behavioral health: A handbook of health enhancement and disease prevention* (pp. 69–90). New York: Wiley.

Jessor, R., Donovan, J. E., & Costa, F. M. (1991). *Beyond adolescence: Problem behavior and young adult development.* New York: Cambridge University Press.

Jessor, R., & Jessor, S. L. (1977). *Problem behavior and psychosocial development: A longitudinal study of youth.* New York: Academic Press.

Jimerson, S., Egeland, B., Sroufe, L. A., & Carlson, E. (2000). A prospective longitudinal study of high school dropouts examining multiple predictors across development. *Journal of School Psychology, 38,* 525–549.

Johnson, J. G., Cohen, P., Smailes, E. M., Kasen, S., & Brook, J. S. (2002). Television viewing and aggressive behavior during adolescence and adulthood. *Science, 295,* 2468–2471.

Jordan, W. J., Lara, J., & McPartland, J. M. (1996). Exploring the causes of early dropout among race-ethnic and gender groups. *Youth and Society, 28,* 62–94.

Kagan, J. (1994). *Galen's prophecy: Temperament in human nature.* New York: Basic Books.

Kagan, S. L. (1999). Cracking the readiness mystique. *Young Children, 54*(5), 2–3.

Kahn, A. J., & Kamerman, S. B. (Eds.). (2002). *Beyond child poverty: The social exclusion of children.* New York: Institute for Child and Family Policy at Columbia University.

Kaiser Family Foundation. (2003a). *Sex on TV 2003: A biennial report to the Kaiser Family Foundation* (Publication No. 3325). Menlo Park, CA: Author.

Kaiser Family Foundation. (2003b). *Zero to six: Electronic media in the lives of infants, toddlers, and preschoolers* (Publication No. 3378). Menlo Park, CA: Author.

Kaiser Family Foundation. (2004). *The role of media in childhood obesity* (Publication No. 7030). Menlo Park, CA: Author.

Kamerman, S. B. (2002a). *Early childhood education and care (ECEC): An overview of developments in the OECD countries.* New York: Institute for Child and Family Policy at Columbia University.

Kamerman, S. B. (2002b). *Social exclusion and children: Background and context.* New York: Institute for Child and Family Policy at Columbia University.

Kamerman, S. B., Neuman, M., Waldfogel, J., & Brooks-Gunn, J. (2003). *Social policies, family types and child outcomes in selected OECD countries* (OECD Social Employment and Migration Working Papers No. 6). Paris: Organisation for Economic Co-operation and Development.

Kandel, D. B., & Wu, P. (1995). The contributions of mothers and fathers to the intergenerational transmission of cigarette smoking in adolescence. *Journal of Research on Adolescence, 5,* 225–252.

Kaplan, G. A., & Keil, J. E. (1993). Socioeconomic factors and cardiovascular disease: A review of the literature. *Circulation, 88,* 1973–1998.

Kaprio, J., Pulkkinen, L., & Rose, R. J. (2002). Genetic and environmental factors in health-related behaviors: Studies on Finnish twins and twin families. *Twin Research, 5,* 366–371.

Karasek, R., & Theorell, T. (1990). *Healthy work: Stress, productivity, and the reconstruction of working life.* New York: Basic Books.

Kawachi, I., & Kennedy, B. P. (1997). Health and social cohesion: Why care about income inequality? *British Medical Journal, 314,* 1037–1040.

Kawachi, I., Kennedy, B. P., & Glass, R. (1999). Social capital and self-rated health: A contextual analysis. *American Journal of Public Health, 89,* 1187–1193.

Keating, D. P., & Hertzman, C. (Eds.). (1999). *Developmental health and the wealth of nations: Social, biological, and educational dynamics.* New York: Guilford Press.

Keating, D. P., & Miller, F. K. (1999). Individual pathways in competence and coping: From regulatory systems to habits of mind. In D. P. Keating & C. Hertzman (Eds.), *Developmental health and the wealth of nations: Social, biological, and educational dynamics* (pp. 220–234). New York: Guilford Press.

Keefe, K. (1994). Perceptions of normative social pressure and attitudes toward alcohol use: Changes during adolescence. *Journal of Studies on Alcohol, 55,* 46–54.

Kelder, S. H., Edmundson, E. W., & Lytle, L. A. (1997). Health behavior research and school and youth health promotion. In D. S. Gochman (Ed.), *Handbook of health behavior research: Vol. 4. Relevance for Professionals and Issues for the Future* (pp. 263–284). New York: Plenum Press.

Kennedy, S. (2003). *The relationship between education and health in Australia and Canada* (SEDAP Research Paper No. 93). Hamilton, Ontario, Canada: McMaster University, Program for Research on Social and Economic Dimensions of an Aging Population.

Kirby, S., & Hurford, J. R. (1997). The evolution of incremental learning: Language, development, and critical periods. *Edinburgh Occasional Papers in Linguistics.* Retrieved November 7, 2004, from http://www3.isrl.uiuc.edu/~junwang4/langev/localcopy/pdf/kirby97theEvolution.pdf

Kisilevsky, B. S., Hains, S. M., Lee, K., Xie, X., Huang, H., Ye, H. H., et al. (2003). Effects of experience on fetal voice recognition. *Psychological Science, 14,* 220–224.

Kohen, D. E., & Hertzman, C. (1998). *Affluent neighborhoods and school readiness* (Report No. W-98-15Es). Ottawa, Ontario, Canada: Human Resources Development Canada.

Kohen, D. E., Hertzman, C., & Brooks-Gunn, J. (1999). Neighbourhood affluence and school readiness. *Education Quarterly Review, 6,* 44–52.

Koivusilta, L. K., Rimpela, A. H., & Rimpela, M. K. (1999). Health-related lifestyle in adolescence: Origin of social class differences in health? *Health Education Research, 14,* 339–355.

Kolar, V. (1999, Autumn). Learning parenting: Intergenerational influences. *Family Matters,* pp. 65–68.

Kolbe, L. J. (1990). An epidemiological surveillance system to monitor the prevalence of youth behaviors that most affect health. *Journal of Health Education, 21,* 44–48.

Korpi, B. M. (2000, December). *Early childhood education and care policy in Sweden.* Paper presented at the international OECD conference Lifelong Learning as an Affordable Investment, Ottawa, Ontario, Canada.

Krieger, N. (2001). Theories for social epidemiology in the 21st century: An ecosocial perspective. *International Journal of Epidemiology, 30,* 668–677.

Krieger, N., & Fee, E. (1994). Social class: The missing link in U.S. health data. *International Journal of Health Services, 24,* 25–44.

Kristenson, M., Eriksen, H. R., Sluiter, J. K., Starke, D., & Ursin, H. (2004). Psychobiological mechanisms of socioeconomic differences in health. *Social Science and Medicine, 58,* 1511–1522.

Kuh, D., & Ben-Shlomo, Y. (Eds.). (2004). *A life course approach to chronic disease epidemiology* (2nd ed.). New York: Oxford University Press.

Kuh, D., Ben-Shlomo, Y., Lynch, J., Hallqvist, J., & Power, C. (2003). Life course epidemiology. *Journal of Epidemiology and Community Health, 57,* 778–783.

Kuh, D., Hardy, R., Langenberg, C., Richards, M., & Wadsworth, M. E. (2002). Mortality in adults aged 26–54 years related to socioeconomic conditions in childhood and adulthood: Post war birth cohort study. *British Medical Journal, 325,* 1076–1080.

Kuh, D., & Smith, G. D. (2004). The life course and adult chronic disease: An historical perspective with particular reference to coronary heart disease. In D. Kuh & Y. Ben-Shlomo (Eds.), *A life course approach to chronic disease epidemiology* (2nd ed., pp. 15–37). New York: Oxford University Press.

Kuhl, P. K. (1993). Early linguistic experience and phonetic perception: Implications for theories of developmental speech-perception. *Journal of Phonetics, 21,* 125–139.

Kulbok, P. A., & Cox, C. L. (2002). Dimensions of adolescent health behavior. *Journal of Adolescent Health, 31,* 394–400.

Kumpfer, K. L., & Turner, C. W. (1990). The social ecology model of adolescent substance abuse: Implications for prevention. *International Journal of the Addictions, 25,* 435–463.

Kunst, A. E., Geurts, J. J., & van den Berg, B. J. (1995). International variation in socioeconomic inequalities in self-reported health. *Journal of Epidemiology and Community Health, 49,* 117–123.

Ladd, G. W., & Price, J. M. (1987). Predicting children's social and school adjustment following the transition from preschool to kindergarten. *Child Development, 58,* 1168–1189.

Lamb, M. E., Bornstein, M. H., & Teti, D. M. (2002). *Development in infancy: An introduction* (4th ed.). Mahwah, NJ: Erlbaum.

Landry, S. H., Smith, K. E., Miller-Loncar, C. L., & Swank, P. R. (1998). The relation of change in maternal interactive styles to the developing social competence of full-term and preterm children. *Child Development, 69,* 105–123.

Landry, S. H., Smith, K. E., Swank, P. R., & Miller-Loncar, C. L. (2000). Early maternal and child influences on children's later independent cognitive and social functioning. *Child Development, 71,* 358–375.

Langer, J. A. (2000). Excellence in English in middle and high school: How teachers' professional lives support student achievement. *American Educational Research Journal, 37,* 397–439.

Lanphear, B. P., Dietrich, K., Auinger, P., & Cox, C. (2000). Cognitive deficits associated with blood lead concentrations >10 microg/dL in U.S. children and adolescents. *Public Health Reports, 115,* 521–529.

Lantz, P. M., House, J. S., Lepkowski, J. M., Williams, D. R., Mero, R. P., & Chen, J. M. (1998). Socioeconomic factors, health behaviors, and mortality: Results from a nationally representative prospective study of U.S. adults. *Journal of the American Medical Association, 279,* 1703–1708.

Lassiter, K. S., & Bardos, A. N. (1995). The relationship between young children's academic achievement and measures of intelligence. *Psychology in the Schools, 32,* 170–177.

Lau, R. R., Quadrel, M. J., & Hartman, K. A. (1990). Development and change of young adults' preventive health beliefs and behavior: Influence from parents and peers. *Journal of Health and Social Behavior, 31,* 240–259.

Lavin, C. (1996). The relationship between the Wechsler Intelligence Scale for Children Third Edition and the Kaufman Test of Educational Achievement. *Psychology in the Schools, 33,* 119–123.

Lawlor, D. A., Ebrahim, S., & Davey, S. G. (2004). Association between self-reported childhood socioeconomic position and adult lung function: Findings from the British Women's Heart and Health Study. *Thorax, 59,* 199–203.

Lawrance, E. C. (1991). Poverty and the rate of time preference: Evidence from panel data. *Journal of Political Economy, 99,* 54–77.

Leave No Child Behind Act of 2003. S. 448, 108th Cong., 1st Sess.

Lee, V. H., & Burkham, D. T. (2002). *Inequality at the starting gate: Social background differences in achievement as children begin school.* Washington, DC: Economic Policy Institute.

Leffert, N., Benson, P. L., Scales, P. C., Sharma, A. R., Drake, D. R., & Blyth, D. A. (1998). Developmental assets: Measurement and prediction of risk behaviors among adolescents. *Applied Developmental Science, 2,* 209–230.

Leidy, L. E. (1996). Lifespan approach to the study of human biology: An introductory overview. *American Journal of Human Biology, 8,* 699–702.

Lempers, J. D., & Clark-Lempers, D. (1990). Family economic stress, maternal and paternal support and adolescent distress. *Journal of Adolescence, 13,* 217–229.

Lerner, R. M., & Benson, P. L. (Eds.). (2003). *Developmental assets and asset-building communities: Implications for research, policy, and practice.* New York: Kluwer Academic/Plenum.

Liu, D., Diorio, J., Day, J. C., Francis, D. D., & Meaney, M. J. (2000). Maternal care, hippocampal synaptogenesis and cognitive development in rats. *Nature Neuroscience, 3,* 799–806.

Lleras-Muney, A. (2002). *The relationship between education and adult mortality in the United States* (NBER Working Paper No. 8986). Cambridge, MA: National Bureau of Economic Research.

Low, B. J. (2001). Association between academic achievement and health status among Hispanic eighth-grade students in Houston (Doctoral dissertation, University of Texas Health Science Center at Houston School of Public Health, 2001). *Dissertation Abstracts International, 62,* 3990.

Low, B. J., Baumler, E., Cardarelli, K. M., Sterner, J. M., & Low, M. D. (2003, November). *Student academic success and health outcomes: Policy implications.* Paper presented at the annual conference of the American Public Health Association, Washington, DC.

Low, M. D., Low, B. J., Baumler, E., Huynh, P., & Cronin, P. (2002, June). *Which American children will succeed? Personal and social determinants of educational attainment and health.* Paper presented at the Annual International Conference on Social Sciences, Honolulu, HI.

Luster, T., & Okagaki, L. (1993). Multiple influences on parenting: Ecological and life-course perspectives. In T. Luster & L. Okagaki (Eds.), *Parenting: An ecological perspective* (pp. 227–250). Hillsdale, NJ: Erlbaum.

Luthar, S. S., Cicchetti, D., & Becker, B. (2000). The construct of resilience: A critical evaluation and guidelines for future work. *Child Development, 71,* 543–562.

Luthar, S. S., & Zigler, E. (1991). Vulnerability and competence: A review of research on resilience in childhood. *American Journal of Orthopsychiatry, 61,* 6–22.

Luxembourg Income Study. (2004, July 7). *Key figures: Relative poverty rates for the total population, children and the elderly.* Retrieved November 12, 2004, from http://www.lisproject.org/keyfigures/povertytable.htm

Lynch, J. W., Kaplan, G. A., Pamuk, E. R., Cohen, R. D., Heck, K. E., Balfour, J. L., et al. (1998). Income inequality and mortality in metropolitan areas of the United States. *American Journal of Public Health, 88,* 1074–1080.

Macintyre, S. (1986). The patterning of health by social position in contemporary Britain: Directions for sociological research. *Social Science and Medicine, 23,* 393–415.

Macintyre, S. (1994). Understanding the social patterning of health: The role of the social sciences. *Journal of Public Health Medicine, 16,* 53–59.

Maggi, S., Hertzman, C., Kohen, D., & D'Angiulli, A. (2004). Effects of neighborhood socioeconomic characteristics and class composition on highly competent children. *Journal of Educational Research, 98,* 109–114.

Margalit, M. (2003). Resilience model among individuals with learning disabilities: Proximal and distal influences. *Learning Disabilities: Research and Practice, 18,* 82–86.

Marmot, M. G. (2002). The influence of income on health: Views of an epidemiologist. Does money really matter? Or is it a marker for something else? *Health Affairs, 21*(2), 31–46.

Marmot, M. G., Bosma, H., Hemingway, H., Brunner, E., & Stansfeld, S. (1997). Contribution of job control and other risk factors to social variations in coronary heart disease incidence. *Lancet, 350,* 235–239.

Marmot, M. G., Feeney, A., Shipley, M., North, F., & Syme, S. L. (1995). Sickness absence as a measure of health status and functioning: From the UK Whitehall II study. *Journal of Epidemiology and Community Health, 49,* 124–130.

Marmot, M. G., Siegrist, J., Theorell, T., & Feeney, A. (1999). Health and the psychosocial environment at work. In M. G. Marmot & R. G. Wilkinson (Eds.), *Social determinants of health* (pp. 105–131). New York: Oxford University Press.

Marmot, M. G., Smith, G. D., Stansfeld, S., Patel, C., North, F., Head, J., et al. (1991). Health inequalities among British civil servants: The Whitehall II study. *Lancet, 337,* 1387–1393.

Marmot, M. G., & Wadsworth, M.E.J. (1997). *Fetal and early childhood environment: Long-term health implications.* New York: Royal Society of Medicine Press.

Martikainen, P., Bartley, M., & Lahelma, E. (2002). Psychosocial determinants of health in social epidemiology. *International Journal of Epidemiology, 31,* 1091–1093.

Masten, A. S. (2001). Ordinary magic: Resilience processes in development. *American Psychologist, 56,* 227–238.

Masten, A. S., Best, K. M., & Garmezy, N. (1990). Resilience and development: Contributions from the study of children who overcome adversity. *Development and Psychopathology, 2,* 425–444.

Mathematica Policy Research. (2002). *Making a difference in the lives of infants and toddlers and their families: The impacts of Early Head Start: Executive summary.* Washington, DC: Administration on Children, Youth and Families, Head Start Bureau.

Mattson, M. P., Duan, W., Wan, R., & Guo, Z. (2004). Prophylactic activation of neuroprotective stress response pathways by dietary and behavioral manipulations. *NeuroRx: The Journal of the American Society for Experimental NeuroTherapeutics, 1,* 111–116.

McAlister, A., Puska, P., Salonen, J. T., Tuomilehto, J., & Koskela, K. (1982). Theory and action for health promotion: Illustrations from the North Karelia Project. *American Journal of Public Health, 72,* 43–50.

McBroom, J. R. (1994). Correlates of alcohol and marijuana use among junior high school students: Family, peers, school problems, and psychosocial concerns. *Youth and Society, 26,* 54–68.

McCain, M. N., & Mustard, J. M. (1999). *Reversing the real brain drain: Early years study: Final report.* Toronto, Ontario, Canada: Ontario Children's Secretariat.

McGinnis, J. M., & Foege, W. H. (1993). Actual causes of death in the United States. *Journal of the American Medical Association, 270,* 2207–2212.

McGroder, S. M. (1990). *Head Start: What do we know about what works?* Washington, DC: U.S. Department of Health and Human Services Office of the Assistant Secretary for Planning and Evaluation.

McIntyre, J. G., & Dusek, J. B. (1995). Perceived parental rearing practices and styles of coping. *Journal of Youth and Adolescence, 24,* 499–509.

McKenzie, F. D., & Richmond, J. B. (1998). Linking health and learning: An overview of coordinated school health programs. In E. Marx, S. F. Wooley, & D. Northrop (Eds.), *Health is academic: A guide to coordinated school health programs* (pp. 1–42). New York: Teachers College Press.

McKnight, J. L. (1999). Two tools for well-being: Health systems and communities. *Journal of Perinatology, 19*(Suppl. 2), 12–15.

McLoyd, V. C. (1998). Socioeconomic disadvantage and child development. *American Psychologist, 53,* 185–204.

Meaney, M. J., Diorio, J., Francis, D., Widdowson, J., LaPlante, P., Caldji, C., et al. (1996). Early environmental regulation of forebrain glucocorticoid receptor gene expression: Implications for adrenocortical responses to stress. *Developmental Neuroscience, 18,* 49–72.

Meisels, S. J. (1999). Assessing readiness. In R. C. Pianta & M. J. Cox (Eds.), *The transition to kindergarten* (pp. 39–66). Baltimore: Brookes.

Micklewright, J., & Stewart, K. (2000). *The welfare of Europe's children: Are EU member states converging?* Bristol, United Kingdom: Policy Press.

Miller, P., Mulvey, C., & Martin, N. (2001). Genetic and environmental contributions to educational attainment in Australia. *Economics of Education Review, 20,* 211–224.

Minister of Public Works and Government Services Canada. (2001). *Federal, Provincial and Territorial Early Childhood Development Agreement: Report on government of Canada activities and expenditures 2000–2001.* Ottawa, Ontario: Health Canada.

Montgomery, S. M., Bartley, M. J., & Wilkinson, R. G. (1997). Family conflict and slow growth. *Archives of Disease in Childhood, 77,* 326–330.

Moore, K. A., Glei, D. A., Driscoll, A. K., Zaslow, M. J., & Redd, Z. (2002). Poverty and welfare patterns: Implications for children. *Journal of Social Policy, 31,* 207–227.

Morison, P., & Masten, A. S. (1991). Peer reputation in middle childhood as a predictor of adaptation in adolescence: A seven-year follow-up. *Child Development, 62,* 991–1007.

Morris, J. A. (1999). Information and redundancy: Key concepts in understanding the genetic control of health and intelligence. *Medical Hypotheses, 53,* 118–123.

Mortimore, P. (1995). The positive effects of schooling. In M. Rutter (Ed.), *Psychosocial disturbances in young people: Challenges for prevention* (pp. 333–363). New York: Cambridge University Press.

Muir, D., & Slater, A. (Eds.). (2000). *Infant development: The essential readings.* Malden, MA: Blackwell.

Mustard, J. F. (2000, April). *What science says about the effects of early intervention: Early child development and the brain: The base for health, learning, and behaviour throughout life.* Paper presented at the World Bank Conference on Investing in Our Children's Future, Washington, DC.

National Center for Health Statistics. (2000). *Health, United States, 2000: Adolescent health chartbook* (DHHS Publication No. PHS 2000-1232-1). Hyattsville, MD: Public Health Service.

National Center for Health Statistics. (2001, June 6). Trends in pregnancy rates for the United States, 1976–97: An update. *National Vital Statistics Report, 49*(4), 1–12. Retrieved May 10, 2005 from http://www.cdc.gov/nchs/data/nvsr/nvsr49/nvsr49_04.pdf

National Center for Health Statistics. (2003a). Births: Final data for 2002. *National Vital Statistics Report, 52*(10), 1–116. Retrieved May 10, 2005, from http://www.cdc.gov/nchs/data/nvsr/nvsr52/nvsr52_10.pdf

National Center for Health Statistics. (2003b). Deaths: Leading causes for 2001. *National Vital Statistics Report, 52*(9), 1–88. Retrieved May 10, 2005, from http://www.cdc.gov/nchs/data/nvsr/nvsr52/nvsr52_09.pdf

National Education Association. (2001, February). *America's top education priority: Lifting up low-performing schools.* Retrieved November 12, 2004, from http://www.nea.org/priority schools/priority.html

National Education Goals Panel, Goal 1 Technical Planning Group. (1995). *Reconsidering children's early development and learning: Toward common views and vocabulary.* Washington, DC.: U.S. Government Printing Office.

National Institutes of Child Health and Development Early Child Care Research Network. (1994). Child care and child development: The NICHD study of early child care. In S. L. Friedman & H. C. Haywood (Eds.), *Developmental follow-up: Concepts, domains, and methods* (pp. 377–396). San Diego, CA: Academic Press.

National Institutes of Child Health and Development Early Child Care Research Network. (2003). Does quality of child care affect child outcomes at age 4½? *Developmental Psychology, 39,* 451–469.

National Institutes of Health. (2002, April 1). *NIH guide: Centers for population health and health disparities* (ES-02-009). Retrieved May 10, 2005, from http://grants1.nih.gov/grants/guide/rfa-files/RFA-ES-02-009.html

National Institutes of Health Working Group on Health Disparities. (n.d.). *Addressing health disparities: The NIH program of action.* Retrieved November 12, 2004, from http://healthdisparities.nih.gov/working.html

National Research Council, Committee on Integrating the Science of Early Childhood Development. (2000). *From neurons to neighborhoods: The science of early child development.* Washington, DC: National Academies Press.

Neiss, M., & Rowe, D. C. (2000). Parental education and child's verbal IQ in adoptive and biological families in the National Longitudinal Study of Adolescent Health. *Behavior Genetics, 30,* 487–495.

Nelson, C. A. (1995). The ontogeny of human memory: A cognitive neuroscience perspective. *Developmental Psychology, 31,* 723–738.

Nelson, C. A., & Bloom, F. E. (1997). Child development and neuroscience. *Child Development, 68,* 970–987.

Neuman, S. B., & Dickinson, D. K. (Eds.). (2001). *Handbook of early literacy research.* New York: Guilford Press.

Neville, H. J., & Bavelier, D. (1999). Specificity and plasticity in neurocognitive development in humans. In M. Gazzaniga (Ed.), *The new cognitive neurosciences* (2nd ed., pp. 83–98). Cambridge, MA: MIT Press.

Nicolopoulou, A. (1993). Play, cognitive development, and the social world: Piaget, Vygotsky, and beyond. *Human Development, 36,* 1–23.

Niedhammer, I., Tek, M. L., Starke, D., & Siegrist, J. (2004). Effort-reward imbalance model and self-reported health: Cross-sectional and prospective findings from the GAZEL cohort. *Social Science and Medicine, 58,* 1531–1541.

No Child Left Behind Act of 2001. Pub. L. No. 107-110, 115 Stat. 1425 (2002).

Offord Centre for Child Studies. (2004, August). *School Readiness to Learn (SRL) Project: Project description.* Retrieved November 5, 2004, from http://www.offordcentre.com/readiness/project.html

Offord, D. R., & Janus, M. (2002). *The School Readiness to Learn Project in Canada.* Retrieved February 24, 2005, from http://www.offordcentre.com/readiness/files/PUB.6.2002_Offord-Janus.pdf

Olson, L. (2002, January 9). Quality counts finds uneven early-childhood policies. *Education Week,* p. 3.

Osler, M., & Prescott, E. (2003). Educational level as a contextual and proximate determinant of all cause mortality in Danish adults. *Journal of Epidemiology and Community Health, 57,* 266–269.

Pappas, G., Queen, S., Hadden, W., & Fisher, G. (1993). The increasing disparity in mortality between socioeconomic groups in the United States, 1960 and 1986. *New England Journal of Medicine, 329,* 103–109.

Perry, B. D., Pollard, R. A., Blakley, T. L., Baker, W. L., & Vigilante, D. (1995). Childhood trauma, the neurobiology of adaptation, and "use-dependent" development of the brain: How "states" become "traits." *Infant Mental Health Journal, 16,* 271–291.

Pfannenstiel, J. C., Lambson, T., & Yarnell, V. (1996, January). The Parents as Teachers program: Longitudinal follow-up to the Second Wave study. Report prepared for the Missouri Department of Elementary and Secondary Education and Parents as Teachers National Center, Inc. Retrieved May 10, 2005, from http://www.parentsasteachers.org/atf/cf/{7A832E5A-3E17-4576-8C7E-F921E4ABDCA5}/2ndwavefollow-up.pdf

Philipson, T., & Soares, R. R. (2001). World inequality and the rise in longevity. In B. Pleskovic & N. H. Stern (Eds.), *Annual World Bank Conference on Development Economics 2001/2002* (pp. 245–259). Washington, DC: World Bank.

Piaget, J. (1952). *The origins of intelligence in children* (M. Cook, Trans.). New York: International Universities Press.

Pickles, A., & Rutter, M. (1991). Statistical and conceptual models of "turning points" in developmental processes. In D. Magnusson, L. R. Bergman, G. Rudinger, & B. Torestad

(Eds.), *Problems and methods in longitudinal research: Stability and change* (pp. 133–165). New York: Cambridge University Press.

Poole, D. L. (1997). The SAFE project: Community-driven partnerships in health, mental health, and education to prevent early school failure. *Health and Social Work, 22,* 282–289.

Potapchuk, W. R., Crocker, J. P., & Schechter, W. H. (1997). Building community with social capital: Chits and chums or chats with change. *National Civic Review, 86,* 129–140.

Power, C., & Hertzman, C. (1997). Social and biological pathways linking early life and adult disease. *British Medical Bulletin, 53,* 210–221.

Power, C., Li, L., & Manor, O. (2000). A prospective study of limiting longstanding illness in early adulthood. *International Journal of Epidemiology, 29,* 131–139.

Power, C., Manor, O., & Fox, J. (1991). *Health and class: The early years.* New York: Guilford Press.

Power, C., Manor, O., & Matthews, S. (1999). The duration and timing of exposure: Effects of socioeconomic environment on adult health. *American Journal of Public Health, 89,* 1059–1065.

Putnam, R. D. (1993). *Making democracy work: Civic traditions in modern Italy.* Princeton, NJ: Princeton University Press.

Putnam, R. D. (1995). Bowling alone: America's declining social capital. *Journal of Democracy, 6,* 65–78.

Quadrel, M. J., Fischhoff, B., & Davis, W. (1993). Adolescent (in)vulnerability. *American Psychologist, 48,* 102–116.

Rakic, P., Bourgeois, J. P., & Goldman-Rakic, P. S. (1994). Synaptic development of the cerebral cortex: Implications for learning, memory, and mental illness. *Progress in Brain Research, 102,* 227–243.

Raphael, B., & Sprague, T. (1996, Winter). Mental health and prevention for families. *Family Matters,* pp. 26–29.

Ratzan, S. C., & Parker, R. M. (2000). Introduction. In C. Selden, M. Zorn, S. C. Ratzan, & R. M. Parker (Eds.), *National Library of Medicine current bibliographies in medicine: Health literacy* (p. iv) (NLM Publication No. CBM 2000-1). Bethesda, MD: National Library of Medicine.

Rehme, G. (2001). *Redistribution of personal incomes, education, and economic performance across countries: Preliminary version.* Helsinki, Finland: World Institute for Development Economics Research.

Reininger, B., Evans, A. E., Griffin, S. F., Valois, R. F., Vincen, M. L., Parra-Medina, D., et al. (2003). Development of a youth survey to measure risk behaviors, attitudes and assets: Examining multiple influences. *Health Education Research, 18,* 461–476.

Repetti, R. L., Taylor, S. E., & Seeman, T. E. (2002). Risky families: Family social environments and the mental and physical health of offspring. *Psychological Bulletin, 128,* 330–366.

Resnick, M. D., Bearman, P. S., Blum, R. W., Bauman, K. E., Harris, K. M., Jones, J., et al. (1997). Protecting adolescents from harm: Findings from the National Longitudinal Study on Adolescent Health. *Journal of the American Medical Association, 278,* 823–832.

Resnick, M. D., Harris, L. J., & Blum, R. W. (1993). The impact of caring and connectedness on adolescent health and well-being. *Journal of Paediatrics and Child Health, 29*(Suppl. 1), 3–9.

Riley, A. W., Green, B. F., Forrest, C. B., Starfield, B., Kang, M., & Ensminger, M. E. (1998). A taxonomy of adolescent health: Development of the adolescent health profile-types. *Medical Care, 36,* 1228–1236.

Roccella, M., & Testa, D. (2003). Fetal alcohol syndrome in developmental age: Neuropsychiatric aspects. *Minerva Pediatrica, 55,* 63–69.

Roisman, G. I., Masten, A. S., Coatsworth, J. D., & Tellegen, A. (2004). Salient and emerging developmental tasks in the transition to adulthood. *Child Development, 75,* 123–133.

Rosenberg, M. L., O'Carroll, P. W., & Powell, K. E. (1992). Let's be clear: Violence is a public health problem. *Journal of the American Medical Association, 267,* 3071–3072.

Rosenfield, D., Folger, R., & Adelman, H. F. (1980). When rewards reflect competence: A qualification of the over-justification effect. *Journal of Personality and Social Psychology, 39,* 368–376.

Ross, C. E., & Mirowsky, J. (1999). Refining the association between education and health: The effects of quantity, credential, and selectivity. *Demography, 36,* 445–460.

Ross, C. E., & Van Willigen, M. (1997). Education and the subjective quality of life. *Journal of Health and Social Behavior, 38,* 275–297.

Ross, C. E., & Wu, C. L. (1995). The links between education and health. *American Sociological Review, 60,* 719–745.

Ross, C. E., & Wu, C. L. (1996). Education, age, and the cumulative advantage in health. *Journal of Health and Social Behavior, 37,* 104–120.

Ross, N. A., Wolfson, M. C., Dunn, J. R., Berthelot, J. M., Kaplan, G. A., & Lynch, J. W. (2000). Relation between income inequality and mortality in Canada and in the United States: Cross sectional assessment using census data and vital statistics. *British Medical Journal, 320,* 898–902.

Rutter, M. (1987). Psychosocial resilience and protective mechanisms. *American Journal of Orthopsychiatry, 57,* 316–331.

Rutter, M. (1989). Pathways from childhood to adult life. *Journal of Child Psychology and Psychiatry and Allied Disciplines, 30,* 23–51.

Rutter, M. (1994). Continuities, transitions and turning points in development. In M. Rutter & D. F. Hay (Eds.), *Development through life: A handbook for clinicians* (pp. 1–25). Boston: Blackwell Scientific.

Rutter, M., & Rutter, M. (1993). *Developing minds: Challenge and continuity across the life span.* New York: Basic Books.

Saluja, G., Scott-Little, C., & Clifford, R. M. (2000, Fall). Readiness for school: A survey of state policies and definitions. *Early Childhood Research and Practice, 2*(2). Retrieved February 9, 2005, from http://ecrp.uiuc.edu/v2n2/saluja.html

Sameroff, A. J., & Fiese, B. H. (2000). Models of development and developmental risk. In C. H. Zeanah (Ed.), *Handbook of infant mental health* (2nd ed., pp. 3–19). New York: Guilford Press.

Scales, P. C., & Leffert, N. (2004). *Developmental assets: A synthesis of the scientific research on adolescent development* (2nd ed.). Minneapolis: Search Institute.

Scandura, T. A., & Lankau, M. J. (1997). Relationships of gender, family responsibility and flexible work hours to organizational commitment and job satisfaction. *Journal of Organizational Behavior, 18,* 377–391.

Schieman, S., McBrier, D. B., & Van Gundy, K. (2003). Home-to-work conflict, work qualities, and emotional distress. *Sociological Forum, 18,* 137–164.

Schunk, D. H. (1987). Peer models and children's behavioral change. *Review of Educational Research, 57,* 149–174.

Seccombe, K. (2000). Families in poverty in the 1990s: Trends, causes, consequences, and lessons learned. *Journal of Marriage and the Family, 62,* 1094–1113.

Sen, A. (2002). Why health equity? *Health Economics, 11,* 659–666.

Seydlitz, R., & Jenkins, P. (1998). The influence of families, friends, schools, and community on delinquent behavior. In T. P. Gullotta, G. R. Adams, & R. Montemayor (Eds.), *Delinquent violent youth: Theory and interventions* (pp. 53–97). Thousand Oaks, CA: Sage.

Shakotko, R., Edwards, L. N., & Grossman, M. (1980). *An exploration of the dynamic relationship between health and cognitive development in adolescence* (NBER Working Paper No. w0454). Cambridge, MA: National Bureau of Economic Research.

Shonkoff, J. P. (2003). Still waiting for the right questions. *American Journal of Preventive Medicine, 24,* 4–5.

Shonkoff, J. P., & Marshall, P. C. (2000). The biology of developmental vulnerability. In J. P. Shonkoff & S. J. Meisels (Eds.), *Handbook of early childhood intervention* (2nd ed., pp. 35–53). New York: Cambridge University Press.

Shore, R. (2003). *Rethinking the brain: New insights into early development* (Rev. ed.). New York: Families and Work Institute.

Siegel, D. J. (1999). *The developing mind: Toward a neurobiology of interpersonal experience.* New York: Guilford Press.

Siegrist, J. (1996). Adverse health effects of high-effort/low-reward conditions. *Journal of Occupational Health Psychology, 1,* 27–41.

Siegrist, J., Klein, D., & Voigt, K. H. (1997). Linking sociological with physiological data: The model of effort-reward imbalance at work. *Acta Physiologica Scandinavica, Supplementum, 640,* 112–116.

Siegrist, J., & Marmot, M. (2004). Health inequalities and the psychosocial environment: Two scientific challenges. *Social Science and Medicine, 58,* 1463–1473.

Siegrist, J., Starke, D., Chandola, T., Godin, I., Marmot, M., Niedhammer, I., et al. (2004). The measurement of effort-reward imbalance at work: European comparisons. *Social Science and Medicine, 58,* 1483–1499.

Simeonsson, N. W., & Gray, J. N. (1994). Healthy children: Primary prevention of disease. In R. J. Simeonsson (Ed.), *Risk, resilience and prevention: Promoting the well-being of all children* (pp. 77–102). Baltimore: P.H. Brookes.

Simeonsson, R. J. (Ed.). (1994). *Risk, resilience and prevention: Promoting the well-being of all children.* Baltimore: P.H. Brookes.

Simons-Morton, B. G., Parcel, G. S., O'Hara, N. M., Blair, S. N., & Pate, R. R. (1988). Health-related physical fitness in childhood: Status and recommendations. *Annual Review of Public Health, 9,* 403–425.

Singer, M. I., Slovak, K., Frierson, T., & York, P. (1998). Viewing preferences, symptoms of psychological trauma, and violent behaviors among children who watch television. *Journal of the American Academy of Child and Adolescent Psychiatry, 37,* 1041–1048.

Smith, G. D., & Kuh, D. (2001). Commentary: William Ogilvy Kermack and the childhood origins of adult health and disease. *International Journal of Epidemiology, 30,* 696–703.

Smith, S. L., & Donnerstein, E. I. (1998). Harmful effects of exposure to media violence: Learning of aggression, emotional desensitization, and fear. In R. G. Geen & E. Donnerstein (Eds.), *Human aggression: Theories, research, and implications for social policy* (pp. 167–202). San Diego, CA: Academic Press.

Smrekar, C., Guthrie, J. W., Owens, D. E., & Sims, P. G. (2001). *March toward excellence: School success and minority student achievement in Department of Defense schools: A report to the National Education Goals Panel.* Washington, DC: U.S. Department of Education, Office of Educational Research and Improvement.

Social Exclusion Unit. (2004). *Tackling social exclusion: Taking stock and looking to the future: Emerging findings.* London: Office of the Deputy Prime Minister.

Sroufe, L. A., & Egeland, B. (1991). Illustrations of person: Environment interaction from a longitudinal study. In T. D. Wachs & R. Plomin (Eds.), *Conceptualization and measurement of organism-environment interaction* (pp. 68–84). Washington, DC: American Psychological Association.

Starfield, B., Riley, A. W., Witt, W. P., & Robertson, J. (2002). Social class gradients in health during adolescence. *Journal of Epidemiology and Community Health, 56,* 354–361.

Stone, R., Cafferata, G. L., & Sangl, J. (1987). Caregivers of the frail elderly: A national profile. *Gerontologist, 27,* 616–626.

Suomi, S. J. (1999). Attachment in rhesus monkeys. In J. Cassidy & P. R. Shaver (Eds.), *Handbook of attachment: Theory, research, and clinical applications* (pp. 181–197). New York: Guilford Press.

Tennant, M., & Pogson, P. (1995). *Learning and change in the adult years: A developmental perspective.* San Francisco: Jossey-Bass.

Teven, J. J. (2001). The relationship among teacher characteristics and perceived caring. *Communication Education, 50,* 159–169.

Thompson, R. A. (1999). Early attachment and later development. In J. Cassidy & P. R. Shaver (Eds.), *Handbook of attachment: Theory, research, and clinical applications* (pp. 265–286). New York: Guilford Press.

Thompson, R. A. (2001). Development in the first years of life. *Future of Children, 11*(1), 20–33.

Thompson, R. A., & Nelson, C. A. (2001). Developmental science and the media: Early brain development. *American Psychologist, 56,* 5–15.

Tolan, P. H., Guerra, N. G., & Kendall, P. C. (1995). A developmental-ecological perspective on antisocial behavior in children and adolescents: Toward a unified risk and intervention framework. *Journal of Consulting and Clinical Psychology, 63,* 579–584.

Tremblay, R. E. (1999). When children's social development fails. In D. P. Keating & C. Hertzman (Eds.), *Developmental health and the wealth of nations: Social, biological, and educational dynamics* (pp. 55–71). New York: Guilford Press.

Tresidder, J., Macaskill, P., Bennett, D., & Nutbeam, D. (1997). Health risks and behaviour of out-of-school 16-year-olds in New South Wales. *Australian and New Zealand Journal of Public Health, 21,* 168–174.

UCLA Center for Healthier Children, Families and Communities. (2004). *Early childhood education* (Building Community Systems for Young Children Policy Brief No. 6). Los Angeles: University of California, California Policy Research Center.

United Nations Children's Fund International Child Development Centre. (2002). *A league table of educational disadvantage in rich nations.* Florence: UNICEF Innocenti Research Centre.

United Nations Development Programme. (2002). *Human development report 2002: Deepening democracy in a fragmented world.* New York: Author.

United Nations Educational, Scientific, and Cultural Organization, Early Childhood and Family Education Section. (2003). *Re-forming education and care in England, Scotland and Sweden* (UNESCO Policy Briefs on Early Childhood No. 12). Paris: Author.

U.S. Census Bureau. (2003a, August 15). *American Community Survey Change Profile, 2001–2002: Table 3. Selected economic characteristics.* Retrieved November 14, 2004, from http://www.census.gov/acs/www/Products/Profiles/Chg/2002/0102/Tabular/010/01000US3.htm

U.S. Census Bureau. (2003b, August). *School enrollment 2000: High school dropouts by race and Hispanic origin: 1990 and 2000.* Retrieved November 14, 2004, from http://www.census.gov/prod/2003pubs/c2kbr-26.pdf

U.S. Department of Education. (1991). *America 2000: An education strategy: Sourcebook.* Jessup, MD: Author.

U.S. Department of Education, National Center for Education Statistics. (1997). *State indicators in education 1997* (Publication No. NCES 1997–376). Jessup, MD: Author.

U.S. Department of Education, National Center for Education Statistics. (2000). *Monitoring school quality: An indicators report* (Publication No. NCES 2001–030). Jessup, MD: Author.

U.S. Department of Education, National Center for Education Statistics. (2001a). *The nation's report card: Fourth-grade reading 2000* (Publication No. NCES 2001–499). Jessup, MD: Author.

U.S. Department of Education, National Center for Education Statistics. (2001b). *Technical report and data file user's manual for the 1992 National Adult Literacy Survey* (Publication No. NCES 2001–457). Jessup, MD: Author.

U.S. Department of Education, National Center for Education Statistics. (2003a). *The condition of education 2003* (Publication No. NCES 2003–067). Jessup, MD: Author.

U.S. Department of Education, National Center for Education Statistics. (2003b, May 29). *The condition of education 2003: Appendix 1 supplemental tables 17-1 and 17-2.* Retrieved November 14, 2004, from http://nces.ed.gov/pubs2003/2003067_App1.pdf

U.S. Department of Health and Human Services. (1991). *Healthy People 2000: National health promotion and disease prevention objectives: Full report, with commentary* (DHHS Publication No. PHS 91-50212). Washington, DC: Author.

U.S. Department of Health and Human Services. (2000). *Healthy People 2010: Understanding and improving health* (2nd ed.). Washington, DC: Author.

U.S. Department of Health and Human Services. (2002). *Healthy People 2010: Understanding and improving health: Objective 11-2: Improvement of health literacy.* Retrieved November 14, 2003, from http://www.healthypeople.gov/document/html/volume1/11healthcom.htm

U.S. Department of Health and Human Services. (2004). *Trends in the well-being of America's children and youth, 2003.* Washington, DC: Author.

U.S. Department of Health and Human Services, Centers for Disease Control and Prevention, National Center for Chronic Disease Prevention and Health Promotion, Office on Smoking and Health. (1994). *Preventing tobacco use among young people: A report of the surgeon general.* Washington, DC: U.S. Government Printing Office.

U.S. Department of Health and Human Services, Health Resources and Services Administration, Maternal and Child Health Bureau. (2002). *Child health USA, 2002.* Rockville, MD: Author.

U.S. Department of Health and Human Services, National Center for Health Statistics. (2004, April 12). *Healthy People 2010: Leading health indicators at a glance.* Retrieved November 5, 2004, from http://www.cdc.gov/nchs/about/otheract/hpdata2010/2010indicators.htm

U.S. Department of Health and Human Services, National Institutes of Health, National Library of Medicine. (2000). Introduction. In C. R. Seiden, M. Zorn, S. Ratzan, & R. M. Parker (Eds.), *Health literacy: January 1990 through October 1999* (p. vi) (NLM Publication. No. CBM 2000–1). Bethesda, MD: Author.

U.S. Department of Health and Human Services, Office of the Assistant Secretary for Planning and Evaluation. (2003a, February 7). Annual update of the HHS poverty guidelines, 68 Fed. Reg. 26, 6456–6458. Retrieved May 10, 2005, from http://www.access.gpo.gov/su_docs/fedreg/a030207c.html

U.S. Department of Health and Human Services, Office of the Assistant Secretary for Planning and Evaluation. (2003b). *Strengthening Head Start: What the evidence shows.* Washington, DC: Author.

U.S. Department of Justice, Bureau of Justice Statistics. (2000). *Correctional populations in the United States, 1997* (Publication No. NCJ-177613). Washington, DC: Author.

Vahtera, J., Pentti, J., & Kivimaki, M. (2004). Sickness absence as a predictor of mortality among male and female employees. *Journal of Epidemiology and Community Health, 58,* 321–326.

Vescio, M. F., Smith, G. D., Giampaoli, S., & MATISS Research Group. (2003). Socio-economic-position overall and cause-specific mortality in an Italian rural population. *European Journal of Epidemiology, 18,* 1051–1058.

Vingilis, E., Wade, T. J., & Adlaf, E. (1998). What factors predict student self-rated physical health? *Journal of Adolescence, 21,* 83–97.

Vondracek, F. W. (1992). The construct of identity and its use in career theory and research. *Career Development Quarterly, 41,* 130–144.

Walker, D., Greenwood, C., Hart, B., & Carta, J. (1994). Prediction of school outcomes based on early language production and socioeconomic factors. *Child Development, 65,* 606–621.

Walker, S. P., Grantham-McGregor, S. M., Himes, J. H., Williams, S., & Duff, E. M. (1998). School performance in adolescent Jamaican girls: Associations with health, social and behavioural characteristics, and risk factors for dropout. *Journal of Adolescence, 21,* 109–122.

Weiss, B. D. (Ed.). (1999). *Twenty common problems in primary care.* New York: McGraw-Hill.

Weiss, B. D., Hart, G., McGee, D. L., & D'Estelle, S. (1992). Health status of illiterate adults: Relation between literacy and health status among persons with low literacy skills. *Journal of the American Board of Family Practice, 5,* 257–264.

Weissberg, R. P., Caplan, M., & Harwood, R. L. (1991). Promoting competent young people in competence-enhancing environments: A systems-based perspective on primary prevention. *Journal of Consulting and Clinical Psychology, 59,* 830–841.

Weller, N. F., Tortolero, S. R., Kelder, S. H., Grunbaum, J. A., Carvajal, S. C., & Gingiss, P. M. (1999). Health risk behaviors of Texas students attending dropout prevention/recovery schools in 1997. *Journal of School Health, 69,* 22–28.

Werner, E. E. (1993). Risk, resilience, and recovery: Perspectives from the Kauai longitudinal study. *Development and Psychopathology, 5,* 503–515.

Werner, E. E., & Smith, R. S. (1982). *Vulnerable, but invincible: A longitudinal study of resilient children and youth.* New York: McGraw-Hill.

Werner, E. E., & Smith, R. S. (1992). *Overcoming the odds: High risk children from birth to adulthood.* Ithaca, NY: Cornell University Press.

Wickrama, K. A., Conger, R. D., Wallace, L. E., & Elder, G. H., Jr. (1999). The intergenerational transmission of health-risk behaviors: Adolescent lifestyles and gender moderating effects. *Journal of Health and Social Behavior, 40,* 258–272.

Wilkinson, R. G. (1999). Health, hierarchy, and social anxiety. *Annals of the New York Academy of Sciences, 896,* 48–63.

Wilkinson, R. G. (2002). Commentary: Liberty, fraternity, equality. *International Journal of Epidemiology, 31,* 538–543.

Williams, M. V., Baker, D. W., Parker, R. M., & Nurss, J. R. (1998). Relationship of functional health literacy to patients' knowledge of their chronic disease: A study of patients with hypertension and diabetes. *Archives of Internal Medicine, 158,* 166–172.

Willis, H. D. (1987). *Students at risk: A review of conditions, circumstances, indicators, and educational implications.* Elmhurst, IL: North Central Regional Educational Laboratory.

Willms, J. D. (1999). Quality and inequality in children's literacy: The effects of families, schools, and communities. In D. P. Keating & C. Hertzman (Eds.), *Developmental health and the wealth of nations: Social, biological, and educational dynamics* (pp. 72–93). New York: Guilford Press.

Willms, J. D. (Ed.). (2002). *Vulnerable children: Findings from Canada's National Longitudinal Survey of Children and Youth.* Edmonton, Alberta, Canada: University of Alberta Press.

Windham, J. (1999, April 9). Giving students a school choice will only help HISD. *Houston Chronicle,* p. A35.

Windle, M., Grunbaum, J. A., Elliott, M., Tortolero, S. R., Berry, S., Gilliland, J., et al. (2004). Healthy Passages: A multilevel, multimethod longitudinal study of adolescent health. *American Journal of Preventive Medicine, 27,* 164–172.

Winick, M., Meyer, K. K., & Harris, R. C. (1975, December 19). Malnutrition and environmental enrichment by early adoption. *Science, 190,* 1173–1175.

Winkleby, M. A., Jatulis, D. E., Frank, E., & Fortmann, S. P. (1992). Socioeconomic status and health: How education, income, and occupation contribute to risk factors for cardiovascular disease. *American Journal of Public Health, 82,* 816–820.

Wolfson, M., Kaplan, G., Lynch, J., Ross, N., & Backlund, E. (1999). Relation between income inequality and mortality: Empirical demonstration. *British Medical Journal, 319,* 953–955.

Woodward, A., & Kawachi, I. (2000). Why reduce health inequalities? *Journal of Epidemiology and Community Health, 54,* 923–929.

Woodward, A. L., & Markman, E. M. (1998). Early word learning. In W. Damon (Ed.), *Handbook of child psychology: Vol. 2. Cognition, perception, and language* (pp. 371–420). New York: Wiley.

Woolcock, M., & Narayan, D. (2000). Social capital: Implications for development theory, research, and policy. *World Bank Research Observer, 15,* 225–249.

World Health Organization. (2000). *The world health report 2000: Health systems: Improving performance.* Geneva: Author.

Worthman, C. M. (1999). Epidemiology of human development. In C. Panter-Brick & C. M. Worthman (Eds.), *Hormones, health, and behavior: A socio-ecological and lifespan perspective* (pp. 47–104). New York: Cambridge University Press.

Wortman, C. B., & Silver, R. C. (1990). Successful mastery of bereavement and widowhood: A life-course perspective. In P. B. Baltes & M. M. Baltes (Eds.), *Successful aging: Perspectives from the behavioral sciences* (pp. 225–264). New York: Cambridge University Press.

Yamada, K., Mizuno, M., & Nabeshima, T. (2002). Role for brain-derived neurotrophic factor in learning and memory. *Life Sciences, 70,* 735–744.

Yancey, A. K., Siegel, J. M., & McDaniel, K. L. (2002). Role models, ethnic identity, and health-risk behaviors in urban adolescents. *Archives of Pediatrics and Adolescent Medicine, 156,* 55–61.

Yoshikawa, H. (1994). Prevention as cumulative protection: Effects of early family support and education on chronic delinquency and its risks. *Psychological Bulletin, 115,* 28–54.

Young, M. H., Miller, B. C., Norton, M. C., & Hill, E. J. (1995). The effect of parental supportive behaviors on life satisfaction of adolescent offspring. *Journal of Marriage and the Family, 57,* 813–822.

Young, T. K. (2005). *Population health: Concepts and methods* (2nd ed.). New York: Oxford University Press.

CHAPTER FIVE

ECONOMIC DEVELOPMENT

Luisa Franzini, J. Michael Swint, Yuki Murakami, Rafia S. Rasu

Chapter Highlights

- A strong association exists between income and health in both developed and developing countries with health improving as income increases and as societal inequalities related to income diminish.
- Economic policies such as taxation; public subsidy and expenditure; and credit, labor market, and trade policies have the potential to affect income.
- Policies that successfully stimulate economic development are likely to reduce poverty, which in turn can improve population health.
- General recommendations regarding the use of economic policy to influence population health are broadly similar in developed and developing countries:

  - Encourage greater recognition of nonmedical determinants of health among policymakers
  - Support research on the impact of economic policies on population health
  - Highlight the health consequences of policies

- **Promote policy development through participatory methods**
- **Strengthen intersectoral collaborations**

- **Specific recommendations include the following:**

  - **Enact health and social policies that provide benefits that counter the negative effects of poverty on population health, such as access to quality health care and good public school systems**
  - **Develop labor market policies that provide minimum-wage incomes; improve entry into the labor force by the young, disabled people, and the most disadvantaged members of society; and improve working conditions in hazardous occupations**
  - **Create trade policies that allow the benefits of globalization and trade to be fairly shared within and between countries**

Introduction

This chapter investigates the relationships between economic factors and health, studying both the impact of economic policies on health and the impact of health on economic development. The term *economic development* refers to the growth of the economy measured, for example, by increases in a nation's real income (excluding price inflation) or gross domestic product (GDP) per capita, as well as a broader concept encompassing factors that reflect a population's quality of life, such as life expectancy and educational attainment.

Research has shown that health improves with income and vice versa in developed and developing countries. Overall, the evidence suggests that income matters to health, that health matters to income, and that both are associated with other factors that affect health.

Policies that affect income will have a substantial influence on health, and health will influence income and related indicators of economic development. Various types of policies have the potential to affect income; prominent among them are economic policies such as taxation; public subsidy and expenditure; and credit, labor market and trade policies.

Overview

In this chapter we first define concepts such as economic factors, economic policies, and economic development. Unlike much of the economics literature, this chapter does not restrict the role of economic development to developing countries, and it draws on evidence from developed countries as well.

Next, the chapter reviews the research on the links between economic factors (e.g., median income or income distribution) and health (e.g., mortality rates or life expectancy) and the direction of causation and the mechanisms involved. It considers two levels: the individual level, with a focus on income and wealth; and the population level, with a focus on income distribution and economic development.

Evidence suggests that health improves with income throughout the income distribution: high-income individuals have better health than do middle-income individuals, who have better health than do low-income individuals. The implication of this gradient is that everyone can benefit from an improvement in income. Two aspects of low income, also denoted as poverty, could explain why income is important for health: poor material conditions and negative psychosocial factors (Lynch et al., 2001; Marmot, 2002). Additionally, health has an effect on income, mainly through the ability to work and its effects on earnings.

This chapter pays particular attention to the effect of income inequality on health. *Income inequality*, as considered in the literature, refers to the dispersion of income. Earlier evidence suggested that, among middle- and high-income countries, it is not the richest countries that have the best health but those with more equal distribution of income (Wilkinson, 1996). More recent research indicates that the income inequality–health association based on cross-country comparisons is dependent on which countries one studies, but countries with more income inequality appear to have a more unequal distribution of health-relevant resources and environmental exposures that are powerful determinants of health (Lynch et al., 2001).

Following a discussion of the evidence, the chapter reviews current economic policies (e.g., monetary, fiscal, and trade policies) and their intended and unintended effects on population health. Studies investigating economic policies and their relationships to population health are reviewed for both developed and developing countries. The economic determinants of health point to the importance of income in affecting population health. Economic policies that successfully stimulate economic development are likely to affect poverty, which in turn can affect health.

Finally, the chapter evaluates the strengths and limitations of economic policies with regard to their influence on population health and the efficiency, effectiveness, and equity of current economic policies. This discussion will focus on various policies that have a strong economic component and for which evidence about health effects is available.

Fields of Study

In order to investigate the links between economic development and population health and the intended and unintended effects of economic policies on population health, key terms need to be defined.

Economics is concerned with the study of how societies make use of scarce resources to produce valued commodities and distribute them among different people (Samuelson & Nordhaus, 2005). Economics uses concepts such as income, prices and inflation, unemployment, the value of the total output produced by a country (gross national product, or GNP) or produced inside a country (gross domestic product, or GDP), and the distribution of income. How these concepts are described, measured, and related to economic outcomes is the subject of *positive economics.* Positive economics is grounded in facts. Questions involving ethics and value judgments are the focus of *normative economics.* For example, positive economics asks questions such as this: What is the level of inflation? How does unemployment affect inflation? Normative economics is concerned with how much inflation should be tolerated.

Economics is further divided into *microeconomics* (which is concerned with individual decision makers, supply and demand in product markets, and various levels of market competition) and *macroeconomics* (which deals with the economy as a whole). Macroeconomics is concerned with the overall level of a nation's aggregate consumption, production, investment, and international trade, as well as inflation and unemployment. The analysis of environmentally responsive corporate decision making in Chapter Three was grounded in microeconomic theory, but macroeconomics provides the principal foundation for the approach used in this chapter.

Economic growth refers to increases in a nation's real income (excluding price inflation) or GDP per capita, whereas *economic development* is a broader concept that includes factors more reflective of a population's quality of life. Traditionally, economists have used measures of total income or economic output to measure social progress. However, as Sen (1970) pointed out, those measures are insufficient because they do not account for distributional issues and because a person's well-being depends on many noneconomic factors. Using social choice theory, Sen (1970, 1976) developed a framework to best measure social progress. He argued that the evaluation of economic efficiency must include general social consequences and that such evaluations require an ethical framework. Based on Sen's work, the United Nations Development Programme (UNDP) (1990) developed a measure of social welfare that goes beyond GDP and captures the different influences on human well-being and opportunities. The resulting human development index, which was introduced in Chapter Four, includes life expectancy and educational attainment as well as income (Gershman, Irwin, & Shakow, 2003). The UNDP has also developed a human poverty index that incorporates mortality, malnutrition, and literacy, as well as access to water, sanitation services, and health services. These indices are used to measure economic development.

Full income per capita is an alternative measurement of economic development that is receiving an increasing amount of attention (Becker, 2003; Bloom, Canning,

& Jamison, 2004; Bourguignon & Morrisson, 2002; Jamison, Sachs, & Wang, 2001; Nordhaus, 2003; Usher, 1973). It incorporates an empirical estimate of the monetary value of a life in a given society, which investigators then use to calculate the positive increment to economic development caused by an increase in life expectancy. The increment is then added to income to yield full income. The benefit of the full-income approach is that it reflects both money income and life expectancy and is therefore a better indicator of economic development. Estimates indicate that in the past fifty years the degree of economic development in developing countries is considerably higher when measured by full income rather than by income per capita. Although the disparity between rich and poor countries has been growing in terms of income per capita, it has actually been decreasing in terms of economic development defined by full income (Bloom et al., 2004).

Sen (1999) further defined the concept of development. He argued (as quoted in Wallace, 2004, p. 7) that

> development should be seen as a process of expanding the real freedoms that people enjoy. Development requires the removal of major sources of unfreedom: poverty as well as tyranny, poor economic opportunities as well as systematic social deprivation, neglect of public facilities as well as intolerance or overactivity of repressive states.

The use of population health (an important component of population quality of life) as a development objective raises the issue of whose health a society wants to improve. For example, focusing solely on the current generation's health may negatively affect the health of future generations. In a very low-income country, resources invested in programs that improve health and the quality of life for the current generation may not contribute adequately to economic growth. The poverty cycle may not be broken, and future generations may have more of the same conditions waiting for them. To a certain extent, there may be an intergenerational trade-off: Sacrifice now for the benefit of future generations' welfare, or sacrifice the welfare of future generations for the benefit of the current generation. Ideally, a society would want to choose strategies that benefit both generations, and indeed, recent evidence indicates that such strategies exist (Bloom et al., 2004).

Policy Domains

Managing the economy is a large part of any government's responsibilities, and economic issues often dominate political agendas. A fundamental goal of economic policies is to foster economic development. *Economic policies* relate to the tools that policymakers use to affect the economy, for example, monetary policies, fiscal policies, business and income policies, and trade policies (Samuelson & Nordhaus, 2005). These policies are largely government macroeconomic policies that target aggregate, national-level economic outcomes. *Monetary policy* is concerned with the supply of money and credit conditions. Monetary policies affect price levels and inflation and influence economic development by affecting employment, the growth of economic output, and the stability of the foreign sector.

Fiscal policy can be defined as the process of shaping taxation and public expenditure. Fiscal policies include determining the types and rates of taxation to be used. *Personal, corporate, and sales taxes* influence the behavior of individuals and businesses as well as raise money for the government. For example, the personal income tax structure affects spending and saving behavior. The mix of progressive taxes (taxes that take a larger fraction of income from high-income people) and regressive taxes (taxes that take a larger fraction of income from low-income people) are major tools for redistributing income among members of society. Taxes on business affect companies' location and hiring practices, which can influence economic development.

Public expenditure is a powerful tool of fiscal policies. Governments can use public expenditures to provide public goods, to redistribute income, and to help ensure minimum standards of health and nutrition. Government spending tends to be higher in high-income countries because affluence brings greater demands for welfare transfers. There are different levels of government expenditures. In the United States, government expenditures are at the federal, state, and local levels (Samuelson & Nordhaus, 2005). Federal spending is mainly for national defense and for entitlement programs that include income security, social security, and Medicare, whereas state and local spending is dominated by spending for education, public welfare, Medicaid, and hospitals.

Income policies, such as wage-price guidelines or mandatory wages (for example, the minimum wage), contribute to wage and salary determination. Business-related policies include regulation of the labor market (through regulation of labor unions and collective bargaining) and other regulation of businesses (for example, antitrust policy).

Trade policies encompass tariffs and quotas, exchange-rate policies, regulation of global competition, foreign aid, and debt relief. *Tariffs* (taxes imposed on imports) and *quotas* (restrictions on the quantity of imports) are controversial. From an economic perspective, tariffs and quotas lead to economic inefficiencies, yet policymakers have advocated restricting trade as a way to protect local industry against foreign competition. Economically developed countries use tariffs and quotas to protect their workforce from competition from cheaper foreign labor, to cater to powerful domestic interest groups, or to maintain a national way of life. Trade policies affect the country implementing the policy as well as its trading partners. Tariffs and quotas result in higher prices for domestic consumers; in effect, domestic consumers subsidize the protected industries.

International organizations have developed to provide a framework for trade. The General Agreement on Tariffs and Trade and the World Trade Organization (WTO), with 130 members who account for 90% of international trade, have provided a framework for reducing barriers to free trade in goods, services, and financial capital for the benefit of developed and developing countries (Samuelson & Nordhaus, 2005). The results of these arrangements have, however, been controversial in terms of the equity of benefit for developed versus developing countries, which this chapter will discuss later.

Because international trade involves the use of different currencies, a well-functioning exchange-rate system to govern financial transactions among nations is crucial to a global economy. After World War II, a group of international economic institutions was created to organize international trade and finance. These include the International Monetary Fund (IMF), with the task of overseeing the exchange-rate system and addressing balance-of-payment difficulties in individual countries; the World Bank, which acts as a lending bank to developing countries; and the Bretton Woods exchange system of stable or adjustable exchange rates, which was replaced in 1971 with a regime of floating exchange rates.

A fixed, or pegged, rate is a rate the government (central bank) sets and maintains as the official exchange rate. A floating exchange rate is determined by the private market through supply and demand. A floating rate is constantly changing. In a floating exchange rate system, the central bank may intervene when it is necessary to ensure stability and to avoid inflation, but it is less likely, in general, to do so (Samuelson & Nordhaus, 2005).

Globalization represents a major trend that has affected and been affected by international trade policies. Stiglitz (2002, p. 9) describes globalization as

> the closer integration of the countries and the peoples of the world which has been brought about by the enormous reduction of costs of transportation and communication, and the breaking down of artificial barriers to the flows of goods, services, capital, knowledge, and . . . people across borders.

It is not a new phenomenon, because exchanges have been occurring for centuries; however, with the reductions in transportation and communication costs, it has accelerated in recent decades. Although globalization has the potential to benefit millions of people, many believe it also has the potential to cause increased suffering to the poor in developing countries (Labonte, 2003; Stiglitz, 2002). Evidence suggests that increased free trade and investment, as it has been implemented, has been associated with increased income inequality in developing countries (Rao, 1999). Increases in income inequality make it less likely that increased economic growth in developing countries will reduce poverty (Labonte, 2003).

The basic relationships between economic policies and population health that will guide our discussion of evidence and policies are illustrated in Figure 5.1.

Economic policies that successfully stimulate economic development are likely to have an impact on income in both developed and developing countries. The nature and the degree to which income and whose income will be affected will in part depend on the type of development that occurs, capital-intensive versus labor-intensive, urban versus rural, and so on, and on the country's degree of economic development. But it also depends on "appropriate macroeconomic and labour-market policies as well as the machinery for good governance" (World Health Organization [WHO], Commission on Macroeconomics and Health, Working Group 1, 2002, p. 88). Increases in income and correlated reductions in poverty are strongly associated with subsequent improvements in population health, particularly in the poorest countries. Improvements in population health will affect economic development by providing a healthier and therefore more productive workforce, and particularly in developing countries, improvements in population health can further reduce poverty by increasing the earning power of the affected individuals.

FIGURE 5.1. RELATIONSHIPS BETWEEN ECONOMIC POLICIES AND POPULATION HEALTH.

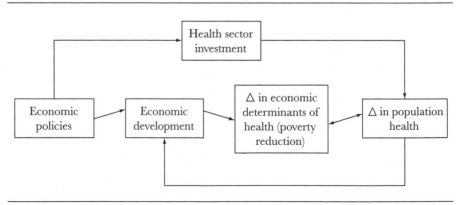

Note. Δ = change.

Evidence Regarding Research on Fundamental Determinants

This section will describe the economic determinants of health in developed and developing countries and investigate the pathways and mechanisms through which economic factors affect population health. Developed and developing countries are considered separately because of fundamental differences in their economic conditions and health problems. Developing countries are characterized by low per capita income, widespread poverty, and typically but not always by inequalities in the distribution of income. Developed countries have adequate per capita income but may be characterized by inequality in the distribution of income. As this section will show, though the economic determinants of health and the pathways through which they operate (see Figure 5.1) are similar in developed and developing countries, their relative importance to health depends on a country's level of economic development.

Developed Countries

Research has shown an association between income and health in developed countries (Berkman & Kawachi, 2000). The association is represented by a gradient, meaning that health improves with income throughout the income distribution, and has been found using different measures of income and of health. Income has been measured at the individual level, the country level, and in different geographical areas, such as neighborhoods, metropolitan areas, counties, and states. The distribution of income across the population of developed countries has also been investigated (Wilkinson, 1996). Health indicators consist of mortality (all-cause and disease-specific mortality, infant mortality, and life expectancy), morbidity, and self-rated health, including quality-of-life indicators.

The Health-Income Gradient. The negative effect of poverty on health has been known for centuries, with references going back to the ancient Greeks and Chinese (Krieger, 2001; Porter, 1998). Several historical records document poorer health among less advantaged populations. For example, Floud and Harris (1996) report that, at the beginning of the 19th century, 14-year-old boys attending the Royal Military Academy at Sandhurst, the elite British military school, were nearly six inches taller than their counterparts in the Marine Society, who came from the lower social classes. Similarly, Rowentree (2001) in 1901 documented an infant mortality gradient based on poverty in areas of York, England.

In recent years an abundant literature has documented a health gradient based on income. The evidence is overwhelming that income and health are associated and that the association is represented by a gradient. Richer individuals have better health than do middle-income individuals, who have better health than do low-income individuals. The gradient implies that as income increases, health steadily increases and not a relationship described by a threshold effect, in which poor people have poor health whereas everyone else has good health.

In the United States, the health gradient was first reported by Kitagawa and Hauser (1973), who merged census and death records and found a relationship between mortality and income and other socioeconomic variables. More recently, Backlund, Sorlie, and Johnson (1996) and Sorlie, Backlund, and Keller (1995) used the National Longitudinal Mortality Study surveys, which represent approximately 500,000 personal or telephone interviews and 40,000 deaths, to describe the relationship between income and mortality. An income-based gradient with declining mortality associated with increasing income exists in all age groups for both males and females, though it is steeper for working-age groups and for males. The gradient flattens but remains when controlling for household size, education, marital status, and employment status, indicating that income has an independent effect on health. Others have found similar gradients in the United States and other countries (McDonough, Duncan, Williams, & House, 1997; Wolfson, Rowe, Gentleman, & Tomiak, 1993).

The gradient is also present with other socioeconomic variables such as wealth, employment grade, education, or social class. The classic Whitehall study of civil servants in the United Kingdom also found a gradient (Marmot, 1986), which was also mentioned in Chapter Four. The top-grade administrative civil servants had a 10-year cumulative mortality rate half that of the next grade professional or executive civil servants, three times lower than the next grade clerical civil servants, and four times lower than civil servants in the lowest grade. The gradient holds for many but not all health outcomes, including cause-specific mortality, morbidity, or self-reported health.

An income-health relationship characterized by the gradient has important policy implications. The implication is that everyone can benefit from an improvement in income. Therefore, the greater effect of policy may be obtained by policies that target the income range that include the majority of the population, that is, the midrange of incomes (Evans, 2002).

The income gradient accounts for some but not all of the persistent racial or ethnic differences in health in the United States. The 2001 age-adjusted death rate for blacks was 1,116.5 per 100,000 compared to 842.9 for whites (National Center for Health Statistics, 2003). Minorities also have lower incomes than whites. According to the U.S. Census Bureau (2004), poverty rates from 2001 to 2002 were higher for blacks (24.1%) and for Hispanics (21.8%) than for whites (8.0%). Although many of the differences in white-black mortality can be attributed to income differences, income does not fully explain mortality differences by race. Complex factors, including discrimination, influence black mortality (Krieger, 2000). These issues are more fully discussed in Chapter Two.

Does Income Affect Health, or Does Health Affect Income? The central question is the degree to which the association between income and health reflects a causal relationship. Does income matter to health, or does health matter to income? Or are both associated with other factors that affect health? The previous section described the effects of income on health.

The evidence of a causal relationship from health to income comes mainly from economists (Deaton, 2002). Health affects income mainly through the ability to work and its effects on earnings. The effects of health as a proximate cause of retirement have been documented (Gruber & Wise, 1999). In countries without universal access to health care, out-of-pocket costs of medical care can have a considerable effect on wealth, though this effect is of relatively small importance overall (Smith, 1999). Finally, health may affect income in subtle ways over a long time frame. As Deaton (2002, p. 16) explains:

> Mother's cigarette smoking during pregnancy predicts teenage educational achievements; height at age seven predicts subsequent unemployment; ill health, even poor prenatal nutrition, decreases the probability of ever being married, itself an aspect of socioeconomic status that is associated with good health; and prenatal nutrition affects cardiovascular disease and Type 2 diabetes in late middle age, exactly the sort of conditions that predict early retirement.

Most of the literature in public health tends to acknowledge the relationship from health to income, referring to it as *reverse causation* or *selection,* and researchers in public health attempt to control for it, for example, through baseline employment or health status (Backlund et al., 1996; Lantz et al., 1998; Marmot et al., 1991).

It seems clear that health and income are mutually determined, as depicted in Figure 5.1. Moreover, some factors are known to affect both health and income; predominant among them is education. It is still controversial whether income and education have separately protective effects on health, though the evidence seems to support independent effects (Backlund et al., 1996). See Chapter Four for a discussion of the impact of education on health. Other factors that may affect both income and health are personality traits and attitudes such as drive, motivation, and the ability to postpone rewards.

In conclusion, the evidence suggests that income matters to health, that health matters to income, and that both are associated with other factors that affect health.

Through What Mechanisms Are Health and Income Related? This section investigates the possible mechanisms through which income influences health.

Risk Factors. A prominent hypothesis about income-based inequalities in health is that the health disadvantage of those who are worse off is due to the higher prevalence of health-risk behaviors and risk factors among those with lower income. However, some studies have shown that although differences in health behaviors and risk factors account for some of the differences in health outcomes, they do not explain most of the health inequalities (Lantz et al., 1998; Rose & Marmot, 1981). Furthermore, one can argue that health behaviors are socially determined, so that risky behaviors are themselves a consequence of low income. In this framework low income leads to poor health behaviors. Also, risky behavior may be neither irresponsible nor irrational given the constraints that poor people face. While those with wealth and education use these assets as sources of income and consumption, for example, by working on Wall Street and enjoying the opera, those with low human and financial capital use their bodies for production and consumption, by working in manual occupations and relieving stress through health-damaging activities, like smoking (Muurinen & LeGrand, 1985).

If health-risk behaviors do not explain much of the relationship between income and health, what can account for this strong association? Two aspects of low income could explain why income is important for health: poor material conditions and negative psychosocial factors (Lynch et al., 2001; Marmot, 2002).

Material Conditions. Material conditions that are necessary for good health include clean water, sanitation, and adequate nutrition and housing. In most developed countries, basic material needs are usually met, which has led some to argue that material conditions do not affect health in rich nations. The line of reasoning is that although clean water is necessary for good health, once water is safe, higher income does not make water more safe (Marmot, 2002). However, even in developed countries, there remain substantial differences in access to material resources because of income. The poor (i.e., individuals with lower incomes) tend to live in poorer quality housing that is substandard and that contributes to a variety of ailments (Bashir, 2002). The poor are also likely to have poorer diets because of the higher cost and the diminished availability of healthier food in poor neighborhoods (James, Nelson, Ralph, & Leather, 1997). Furthermore, individuals with low income are more likely to work in dangerous occupations such as construction or mining, where they may be exposed to occupational and environmental health hazards (Johnson & Hall, 1995). In countries without a universal health care system, as is the case in the United States, low income strongly influences access to preventive and therapeutic health care with negative consequences for health. Technical progress in medicine tends to spread faster among the rich and slower among the poor, thereby making an existing gradient steeper or creating one where none existed (Deaton, 2002).

Poverty may also affect health through the effect of low income on social participation (Marmot, 2002). Having a low income can mean not being able to have a meaningful leisure activity, not having friends and family over for a meal, or not having access to a safe place for exercising or swimming. In some subtle but meaningful ways, low income affects the ability of individuals to lead a healthy lifestyle that includes participating socially, politically, and emotionally in the life of their community. The negative health effects of social exclusion and lack of social support are well documented (Berkman & Glass, 2000).

Living in a low-income neighborhood has deleterious effects on health, independent of individual income. Poor neighborhoods lack the resources and the physical and social infrastructure that promote good health. For example, residents of poor neighborhoods are more likely to be exposed to toxic environments, to have lower availability of healthy foods, to live in poor quality housing, and to have less access to health and educational resources in their neighborhoods (Leventhal & Brooks-Gunn, 2000; Macintyre, Ellaway, & Cummins, 2002).

Psychosocial Mechanisms. The proponents of the psychosocial explanation of the relationship between income and health argue that it is not income per se, or the access to the material resources that it entails, that influences health. They propose that income is a marker for social position because income defines perceptions of an individual's relative position in the social hierarchy. Such perceptions produce negative emotions such as shame, distrust, and stress, which have negative biological consequences through psycho-neuroendocrine mechanisms and that induce health-damaging behaviors such as smoking (Wilkinson, 1996, 2001). Wilkinson hypothesized that chronic anxiety tends to increase as income decreases. Though lower-income individuals tend to have more material problems, making it difficult to separate the effects of absolute material deprivation from that of relative deprivation, Wilkinson (1997) argued that it is not so much the absolute living standards that affect health but the chronic stress due to the pressure to consume in order to maintain one's self-respect and social position relative to the social standards of developed societies. These biological pathways trace the mechanisms for the embodiment of the social environment in which individuals live by explaining how lived experiences are biologically incorporated (Krieger, 2001).

Chronic social anxiety associated with relative lower income triggers a stress response known as the fight-or-flight mechanism. The body mobilizes energy for the muscles while reducing resources for other functions that are not essential when facing a brief emergency like tissue maintenance and repair, digestion, immunity, growth, and reproductive functions (Sapolsky, 1998). Once the emergency passes, everything goes back to normal, and there are no long-term consequences. However, if the anxiety and the resulting stress response last for long periods of time, the constant high-alert status of the body causes a wide range of possible negative health consequences (Uno, Tarara, Else, Suleman, & Sapolsky, 1989). The results of chronic stress may look like rapid aging and provide something like general vulnerability, which has been implicated in the socioeconomic gradient because it is consistent with the all-causes mortality gradient, a gradient that persists despite changes in causes of death over time or in different countries (Marmot, Shipley, & Rose, 1984). Although much of the biological research of relative position on health has been carried out among primates (Sapolsky, 1998; Shively, Laber-Laird, & Anton, 1997), Wilkinson (2001) suggests that similar mechanisms operate in humans. However, recent research shows that there is no consistent relationship between social rank and stress response among primates. The different relationship between social rank and stress response among primate species may be explained by crucial differences in social behavior and organization (mainly the frequency at which subordinates are subjected to stressors and social support available to subordinates) between primate societies, making generalizations to humans problematic (Abbott et al., 2003).

Several rich countries have adopted the approach of focusing on relative income (income relative to others) rather than absolute income. For example, the European Union defines poverty in relative rather than absolute terms. The psychosocial explanation of the relationship between social determinants and health has, however, been criticized for not taking into account the de facto economic and political sources of the social structure in which those determinants arise (Krieger, 2001; Lynch et al., 2001).

How Important Are Income Inequalities to Health? Although it is well accepted that overall income levels and health are related, the relationship between relative income inequalities and health is controversial. *Income inequality*, as this literature considers it, refers to the dispersion of income within a society, measured so as to be unaffected by average income. This implies that two societies with very different median incomes can have the same degree of income inequality. A society with more income inequality is characterized by greater concentration of income among those with the highest incomes. Income inequality is usually measured by the Gini coefficient, a statistical construct that ranges between 0 and 1, with higher values indicating greater inequality. However, investigators have used several measures of income inequality with similar results (Kawachi, 2000).

The field of income inequality and health has seen an explosion in the last decade (Kawachi & Kennedy, 1999; Lynch et al., 1998, 2004; Subramanian & Kawachi, 2004; Wilkinson, 1996). The investigation into the relationship between income inequality and health arose from the realization that, among developed nations, it is not the richest countries that have the best health but those with the more equal distribution of income (Wilkinson, 1996). Early evidence from Rodgers (1979) indicated strong correlations between income distribution and life expectancy at birth, life expectancy at age five, and infant mortality in cross-country comparisons. Using 1970 and 1980 data, Wilkinson (1992) observed strong negative associations between life expectancy and income inequality in nine of the Organisation for Economic Co-operation and Development (OECD) countries, meaning that as income inequality increased, life expectancy decreased.

However, the limitations of those studies, mainly because of data from different countries that was not comparable in terms of quality or reliability, led researchers to investigate variations in income distribution within countries. Investigators (Kennedy, Kawachi, & Prothrow-Stith, 1996; Kaplan, Pamuk, Lynch, Cohen, & Balfour, 1996) examined the correlations between household income inequality and all-cause and cause-specific mortality in the 50 U.S. states. Both studies found that states with greater inequality had higher mortality. These findings have been extended to U.S. metropolitan areas (Lynch et al., 1998) and to large counties in Texas (Franzini, Ribble, & Spears, 2001). In multilevel models that adjust for a comprehensive set of individual characteristics (including race, income, education, smoking, obesity, and health insurance) and for other contextual factors (such as median state income or state racial composition), Kawachi and colleagues reported that income inequality affects self-rated health in the United States (Blakely, Kennedy & Kawachi, 2001; Blakely, Lochner & Kawachi, 2002; Kennedy, Kawachi, Glass, & Prothrow-Stith, 1998; Subramanian & Kawachi, 2003, 2004; Subramanian, Kawachi, & Kennedy, 2001). This evidence strongly supports an association between income inequality and health in the United States.

Scholars have proposed several mechanisms through which income inequality may affect health (Gravelle, 1998; Kawachi, 2000; Kennedy et al., 1998; Lynch, Smith, Kaplan, & House, 2000; Lynch et al., 2004; Subramanian & Kawachi, 2004). The main mechanism focuses on the psychosocial environment and postulates that income inequality may affect health by leading to underinvestment in human capital, for example, through reduced social spending on education, by disrupting the social fabric and lowering social capital and cohesion, and through psychosocially mediated effects of relative deprivation, in particular those due to the chronic stress of being of low rank (e.g., distrust, envy, feelings of being disrespected, and shame at not being able to conform to a community-defined decent standard of living) (Kawachi, 2000; Wilkinson, 1996).

Many studies have challenged the relationship between income inequalities and health (Judge, 1995; Judge, Mulligan, & Benzeval, 1998; Lynch et al., 2001, 2004; Wolfson, Kaplan, Lynch, Ross, & Backlund, 1999). By including more countries, such as the 23 countries in the Luxembourg Income Study, the studies produced different results: all-cause and most cause-specific mortality were not associated with income inequality (Lynch et al., 2001). Similarly, a comparison of U.S. states and Canadian provinces indicates that the association between income inequality and mortality did not hold in the Canadian provinces (Ross & Wolfson, 1999).

Thus, it now appears that the income inequality–health association based on cross-country comparison is dependent on which countries are included. Also, though the income inequality–health association in the case of the United States seems strong (Blakely et al., 2001; Kennedy et al., 1998; Subramanian & Kawachi, 2003, 2004; Subramanian et al., 2001), it seems to apply to some countries but not all. Subramanian and Kawachi (2004), in their excellent review of multilevel studies of income inequality and health, point out that there is support for the relation in countries more unequal than the United States but not in countries more equal than the United States, indicating a possible threshold effect of inequality on health.

Several debates are still unresolved in the investigation of the relationship between income inequality and health, including separating the pathways from the confounders (e.g., is aggregate educational attainment controlled for, or is it a pathway through which income inequality operates?), determining the geographic scale at which income inequality should be measured, identifying the mechanisms through which income inequality affects health, and discovering for whom income inequality is most harmful (Subramanian & Kawachi, 2004). Lynch et al. (2004) argue that, to affect health, income inequality must be correlated with the social distribution of risk factors for specific health outcomes. However, the distribution of risk factors is influenced not only by income inequality but also by other factors, such as culture and history.

These results underscore the importance of income inequality for population health. The distribution of income in a country is likely to reflect the distribution of private health–relevant resources (such as housing, healthy food, and medical care) and public health–relevant resources (such as availability of health care, education, and income supplementation; and environmental and health regulations) that particularly affect the health of those with lower incomes. Thus, the association between income inequality and health could in part be modified, depending on the distribution of population health–relevant resources (Lynch et al., 2001, 2004).

Developing Countries

This section will discuss the relationships depicted in Figure 5.1 that operate in developing countries. Poverty has a strong positive correlation with infant, child, and adult mortality rates and a strong negative correlation with life expectancy at birth (Bhargava, Jamison, Lau, & Murray, 2001; WHO, Commission on Macroeconomics and Health, 2002; WHO, 1999). According to the World Bank Group (2004), 2.8 billion people are living on less than $700 a year; of these, 1.2 billion earn less than $1 a day. This is the cause of an estimated 33,000 children dying every day in developing countries. Although much progress was made in Asia during the period from 1990 to 1998, poverty actually increased in much of the rest of the world. Defining *absolute poverty* as living on less than $1 per day, in 1998 46% of the population in sub-Saharan Africa, 16% of the people in Latin America, and 15% of people in the former Soviet Union lived in absolute poverty (Stiglitz, 2002; World Bank Group, 2004). Thus, policies that have disproportionately lowered trade barriers in developing countries relative to developed countries have not succeeded in reducing poverty in much of the world. Poverty is the most fundamental problem to address when examining the relationship between economic development and health in developing countries.

The Impact of Economic Development on Health. In this section we present evidence of the influence of economic development on population health in developing countries.

Income Levels. Cross-country data from the World Bank for the year 2000 indicate the relationship between GDP per capita and life expectancy. This is illustrated in Figure 5.2. For the poorest countries, as GDP per capita rises, there is a very strong positive correlation with increased life expectancy. Increases in income provide improved access to and quality of health services, better nutrition, clean water, sanitation, and housing (Bloom & Canning, 2000; Bloom et al., 2004; Hobdell, 2001; Preston, 1975). In countries with widespread malnutrition, increases in income have direct causal, positive impacts on health (Deaton, 2003). However, the relationship weakens as GDP per capita rises above a threshold level; after that level, only modest increases in life expectancy are associated with gains in GDP per capita (World Bank Group, 2004).

Income Distribution. Studies conducted in less developed countries show a strong relationship between the distribution of income and life expectancy, suggesting that the larger the inequality in income distribution, the lower the average life expectancy

FIGURE 5.2. LIFE EXPECTANCY AND GROSS DOMESTIC PRODUCT (GDP) PER CAPITA, 2000.

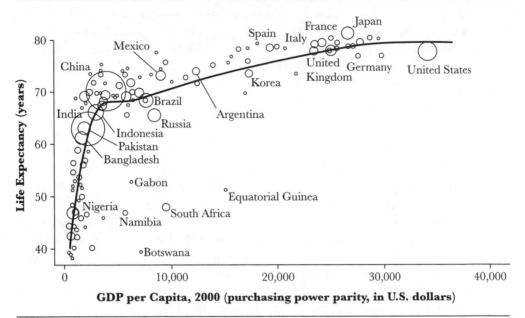

Note. Circles are proportional to population, and some of the largest (or most interesting) countries are labeled. The solid line is a plot of a population-weighted nonparametric regression. Luxembourg, with per capita GDP of $50,061 and life expectancy of 77.04 years, is excluded. From "Health, Inequality, and Economic Development," by A. Deaton, 2003, *Journal of Economic Literature, 41*, p. 116, fig. 1. Used with permission of the American Economic Association.

(Jack, 1999). Kawachi and Kennedy (2002) found that when countries have the same per capita income, the country with the most unequal income distribution has the highest mortality rate. Some poor countries show unexpectedly high levels of health achievement for their level of income per capita (Subramanian, Belli, & Kawachi, 2002).

Between-country comparisons show that disparities between poor and nonpoor groups of a population vary enormously across countries and across regions. Analyzing inequalities in mortality, malnutrition, and incidence of diarrhea and acute respiratory disease in infants and children under the age of five, Subramanian, Belli, and Kawachi (2002) found that children born in the lowest household income quartile are roughly twice as likely to die as are children born in the highest household income quartile. Evidence also implies that the redistribution of income from rich to poor will increase the average life expectancy in the population (Kawachi & Kennedy, 1999).

The Impact of Health on Economic Development. Health is necessary for job productivity and for the ability to learn in school; it is therefore a form of human capital and an input in the growth process, as well as an end in itself. A healthy population is a critical ingredient for economic growth and plays an important role in poverty reduction and economic development (Smith, 1999; WHO, Commission on Macroeconomics and Health, 2002). Countries with unhealthy populations are finding it more difficult to achieve sustained economic growth than are countries with better population health (Bhargava et al., 2001; Bloom et al., 2004; WHO, Commission on Macroeconomics and Health, 2002). Thirty-five of 36 countries high in human development enjoyed rising living standards and experienced an average 2.3% income growth rate per year from 1990 to 1998 (WHO, 2001). Seven of 34 countries with middle human development experienced declines in their living standards and had an average 1.9% growth rate per year during the same period. The countries with the lowest human development had close to zero economic growth (Subramanian et al., 2002; WHO, 2001).

The Influence of Life Expectancy. Evidence confirms the relationship between population health and economic development in Figure 5.1, because income grows much more slowly in countries with high rates of infant mortality. The Commission on Macroeconomics and Health (WHO, 2001) found that within the group of countries with income per capita of $750 and below in 1965, those with lower rates of infant mortality experienced higher per year growth of income per capita for the years 1965 through 1994. Similar patterns were found in countries with income per capita between $750 and $1,500 in 1965.

Barro (1997) has shown that increases in life expectancy are significantly correlated with subsequent economic growth, with a 10% increase in life expectancy resulting in a 0.3 to 0.4% increase in the annual economic growth rate. This results in a 1.6% annual economic growth differential in favor of a typical developed country as compared to a typical developing country, which results in an enormous difference in aggregate economic growth over time.

Bhargava et al. (2001) found that in low-income countries increased adult survival rates have a positive effect on GDP growth rates. Also, studies in Mexico found that if male life expectancy increased by one year, the gross domestic product would increase an additional 1% within fifteen years (WHO, 1999). The overall contribution of health to economic growth suggested that a one-year increase in life expectancy is associated with a 4% increase in GDP per capita (Bloom et al., 2004).

The Influence of Nutrition. Fogel (1991, 1997, 2000) has shown that available food supply per capita, a proxy for income per capita in developing countries, is critical for long-term labor productivity growth. He estimated that 30% of Britain's income per capita growth over the last 200 years was due to the increases in the availability of caloric intake. A study by Subramanian et al. (2002) estimates that about 40% of economic growth in a developing country can be attributed to its improving health and nutritional status.

Inadequate nutrition levels result in deficiencies in iodine and vitamin A. Throughout the world 740 million people suffer from disorders including mental retardation and delayed motor development, 49.5 million people suffer from brain damage, and 2 billion people are anemic ("Nurturing Economic Growth Through Nutrition," 2001). These deficiencies influence economic development by reducing labor market participation and productivity.

The Influence of Fertility. High rates of fertility are very common in developing countries (Bhargava et al., 2001). According to the Global Health Council, from 1995 to 2000, 1.4 billion women aged 15 to 46 were expected to have 1.2 billion pregnancies, and 338 million (28%) of them were unintended or unwanted. Unintended or unwanted pregnancies tend to be higher-risk pregnancies that are associated with higher rates of mortality and morbidity. Women in the childbearing years are at the peak of their economically productive lives.

Unwanted fertility also adversely affects a household's resource allocation decision in developing countries (Bhargava et al., 2001). Total fertility rates have a negative relationship with economic growth because high fertility leads to diminishing resource availability for health care and education (Bhargava et al., 2001). Women who have control over their own fertility have a greater likelihood of obtaining an education and contributing to the economic well-being of the community.

The Influence of Specific Diseases. Tuberculosis, malaria, and HIV/AIDS have had major population health and economic impacts in many countries.

Tuberculosis. Tuberculosis (TB) is the world's most common infectious human disease, killing about 2 million people per year, disabling many more, and the epidemic is growing. Its incidence is positively correlated with poverty, and its coexistence with AIDS in sub-Saharan Africa makes its impact even worse (WHO, Commission on Macroeconomics and Health, 2002). The loss in productivity and income to the poor per year globally is estimated to be enormous (WHO, Stop TB Partnership Secretariat, 2002).

Malaria. Malaria represents a significant cost in terms of long-term economic growth and development. It is associated with poverty and kills more than 1 million people per year throughout the world, with 90% of those in sub-Saharan Africa (WHO, Commission on Macroeconomics and Health, 2002). The Macroeconomic Commission on Health estimated that in 1999 malaria was responsible for 36 million disability-adjusted life years (DALYs) in sub-Saharan Africa; using a range of economic values for a DALY, the commission estimated that this loss ranged from 5.8 to 17.4% of the region's GNP (WHO, 2001).

Gallup and Sachs (2000) found that the growth of income per capita since the mid-1960s was lower in countries with severe malaria compared to countries with a low prevalence of the disease. When the incidence of malaria is sufficiently high in a region, businesses may not be willing to invest in it, and arable land can be left unused by the population.

HIV/AIDS. Unfortunately, the HIV/AIDS epidemic in Africa is providing growing evidence of the negative impact of reductions in health on economic growth. It is estimated that this epidemic in Africa will reduce the total national wealth of the most heavily affected countries by as much as 20% in the next ten years (Afrol News, 2000). In South Africa, where an estimated 20% of the population is infected with HIV/AIDS, GDP will decrease significantly in the next decade (Afrol News, 2000); and predictions are that life expectancy will fall by as much as 25 years below its former level (Arndt & Lewis, 2000). Theodore (2001) concludes that if HIV/AIDS trends continue in the Caribbean, there will be a significant loss of GDP. Although the AIDS epidemic is in a relatively early phase in China and India, there are reports of increasing rates of HIV infection; and without serious, effective interventions, the health and economic consequences could be disastrous (WHO, 2001).

With successful economic development, countries begin to shift from a population health perspective toward a medical care perspective as they transition out of poverty. It appears that the functional definition of *health* changes along that continuum as well. That is, the empirical literature is primarily focused on mortality in low-income countries; but as countries develop economically, with the demographic transition toward lower mortality rates, higher life expectancies, and lower birth rates, there is relatively less to be gained by focusing on mortality reduction. Countries that have gone through the epidemiologic transition from communicable to chronic diseases begin to allocate relatively more health sector resources toward interventions directed toward improvements in the quality of life (lower morbidity, reduced pain and suffering, and lower anxiety). In the next section, we discuss policies that address the economic determinants of health in both developed and developing countries.

Current Policies That Address Fundamental Determinants

Evidence regarding the economic determinants of health points to the importance of income in affecting population health and vice versa. It follows that policies that affect income will have a substantial influence on health and that health will influence income and related indicators of economic development. This section discusses policies that affect income and related indicators of economic development and that have an impact on population health in developed and developing countries.

Policies of Developed Countries

Several policies have the potential to affect income-related indicators of economic development; prominent among them are economic policies, such as taxes and subsidies, labor market policies, and trade policies. The focus on population health as a legitimate outcome of economic policy, the awareness of a population health perspective on the part of policymakers in the finance sector, and the implementation of economic policies based on these ideas vary greatly among developed countries. In this section we discuss when and how governments of selected developed countries have attempted to incorporate population health concerns into the development of economic policies.

Canada. Since the Lalonde report (1974) addressing nonmedical determinants of health, Canada has included economic determinants in discussions of health. Canadian researchers have been active in the field of population health, and the Population Health Program of the Canadian Institute for Advanced Research has been one of the leaders in nonmedical determinants research as well as in disseminating that research to policymakers and the public (Huynh, 2002). It may appear that Canada has attempted, more or less successfully, to incorporate nonmedical determinants in policymaking. However, a closer analysis reveals a different situation. When interviewed, several of the Population Health Program members agreed that familiarity and acceptance of the ideas had expanded, but they could not point to specific policy changes. They instead reported that policymakers used the nonmedical determinants ideas to justify decreasing spending on health care but did not heed the message to increase spending on nonmedical determinants. There was, however, an increase in research funding for population health and the creation of population health departments or divisions in universities and government organizations (Huynh, 2002).

Lavis et al. (2002) report that changes in the level and distribution of health status in Canada from the early 1970s to mid-1990s were consistent with a growing acceptance of population health ideas, but a closer analysis reveals that non-medical determinants of health have not had an influence on setting the agenda or on policy development outside the health care sector. A survey of federal and provincial civil servants in the departments of finance, labor, social services, and health indicated that efforts to spread the nonmedical determinants ideas to policymakers have not been successful in the economic and finance sectors, where much of the potential lies (Lavis et al., 2003). Lavis et al. (2002) conclude that changes in the level and distribution of health in Canada over the last decades cannot be attributed to policies based on nonmedical determinants of health. On the contrary, most policy aimed at health in Canada remains health policy.

However, even if not guided by health considerations, Canadian tax policy and income transfer programs have been successful in reducing poverty, especially among seniors and children, through more progressive rather than regressive distributional policies (Canadian Institute for Health Information, 2004). Though no researcher has evaluated the health impact, these policies have likely had significant health consequences.

On a smaller scale, a controlled, earning incentives experiment in Canada demonstrated health effects. The Self-Sufficiency Projects (SSP) in British Columbia and New Brunswick used a randomized control trial design to study the effects of earning supplements to single parents on income assistance. A monthly income supplement was paid on top of earnings from employment for up to three years if the person remained fully employed. Because the focus of the experiment was work effort, only limited health outcomes were collected. However, besides beneficial effects on income and employment, researchers documented positive effects on children's behavioral and emotional well-being as well as on maternal well-being and depression (Social Research and Demonstration Corporation, 2002, 2003). See the discussion of the evaluation of the SSP program later in the chapter.

Britain. Britain has a long history of interest in nonmedical determinants of health. The Black report (1980; Townsend & Davidson, 1992), prompted by the failure of the National Health Service to remove the health-income gradient, investigated the relationship between social class and health. However, the Black report did not find any policy outlet in the Thatcher administration. The Blair Labor government revived the issue and commissioned the Acheson report (1998) to identify social policy recommendations associated with nonmedical determinants. The Acheson report was followed by *From Vision to Reality* (Department of Health, 2001), which summarizes subsequent actions and proposals. International comparisons suggest that Britain is ahead of most developed countries in implementing nonhealth, especially economic, policies with the intent to influence health

(Mackenbach, Bakker, & European Network on Interventions and Policies to Reduce Inequalities in Health, 2003).

The recommendations of the Acheson report (1998) focus on alleviating poverty and disadvantage but fail to heed the main implication of the gradient, that everyone can benefit from an improvement in income so that the greater effect may be obtained by policies that target the population with incomes in the midrange (Evans, 2002). The recommendations also have been criticized for being too vague and for lacking a strong theoretical or empirical basis and for not addressing the effectiveness of the recommended policies (Evans, 2002; Macintyre, Chalmers, Horton, & Smith, 2001). Many of the policies are concerned with economic policies, including general income support policies such as family and child tax credits and increases in the minimum wage (Deaton, 2002). Several of those recommendations have been implemented, for example, policies to reduce child poverty (that include tax and benefit reform including a tax credit for low-income families with children), policies to reduce poverty through a national minimum wage and a minimum income guarantee, and employment policies to improve entry into the labor force by young and disabled people (Exworthy, Stuart, Blane, & Marmot, 2003). This has resulted in an active program of research on health inequalities reduction in the United Kingdom as well (see Table 5.1). Further, the Acheson report (1998) supports the use of health impact assessments for nonhealth policies.

On the other hand, the more recent *From Vision to Reality* (Department of Health, 2001) emphasizes reforms in the National Health Service, again focusing on policies concerned with health and away from economic policy (Evans, 2002).

Continental Europe. European countries are at varying stages of awareness, of willingness to take action, and of implementation of policies that address nonmedical determinants of health. The European Network on Interventions and Policies to Reduce Inequalities in Health (Mackenbach et al., 2003) has assessed policy developments in nine countries. The time line for policy developments in nine European countries is reproduced in Table 5.1.

Greece is the only European country that has not had any activity in this area. Spain has produced a document, often referred to as the Spanish Black report (Navarro, Benach, & Scientific Commission for the Study of Health Inequalities in Spain, 1996, as cited in Mackenbach et al., 2003) on inequalities in health, but has not moved into the policy arena. In France (Leclerc, Fassin, Grandjean, Kaminski, & Lang, 2000, as cited in Mackenbach et al., 2003) and Italy (Costa & Faggiano, 1994, as cited in Mackenbach et al., 2003), reports on health inequalities have been published, and policymakers are concerned about the issue. Lithuania is ready to take action (WHO, National Board of Health, & Kaunas

TABLE 5.1. TIME LINE: CONCURRENT POLICY DEVELOPMENT IN NINE EUROPEAN COUNTRIES.

Country	Time Line				
	1980–1984	1985–1989	1990–1994	1995–1999	2000–2002
Finland				○	*§
France				○	**
Greece					
Italy			*○	§	○Δ
Lithuania				*§	
Netherlands		*○Δ		○§	Δ
Spain		*		Δ	
Sweden				○	Δ
United Kingdom	Δ	*		*○○ΔΔ§§	§

Note. Adapted from "Tackling Socioeconomic Inequalities in Health: Analysis of European Experiences," by J. P. Mackenbach, M. J. Bakker, & European Network on Interventions and Policies to Reduce Inequalities in Health, 2003, *Lancet, 362,* p. 1410. Used with permission of Elsevier.

*High-profile independent report recommending policy action on health inequalities.

○ Start of national research program on health inequalities.

Δ Report of government advisory commission focusing on health inequalities reduction.

§ Government policy document focusing on health inequalities reduction.

University of Medicine, 1998, as cited in Mackenbach et al., 2003). Finland (Ministry of Social Affairs and Health, 2001, as cited in Mackenbach et al., 2003), the Netherlands (Scientific Council for Government Policy, 1987, as cited in Mackenbach et al., 2003), and Sweden (Ministry of Health and Social Affairs, 2000, as cited in Mackenbach et al., 2003) have produced documents describing health inequalities and have developed recommendations. Britain is the most advanced European country in this process, as the previous subsection described.

Political will and at times the strength of the economy have influenced progress toward the concern for and action related to health inequalities. Mackenbach et al. (2003) identified five types of approaches for tackling socioeconomic inequalities in health: policy-steering mechanisms, labor market and working conditions, health-related behaviors, health care, and territorial approaches. The five approaches are described in Exhibit 5.1. Two of them, policy-steering mechanisms and labor market and working conditions, specifically include economic policies.

In Sweden a committee of scientists, representatives of political parties, and advisers from governmental and nongovernmental organizations developed a new health policy that was concerned with nonmedical determinants of health (Ministry of Health and Social Affairs, 2000, as cited in Mackenbach et al., 2003).

EXHIBIT 5.1.   APPROACHES FOR ADDRESSING
SOCIOECONOMIC INEQUALITIES IN HEALTH.

Possibly Effective and Innovative Approaches for Tackling Socioeconomic Inequalities
in Health, Developed During the 1990s in Various European Countries

Policy-steering mechanisms
Quantitative policy targets
- Netherlands: reduction of inequalities in 11 intermediate outcomes (poverty, smoking, working conditions, etc.)

Health inequalities impact assessment
- Sweden: qualitative assessment of effect on health inequalities of European Community agricultural policy

Labour market and working conditions
Universal approaches
- Sweden: strong employment protection and active labour market policies for chronically ill citizens
- France: occupational health services offering annual check-ups and preventive interventions to all employees

Targeted approaches
- Netherlands: job rotation among dustmen (trashmen)

Health-related behaviours
Universal approaches
- Finland: serve low-fat food products through mass catering in schools and workplaces

Targeted approaches
- UK: multimethod intervention to reduce smoking in women on low income

Health care
Improving quality of care
- Netherlands: nurse practitioners to lend support to family doctors working in deprived areas

Working with other agencies
- UK: community strategies led by local government agencies, but integrating care across all the local public sector services, including health

Territorial approaches
Comprehensive health strategies for deprived areas
- UK: health action zones
- Spain: municipal health policy towards Ciutat Vella, Barcelona

Approaches were labelled innovative if they had been developed or implemented during the 1990s. Approaches were labelled possibly effective if evidence was obtained with an appropriate evaluation design—e.g., a time-series analysis, a before and after comparison of process or outcome indicators between one or more experimental and control groups, or a full randomised controlled trial, depending on the policy or intervention to be assessed—and showed an absolute improvement in lower socioeconomic groups. This selection criterion did not apply to the more complex approaches (policy steering mechanisms, working with other agencies, health action zones).

Note. From "Tackling Socioeconomic Inequalities in Health: Analysis of European Experiences," by J. P. Mackenbach, M. J. Bakker, & European Network on Interventions and Policies to Reduce Inequalities in Health, 2003, *Lancet, 362,* p. 1411, panel 1. Used with permission of Elsevier.

The recommendations included a reduction of inequalities in income and other socioeconomic factors through antipoverty measures and benefits to counter the health effects of poverty. The committee also recommended strong employment protection and active promotion of labor market participation by those with chronic illnesses. Additional policies related to import barriers on food products and subsidies for farmers (which raise the price of fresh fruits and vegetables, contributing to reduced consumption in low socioeconomic groups) (Dahlgren, Nordgren, & Whitehead, 1996). Strong involvement by policymakers characterized the Swedish approach.

In the Netherlands a six-year research program assessed the effectiveness of various attempts to address inequalities in health such as interventions to reduce inequalities in education and income and the creation of benefits to counter the health effects of poverty (Programmacommissie Sociaal-Economische Gezonheids Verschillen, Tweede Fase, 2001, as cited in Mackenbach et al., 2003). Most implemented interventions were small-scale and did not directly address the economic determinants of health, though the government has adopted some policies aimed at reducing poverty and improving working conditions.

Overall, the European approaches to addressing health inequalities did not emphasize economic and financial policies. The Copenhagen Declaration on Reducing Social Inequalities in Health (International Conference on Reducing Social Inequalities in Health, 2002), which was put forward by policymakers, researchers, and decision makers at the community level, listed European approaches and actions to improving health in the following areas: health care services, the workplace, local communities and families, and urban development (Krasnik & Rasmussen, 2002). The document made no mention of economic policies. Similarly, although the WHO has made the fight against health inequalities a priority in Europe, its recommendations do not include economic policies, except for a brief mention supporting health impact assessments (Zollner, 2002). Britain is somewhat unique in its inclusion of taxation and social security in its policy recommendations to address health issues.

The United States. Although the United States has the highest health care spending, it ranks in the middle to the bottom on health indicators among developed countries, showing that high investment in health care does not translate into desired health outcomes (Lurie, 2002). This evidence should point not only toward improvements in the health care delivery sector but also toward considering allocating resources to nonmedical determinants of health that may have a greater impact on population health. Some academics, for example George Kaplan, have argued that "economic policy is health policy and should be considered as such" (as cited in Lurie, 2002, p. 94). However, the population health implications rarely come up in economic and social policy debates; and policymakers at the federal level do not prominently recognize the ideas of nonmedical determinants of health, though policymakers at the state and local level have begun to discuss them (Lurie, 2002). The lack of economic and social policies that explicitly buffer the market and redistribute resources discourages implementation of the nonmedical determinants agenda in the United States (Syme, Lefkowitz, & Krimgold, 2002).

At this time the best hope for implementing the population health approach in the United States lies at the state and community levels. For example, the Minnesota Department of Health, in a study to address health disparities, highlighted the need for interventions targeting nonmedical determinants to improve population health (Minnesota Health Improvement Partnership Social Conditions and Health Action Team, 2001). The Minnesota Family Investment Program (MFIP) was part of the Minnesota welfare reform. MFIP offered financial incentives to encourage work and required participation in employment services to improve skills. The goal of the program was to increase employment and earnings and to decrease dependence in single-parent long-term welfare recipients. The research design consisted of two randomized groups, one receiving the incentives and one receiving the standard program that reduces benefit amounts as employment earnings increase. Though the main intent of the program was not to improve health, investigators evaluated selected health outcomes. Participants in the program not only obtained clear economic benefits, but MFIP also had positive effects on family life, child well-being, and participants' health. The evaluation concluded that financial incentives accounted for nearly all of the program's beneficial effects on marriage, domestic abuse, and mothers' depression, as well as for the positive effects on children, such as less problem behavior and better performance at school (Manpower Demonstration Research Corporation, 2000a, 2000b, 2000c). Later, this chapter presents evidence evaluating the MFIP.

Policies of International Organizations

Policies of the governments of OECD countries deal with foreign aid, debt relief, trade barriers, subsidies of agricultural exports to low-income countries, and sales below production costs (or dumping) (WHO, 2001). Many of the policy preferences of high-income countries that importantly affect developing countries are forged by international policymaking organizations. We will discuss relevant policies in this context.

The World Health Organization. Many specific policies have successfully improved health conditions in low-income countries with respect to specific diseases and health conditions. WHO (2000) has published a compilation of a wide range of successful interventions, and thus of the policy decisions to allocate resources against specific diseases in specific low-income countries. These case studies include successes against TB, malaria, and HIV/AIDS, as well as childhood and other diseases, resulting in significant improvements in population health. Few studies estimate the economic consequences of improved health at the individual level in low-income countries; however, the evidence at the aggregate level is strong.

Policies to allocate resources to the worldwide eradication of specific diseases have also been successful. Smallpox has been eradicated, and the incidence of polio has been greatly diminished. The WHO is pursuing efforts to eradicate or substantially diminish seven other diseases, such as polio, that heavily affect low-income countries. These efforts are being supported by funds from nongovernmental organizations and the pharmaceutical industry (WHO, 2001).

Although there is little evidence that economic development policies in the past have been formulated to improve population health in an effort to achieve gains in economic development, this may change. The WHO Millennium Development Goals for developing countries (Annan, 2000) call for significant reductions in poverty and improvements in population health by 2015. Recognizing increased global interdependence, WHO's Commission on Macroeconomics and Health (WHO, 2001) has recommended a bold, detailed, and comprehensive set of policies to invest in population health. The recommendations are based on the links between economic development, investment in the health sector, and population health that are represented in Figure 5.1.

The commission's proposal (WHO, 2001) considers a wide range of issues and the associated policies needed to deal with them. Here is a selection:

- Policies to encourage labour absorption with respect to the "demographic dividend" (labour-using technology).
- Policies to increase the level of foreign aid going to poor countries to fund increased access to medicines.
- Policies to encourage research into prevention and treatment of diseases that primarily impact the populations of developing countries (known as Type III diseases).
- Policies to change the composition of foreign aid to increase the emphasis on health-oriented public good activities.
- Policies to encourage differential pricing of patented drugs in low income countries and to encourage production of generics in these countries.
- Policies to encourage differential pricing of non-patented drugs through compulsory licensing of other third world countries.
- Policies to lower poor country tariffs on non-patented drugs.

Each country would have to define its program of essential interventions. The commission suggested four selection criteria: interventions should be efficacious and practical; targeted diseases should impose a heavy burden on society, including social and economic spillovers; benefits should exceed costs; and the needs of the poor should be stressed. This partnership between developing and developed countries would entail a significant increase in resources allocated to the health sector in poor countries, financed by both low- and high-income countries. The objective is to intervene against the conditions underlying the main causes of avoidable deaths in low-income countries: HIV/AIDS, TB, malaria, childhood infectious diseases, maternal and perinatal conditions, nutritional deficiencies, and tobacco-related illnesses. The improvements in health are likely to lead to higher incomes, higher economic growth, and reduced population growth (WHO, 2001).

The commission (WHO, 2001) estimated that by the year 2010 the actions of these proposed policies could save 8 million lives per year. The disease burden in developing countries would be greatly reduced and in doing so not only improve population health but also result in very significant gains in economic development in low- and middle-income countries. The increased strength of these global trading partners would increase trade and thus benefit high-income countries as well.

The costs of these policies would be substantial, but they would be more than offset by the subsequent population health and economic consequences. The targeted countries (those with 1999 GNP per capita of less than $1,200, plus the few sub-Saharan countries with per capita incomes above $1,200) would have to increase their annual health sector expenditures, and donor countries would have to increase their health sector assistance in these countries. In addition to the 8 million lives being saved annually by 2015, the commission conservatively estimated the direct economic benefit from this at $186 billion, versus the $94 billion in program costs. The benefit estimate does not include the positive impact of improved population health on economic growth (WHO, 2001).

Although we are stressing the significance of improvements in population health as a mechanism to achieve gains in economic development, there is significant evidence that improvements in education in low-income countries also have a positive impact on economic health (Bloom et al., 2004; Deaton, 2003; WHO, 2001). The contribution of education to health is discussed in detail in Chapter Four. The commission (WHO, 2001) recommends that nations make additional investments in education, as well as in water and sanitation systems.

The International Monetary Fund. International Monetary Fund (IMF) policies are often controversial. Policies that are oriented toward long-term economic growth are often accompanied by short-term sacrifices. The short-run consequences can be severe. When a country is in economic trouble (high inflation, high unemployment, a large foreign debt) and cannot pay its debts, the IMF must sometimes intervene. Although the IMF may help relieve or restructure the debt, the accompanying policy prescription can be painful, as the agency requires an increased degree of economic austerity such as reduced government spending associated with a limit on the level of allowable federal budget deficits.

Stiglitz (2002) contends that the IMF has based much of its policy to stabilize economies in developing countries on incorrect assumptions about the ability of free markets alone to accomplish IMF objectives; he believes that this has resulted in unnecessarily severe levels of suffering by the poor. This chapter will later discuss the pros and cons of globalization.

The World Bank. Two institutions make up what is commonly called the World Bank: the International Bank for Reconstruction and Development (IBRD) and the International Development Association (IDA). According to the World Bank Group (2004), the World Bank is committed to fighting global poverty and "centers its efforts on reaching the Millennium Development Goals . . . aimed at sustainable poverty reduction."

The IBRD loans money to higher-income developing countries that are given more time to repay the loans (15 to 20 years) than commercial lenders would allow. The IBRD also give borrowing countries a three- to five-year grace period before repayment begins. Countries borrow for poverty reduction programs as well as to promote economic growth to improve the standard of living, social services, and environmental programs. In 2002, 40 countries borrowed a total of $11.5 billion from the IBRD.

The IDA is the part of the World Bank that helps the world's poorest countries by providing grants, interest-free loans, and technical assistance. The IDA gives them 35 to 40 years to repay the loans, with a 10-year grace period. In 2002 it provided $8.1 billion to 62 very low-income countries. Forty developed countries make contributions every four years to replenish the IDA's funding resources. Descriptions of two World Bank initiatives that illustrate the relationships between economic policies and health in developing countries follow.

Heavily Indebted Poor Countries Initiative. The financial consequence of a low-income country having a large foreign debt is the reduced availability of funding for poverty reduction and other economic development efforts. Payment of interest on the debt (debt service) and repayment of the debt itself are often onerous burdens. In response to this, in 1996 the World Bank and the IMF jointly sponsored the Heavily Indebted Poor Countries Initiative to reduce the debt burden in developing countries. In 1999 they expanded the program, and thus far "26 countries have received debt relief which will save them $41 billion over time. The money these countries save in debt repayments instead will be put into housing, education, health, and welfare programs for the poor" (World Bank Group, 2004).

Microcredit and Microfinance Initiatives. The majority of population in the world's low-income countries lives in rural areas, often not participating in the formal economy and without adequate access to credit services. Bangladesh pioneered an innovative approach to reach those hard-to-reach very poor groups that has since spread to other countries. In 1976 a three-year demonstration and research project in Bangladesh determined the feasibility of a banking credit system for the rural poor. With the sponsorship of the Bangladesh Central Bank and support from nationalized commercial banks, the program expanded to other rural areas in Bangladesh and converted into the independent Grameen Bank (*Grameen* means "rural" in the Bangla language) (Grameen Communications, 1998). The initial focus was on providing *microcredit*, very small, nonsecured loans (to stimulate production) to rural poor individuals. Ninety-five percent of the borrowers in the Grameen Bank program are women (Asian Development Bank, 2004).

There has been a surge of interest in microfinance services, such as insurance and savings services, to be made available for the poor as well as in policies to support these services. These services are important elements of poverty reduction strategies in rural areas. Microfinance services are now supported by international organizations, as well as private- and public-sector institutions (Asian Development Bank, 2004).

However, although microcredit and microfinance have helped reduce poverty for many poor people, an Asian Development Bank study (2004) found that 95% of the poor in rural Asia still have little access to needed credit and other financial services. Clearly, a great deal remains to be done.

The World Trade Organization. The World Trade Organization (WTO) deals with the rules of international trade. It has a direct impact on the lowering of barriers between countries and the resulting increased movements of information and culture, people, financial capital, consumer goods, and physical capital goods (Navarro, 2000; WHO, 2001). The result is increased global interdependence and in particular a more integrated global market. However, although WTO negotiations to further reduce trade barriers have the potential to continue to stimulate economic growth, they also have the potential to cause significant harm (Deaton, 2002; Stiglitz, 2002; WHO, 2001; WHO, Commission on Macroeconomics and Health, 2002; Yach & Bettcher, 1998). Stiglitz (2002, p. 5) maintains, "Those who vilify globalization too often overlook its benefits. But the proponents of globalization have been, if anything, even more unbalanced." The discussion that follows reviews the pros and cons of globalization.

Globalization. Globalization has affected economic development and population health in developed and developing countries. It offers enormous potential for economic growth with the efficiency gains associated with the comparative advantages of freer trade. OECD countries would likely not have developed economically as successfully as they have without significant involvement in foreign trade. Globalization also offers potential health benefits because a more integrated global market is likely to increase rates of innovation and diffusion of technological change, the amount of trade in health services, the availability of information on evidence of alternatives, and the exchange of experiences (WHO, Commission on Macroeconomics and Health, 2002). In 2005 all WTO member countries were required to put in effect a patent protection system that will be more effective than the current system. Low-income countries generally cannot afford price-protected drugs; however, this affirmation of intellectual property rights will likely strengthen research-based pharmaceutical industries in Brazil, China, India, and South Africa, which may be more attuned to the special needs of the developing countries.

On the other hand, globalization has had negative effects on developing countries. WTO and developed country policies affecting the globalization process do not explicitly concern themselves with certain equity considerations. There are at least two areas of concern: the potential lack of equity in the impact of these policies on the growth and distribution of income both within and between countries and the lack of equity in the process of policy development itself. The governments of many developing countries maintain that OECD countries dominate the WTO and have forced disproportionate tariff and quota reductions in developing countries, while at the same time refusing to eliminate import barriers to agricultural products from developing countries.

In addition, some developed countries, such as the United States, have policies that provide production subsidies and thus a competitive pricing advantage for some commodities that their producers export to developing countries. The increased competition that producers in developing countries face due to policies that reduce trade protection and subsidize competition from developed countries can result in increased unemployment and poverty. Even with long-run benefits from globalization, the system as it is currently being managed will likely create negative consequences that will weigh heavily on the poor in developing countries.

Another major concern is that lower tariffs and quotas and the loss of protection will retard the development of infant industries in developing countries, that is, industries newly introduced in the country. It is unlikely that the many currently developed countries would have developed as successfully as they did without such protection. Poor countries face other challenges with globalization. It intensifies the problem of the brain drain; for example, in 20 poor African countries, more than 35% of those with university degrees now live abroad (WHO, Commission on Macroeconomics and Health, 2002). Increased international competition for mobile financial capital may cause governments to lower taxes in an effort to compete for capital. The resulting loss of government revenue would reduce the ability to fund expenditures for health and economic development projects. Another concern is that globalization and the associated increases in tourism, migration, and business travel are increasing the rate of transmission of diseases such as HIV/AIDS, SARS, and avian flu.

Finally, there is concern that globalization is undermining many local economies and cultures. The effects of globalization reach, for example, inner cities and rural areas of the United States, as documented in Appendix 5.1.

Strengths and Limitations of Current Policies

This section will review the barriers to using economic policies to affect population health, the tools available to evaluate the health impact of economic policies, and the criteria used to evaluate the health effect of economic policies. Finally, it will illustrate the evaluation of selected economic interventions on health.

Barriers to the Use of Economic Policies to Affect Population Health

Usually, economic policies have the intent of affecting economic factors such as income levels and income distribution. Only rarely do policymakers take into account their effects on population health, and even more rarely do policymakers formulate policies with the explicit intention of influencing population health. When economic policies are motivated by health considerations, it is usually within the context of reducing health inequalities.

There are several reasons for this lack of attention to population health in formulating economic policies. First, although there is strong evidence regarding the association between income and health, and although research has found some identifiable mechanisms through which income affects health, there is no clear scientific or political consensus of how the mechanisms operate (Deaton, 2002).

Second, there is scant specific evidence regarding which economic policies or interventions are effective in improving population health or reducing health inequalities (Evans, 2002; Krasnik & Rasmussen, 2002). The development of policies is hindered by divergent views on how to evaluate the impact of policies (Bennett, 2003). Randomized control trials are obviously not feasible in policy evaluation; therefore, isolating the effect of policy factors that affect health is difficult. It is likely that there are long lag times between an economic intervention and its effect on health, depending on the health outcome, making evaluation even more problematic. In practice, we do not know how to use economic policy directly to reduce health inequalities.

Third, policies that affect population health must be intersectoral policies because they are characterized by explicit concern for health in all areas of policy, including finance, employment, social services, health care, education, and the environment (Bennett, 2003). The need for intersectoral policies further complicates the measurement of resource use and the evaluation of programs originating in different departments.

Finally, there may not be the political will to address the population health issue, and sectors that do not see health as a legitimate player in their policy environment may sometimes find the expectation of incorporating health issues in policy development as health imperialism (Bennett, 2003).

Income Redistribution Policies. Particularly controversial among economic policies that might affect population health are income redistribution policies. Though a social justice public health perspective often implicitly favors such policies, health economists have expressed numerous reservations. First, economists challenge the evidence of a causal relationship between income distribution and health outcomes. Deaton (2003) and others (Lynch et al., 2001) recognize the importance of inequalities to health, but they question whether it is income inequality rather than other types of inequality (for example, inequalities in health-related resources) that matters. Second, economists point to the negative impact on incentives to work and on the deadweight loss associated with redistribution. *Deadweight loss* refers to the administrative costs associated with redistributing income, which results in the better off losing more than $1 for each dollar allocated to the worse off in the redistribution of income or wealth through taxation (Deaton, 2002). For this reason, economists tend to favor policies that affect both income and health, such as educational policies, rather than policies aimed at income redistribution. However, some economists recognize that funds spent on income provision to the poor can improve population health more than can similar funds spent on health care delivery (Case, 2001).

Health Impact Assessment

One possible tool for explicitly considering health impacts in the evaluation of policies in all sectors, including the economic and finance sectors, is the health impact assessment (HIA). Similar in concept to the environmental impact assessment that U.S. law mandates under certain conditions, the HIA considers a policy's likely intended and unintended consequences for health and includes that information in the policymaking process. It enhances recognition of societal and economic determinants of health and the intersectoral responsibility for health among a broad public, as well as increasing the transparency and accountability in policymaking (Krieger et al., 2003). Though methodological difficulties may lead to the erroneous impression that impacts can be exactly measured, HIA has the potential for promoting inclusion of health considerations in economic policy development. HIA has not been widely developed and used in the United States, particularly in evaluating the health impacts of policies outside the health sector. HIA has, however, been used in formulating transportation policy in Scotland (Gorman, Douglas, Conway, Noble, & Hanlon, 2003), in agriculture and food policy in Slovenia (Lock et al., 2003), and in international development assistance (Mercier, 2003).

Definition of Criteria

This section reviews, adapts, and applies three policy evaluation criteria (i.e., effectiveness, efficiency, and equity) with the aim of evaluating the strengths and limitations of economic policy in improving population health. Conventionally, all these criteria deal with resource allocation among alternate uses, for example, the distribution of goods and services among the different groups of society (Bromley & Paavola, 2002; Heyne, Boettke, & Prychitko, 2005).

We consider two approaches to the definition of efficiency. First, Aday, Begley, Lairson, and Balkrishnan (2004) define efficiency in evaluating the medical care system in the health care field. Chapter One presents these issues in detail. Second, the traditional welfare economics approach defines technical (production) efficiency in terms of producing a given output at the least possible cost or with fixed inputs to maximize output. The outputs produced are intermediate outcomes. The final outcome is total utility achieved. *Utility* is an economic term to denote the total satisfaction derived from the consumption of goods and services. *Allocative efficiency* is then defined as producing the mix of intermediate outcomes (the mix of goods and services for consumers) that will result in maximizing total utility.

Thus, both of these approaches define technical (production) efficiency in terms of least-cost production of intermediate outcomes, and they define allocative efficiency in terms of achieving the right mix of intermediate outcomes to maximize the value of their objective function. In the case of health care, the objective to be maximized was health improvements; and in welfare economics, the objective to be maximized was total utility.

Figure 5.3 summarizes our approach to the evaluation of economic policies in the context of population health outcomes. In population health research, the

FIGURE 5.3.   EVALUATION OF ECONOMIC POLICIES.

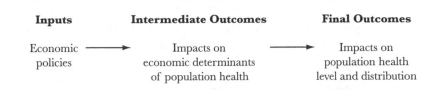

value to be maximized is population health. In the framework of welfare economics, it is equivalent to maximizing utility when total utility depends only on population health. The utility function allows both the aggregate-level population health and the equity of the distribution of health in the population to be included. Economists, on the other hand, include other measures of well-being besides health in the utility function, such as income and wealth, employment, or education. From an economic viewpoint, health is only one of the items that confers utility. Therefore, from an economist's point of view, the issue is not to maximize population health but to find the optimal mix of health, income and wealth, education, and other factors that maximize aggregate utility.

In the context of this chapter, the value of efficiency, both technical and allocative, is affirmed if efficiency improves population health; and equitable distribution would mean that the range of inequality is limited. Consequently, economic factors (e.g., income and wealth and income inequality) are here considered as the intermediate outputs because they are among the fundamental determinants of population health but are not present in the final total utility to be maximized.

In the evaluation of economic policies in improving population health, one can address the concepts of effectiveness, efficiency, and equity as follows:

- How effective is an economic policy in terms of achieving improvements in the level and distribution of population health?
- How technically efficient (production efficiency) is a policy or set of policies in terms of using the fewest resources to produce the intermediate economic outcomes (i.e., the economic determinants of population health)?
- What mix of intermediate outcomes (economic determinants of population health) is allocatively efficient in terms of maximizing population health improvement, given resource constraints?
- How equitable is a policy or mix of policies in terms of the distribution of both its costs and in terms of its population health benefits?

Issues of intergenerational equity are of particular concern to developing countries. Deliberative justice may be less relevant in this setting because many economic policies are set at the highest government levels, with participation of the affected parties mainly through representation rather than direct participation.

Evaluation of Selected Economic Policies

As discussed earlier, the effectiveness of economic policies in directly improving population health is difficult to establish (Bennett, 2003; Deaton, 2002; Evans, 2002; Krieger et al., 2003). The literature on evaluating the effectiveness, the technical and allocative efficiency, and the equity of economic policies in improving population health is scant because researchers have conducted few formal studies of effectiveness. This is due partly to the rarity of the use of economic policies to influence population health and partly to the recentness of the few attempts made. But evidence exists of the effectiveness of economic policies in addressing economic determinants of health such as income and employment (Samuelson & Nordhaus, 2005).

Because of the lack of necessary information to evaluate the impact of broad economic policies on population health, we focus on more limited policies that have a strong economic component and that others have evaluated with respect to health effects. We discuss two economic policy interventions in developed countries and two in developing countries.

The Self-Sufficiency Projects in Canada. The Self-Sufficiency Projects (SSP) in British Columbia and New Brunswick used a randomized control-trial design to study the effects of earning supplements to single parents on income assistance. Evaluation indicated that the SSP were effective in that they significantly increased full-time employment, employment earnings, and income and reduced poverty (Social Research and Demonstration Corporation, 2002, 2003). The SSP were also effective in that there was some evidence of positive effects on children's academic functioning and behavioral and emotional well-being as well as on maternal well-being and depression. Evaluating their production efficiency and their allocative efficiency is not possible because there is no information on whether the minimum amount of resources was used to achieve these effects or on whether an alternative approach (instead of supplementing income) would cause stronger effects on health outcomes.

SSP can be considered equitable in that the program allocated supplemental income to disadvantaged individuals with the effect of improving the distribution of income and health. The program satisfies the criteria of intergenerational justice by improving disadvantaged children's well-being and academic achievement, of social justice by improving the health of disadvantaged individuals and therefore minimizing health disparities among groups, and of distributive justice by distributing more fairly the benefits and burden across groups. Whether it meets deliberative justice criteria is unknown, because it is not clear how involved the recipients of the program were in developing the intervention.

The Minnesota Family Investment Program. As discussed earlier, the Minnesota Family Investment Program (MFIP) offered financial incentives to encourage work and required participation in employment services to improve skills as part of welfare reform. Evaluation indicated that MFIP was effective in achieving its goals in that participants were more likely to be employed, had lower poverty rates, and higher earnings (Manpower Demonstration Research Corporation, 2000a, 2000b, 2000c). The program was also effective in improving participants' well-being as documented by the participants being more likely to be married after three years, to experience a reduction in domestic abuse, and to be less likely to use harsh parenting techniques. MFIP children had less problem behavior, better performance in school, and more engagement in school. The program was also effective from a health point of view because participants were 8% less likely to be at risk for clinical depression. Evaluating the technical and allocative efficiency of MFIP is not possible because no data exist on whether it used the fewest possible resources to produce improvements in employment and earnings, nor are there data on whether another mix of economic improvements would have led to better health outcomes.

The program was equitable in the social justice sense; welfare recipients have higher rates of depression than does the general population, so a reduction in their rates of depression reduces health disparities among groups. It was equitable in the distributive sense in that providing more economic and health resources to long-term welfare recipients implies a fairer distribution of benefits across social groups. And it was equitable in the intergenerational sense in that resources and benefits were shifted to children. It is unclear whether the affected parties participated in the decision-making process.

The Grameen Bank Project in Bangladesh. Evaluation of the Grameen Bank project, a microcredit project described earlier, indicated that it has been effective in achieving its objective of making credit available to many poor, rural people in Bangladesh and that many people who participated have improved their economic welfare, quality of life, and health. To be productively efficient requires that the least possible amount of resources be used to achieve the stated objectives. Because the project is a nonprofit, self-sustaining operation, which is 90% owned by the rural poor who are also its beneficiaries, the poverty-reducing benefits of this project relative to the level of societal resources invested in it are likely to be substantial. Thus, this project is productively efficient.

With respect to allocative efficiency, the success of the Grameen Bank project engendered the development of a wide variety of other microfinance programs in the following two decades. (Some of these were described earlier.) Many have also been effective in achieving poverty reduction objectives. Data are not available to determine what combination of these projects would produce the maximum reduction in poverty and improvement in population health. In fact, the appropriate combination of available microfinance interventions in different situations currently is the subject of many economic development policy discussions. As such, although it is not possible to know whether it would have been more allocatively efficient to use other types of interventions in combination with the Grameen Bank project, the issue is being tested as more and more microfinance projects are being implemented.

The microcredit program can be considered equitable because its objective, which it successfully achieved, was to reduce poverty and improve the quality of life among the very poor and disadvantaged in rural areas and thereby improve the distribution of income and health. It satisfies the criteria of intergenerational justice by helping the very poor, many of whom are children, and by breaking the vicious cycle of poverty, which will benefit future generations. It satisfies the criterion of social justice by improving the economic welfare, quality of life, and health of the disadvantaged and thus reducing health disparities. Ninety-five percent of program borrowers from the Grameen Bank are women, often single and with children. The project satisfies the criterion of distributive justice by distributing the availability of credit across groups in society; and it satisfies the criterion of deliberative justice, given the borrowers' input in the early phases of the project's development and by the fact that the rural poor now own 90% of the Grameen Bank.

The Heavily Indebted Poor Country Initiative of the World Bank and the IMF.

As described earlier, the Heavily Indebted Poor Country Initiative (HIPC) of the World Bank and the IMF is designed to reduce the onerous burden of debt and debt service of very poor countries. Given that it has achieved debt reductions that will amount to $41 billion over time for 26 low-income countries and that these savings instead will be put into housing, education, health, and welfare programs for the poor (World Bank Group, 2004), the HIPC presumably has been effective in achieving some poverty reduction and population health objectives. However, the situation is too complex to understand whether the HIPC is either productively or allocatively efficient—that is, whether the impacts could have been achieved with fewer resources or whether an alternative set of policies might have resulted in even greater benefit, given resource constraints.

The HIPC is equitable in that it has shifted interest and debt payment to developed countries and the World Bank and IMF to health, education, housing, and welfare services for the poor in low-income countries. It thus meets the social justice, intergenerational, and distributive justice criteria; and although the poor themselves were not involved in development of the program, leaders and representatives of low-income countries were involved, and in that sense the HIPC also meets the deliberative justice criterion.

Recommendations

Recommendations on the use of economic policy to influence population health are broadly similar in developed and developing countries. Policies that stimulate economic development and improve the distribution of income are likely to have a beneficial effect on the health of the population. The authors' recommendations include general recommendations as well as more specific policy recommendations.

General Recommendations

Our general recommendations propose actions to increase public and policymaker awareness of the influence of economic policies on population health and encourage participation in policy development by all stakeholders. These include encouraging greater recognition of nonmedical determinants of health among policymakers, supporting more research on the impact of economic policies on population health, highlighting the health consequences of policies, promoting policy development through participatory methods, and strengthening intersectoral collaboration.

Encourage Greater Recognition Among Policymakers of Nonmedical Determinants of Health. As we have discussed, a few countries have already developed economic policies with the intent of affecting population health. However, these policies are very limited. We would like to see a greater recognition at the policy level of the influence of nonmedical determinants of health, in particular economic determinants, which should lead to more support for the use of economic policies to improve population health. In the United States, Lurie (2002) suggests some steps that the U.S. federal government could take, such as providing leadership (through the surgeon general, the Centers for Disease Control, or the Veterans Administration) to educate the public and policymakers on economic and social determinants. The federal government can play an important role in monitoring and reporting on nonmedical determinants, for example, by explicitly listing nonmedical determinants as objectives in the Healthy People agenda, the process that sets and monitors health objectives for the nation.

Support More Research on the Impact of Economic Policies on Population Health. Our recommendations include more research on the mechanisms through which economic factors affect health, on the effectiveness and efficiency of using economic policies to affect health, and on the cost-effectiveness of different economic tools to improve population health. The government could take the lead in funding the research necessary to evaluate nonmedical interventions for health, for example, the examination of the health effects of economic policies such as minimum wage, income tax credit, or investments in low-income communities. In the United States, for example, decision makers base policies on market values and pragmatic considerations rather than on notions of equity (Syme et al., 2002). Demonstration of cost-effectiveness may convince some policymakers of the potential of the nonmedical determinants approach.

Highlight the Health Consequences of Policies. We recommend highlighting the health consequences of policy decisions in the economic realm using tools such as health impact assessments (HIA). The Acheson report (1998) also supports the use of HIAs for policies that are not direct health policies.

Promote Policy Development Through Participatory Methods. We support Nobel-laureate economist Sen (1999) in emphasizing the importance of public discussions. Democracy is not just about elections but also about public discussions. Following Sen, we recommend more public discussion of issues that require a participatory process, for example, those related to health and public spending, and greater participation in those public discussions by the people who are often excluded because of illiteracy, poor health, or poverty (Wallace, 2004). We strongly support the trend apparent in some European countries of developing policies to address health disparities through a process of participation by local and national policymakers, researchers, and the communities affected. Such policies are more likely to meet the needs of the populations involved and to be acceptable to all stakeholders, while being based on sound scientific evidence.

Strengthen Intersectoral Collaboration. Organizational barriers to a nonmedical approach to population health include the lack of collaboration among multiple agencies, congressional committees, and academic disciplines. There is a need for better coordination and cross-cutting initiatives at the policy and the academic levels. In the United States, the public health community is segmented and lacks the tradition of involvement in social medicine that is present in Canada or Europe, though recent developments speak of greater involvement (Institute of Medicine, Committee on Assuring the Health of the Public in the 21st Century,

2003). In order to actively promote the population health approach, a larger constituency of public health researchers and practitioners must be engaged (Syme et al., 2002).

Specific Policy Recommendations

Policy recommendations include the major specific economic policies that are known to affect population health. These include targeted programs to reduce poverty and selected labor market and trade policies.

Policies to Reduce Poverty. We recommend economic policies that reduce poverty in order to improve population health. The HIPC of the World Bank and the IMF and policies supporting the extension of credit availability to very low-income individuals (microcredit) are examples of economic policies directed toward improving population health in low-income countries. The package of policies proposed by the WHO's Commission on Macroeconomics and Health (2002) contains recommendations for the use of economic policy to improve population health in low-income countries on a massive scale. These policies focus on reducing poverty as a means of improving population health and also on direct improvements of population health, which in turn can facilitate economic growth and reduce poverty. In developed countries economic policies that reduce poverty with the intent of improving population health have been recommended in selected cases. For example, the recommendations of the Acheson report (1988) focused on alleviating poverty and disadvantage. Many of the recommended policies are economic policies, including child tax credits, increases in the minimum wage, and unemployment benefits. Finally, for all countries, we recommend policies that provide benefits that counter the negative effects of poverty on population health, such as providing access to quality health care, excellent public school systems, and a minimum income guarantee, including policies addressing the minimum wage and unemployment and disability benefits.

Labor Market Policies. Labor market policies can have a significant impact on population health. We recommend employment policies similar to those proposed or implemented in the United Kingdom, Sweden, and France to improve entry into the labor force by young and/or disabled people and to improve working conditions, for example, strong employment protection and active promotion of labor market participation by those with chronic illnesses. In developing countries we recommend policies to improve working conditions and access to employment for the most disadvantaged members of society. These include economic policies as well as educational and training policies, health care policies, and transportation policies. Examples would be universal primary school, vocational training for adolescents, a national universal health care system, and the provision of public transportation.

Trade Policies. We recommend trade policies that allow the fair sharing of benefits of globalization and trade between countries and within countries. This includes reducing agricultural subsidies in developed countries and eliminating the practice of forcing tariff reductions in developing countries for products exported by developed countries while maintaining import barriers in developed countries for products exported by developing countries. Trade negotiations must address the unique needs of developing countries. For example, these must reach a fair approach to the issues of patent protection, in particular in the pharmaceutical field, and of the brain drain. Finally, as mentioned earlier in the context of more participatory models of decision making, developing countries should be able to sit at the negotiation table as equal partners.

An editorial in the *American Journal of Public Health* posed the provocative question, "Is economic policy health policy?" (Kaplan & Lynch, 2001). The answer provided by the policies and evidence reviewed in this chapter is a resounding yes. Both a gradient and gaps in health exist between those with the most and least incomes. The precise mechanisms through which this relationship operates are still being explored. Further, inequalities in the distributions of incomes between communities, states, and countries that appear to be correlated with inequalities in health across areas may be due to other compositional, contextual, or policy factors (e.g., racial or ethnic composition, history and patterns of residential segregation, or tax or income transfer policies that support more extensive education, public health, and social services). Considerable and convincing evidence, however, documents that individuals and families that have greater economic resources have better health. Policies that affect the economic well-being of individuals and families are also quite likely to affect their physical health and well-being.

This chapter has explored the population health consequences of macroeconomic factors and policies. Chapter Six points out the important role of local economies and communities in promoting population health and well-being.

References

Abbott, D. H., Keverne, E. B., Bercovitch, F. B., Shively, C. A., Medoza, S. P., Saltzman, W., et al. (2003). Are subordinates always stressed? A comparative analysis of rank differences in cortisol levels among primates. *Hormones and Behavior, 43,* 67–82.

Acheson, D. (1998). *Independent inquiry into inequalities in health report.* London: Stationery Office.

Aday, L. A., Begley, C. E., Lairson, D. R., & Balkrishnan, R. (2004). *Evaluating the healthcare system: Effectiveness, efficiency, and equity* (3rd ed.). Chicago: Health Administration Press.

Afrol News. (2000, July 11). *AIDS seriously hinders economic growth.* Retrieved August 3, 2004, from http://www.afrol.com/html/Categories/Health/health007_aids_hinders_growth.htm

Annan, K. A. (2000). *We the peoples: The role of the United Nations in the 21st century.* New York: United Nations.

Arndt, C., & Lewis, J. D. (2000). The macro implications of HIV/AIDS in South Africa: A preliminary assessment. *South African Journal of Economics, 68,* 856–887.

Asian Development Bank. (2004). *Microfinance development strategy: Introduction 2004.* Retrieved August 16, 2004, from http://www.adb.org/Documents/Policies/Microfinance/microfinance0100.asp?p=policies

Backlund, E., Sorlie, P. D., & Johnson, N. J. (1996). The shape of the relationship between income and mortality in the United States: Evidence from the National Longitudinal Mortality Study. *Annals of Epidemiology, 6,* 12–20.

Barro, R. J. (1997). *Determinants of economic growth: A cross country empirical study.* Cambridge, MA: MIT Press.

Bashir, S. A. (2002). Home is where the harm is: Inadequate housing as a public health crisis. *American Journal of Public Health, 92,* 733–738.

Becker, E. (2003, September 9). Western farmers fear third-world challenge to subsidies. *The New York Times,* p. A1.

Bennett, J. (2003). *Investment in population health in five OECD countries* (OECD Health Working Papers No. 2). Paris: Organisation for Economic Co-operation and Development.

Berkman, L. F., & Glass, T. (2000). Social integration, social networks, social support, and health. In L. F. Berkman & I. Kawachi (Eds.), *Social epidemiology* (pp. 137–173). New York: Oxford University Press.

Berkman, L. F., & Kawachi, I. (Eds.). (2000). *Social epidemiology.* New York: Oxford University Press.

Bhargava, A., Jamison, D. T., Lau, L. J., & Murray, C.J.L. (2001). Modeling the effects of health on economic growth. *Journal of Health Economics, 20,* 423–440.

Black, D. (1980). *Inequalities in health: Report of a research working group.* London: Department of Health and Social Security.

Blakely, T. A., Kennedy, B. P., & Kawachi, I. (2001). Socioeconomic inequality in voting participation and self-rated health. *American Journal of Public Health, 91,* 99–104.

Blakely, T. A., Lochner, K., & Kawachi, I. (2002). Metropolitan area income inequality and self-rated health: A multi-level study. *Social Science and Medicine, 54,* 65–77.

Bloom, D. E., & Canning, D. (2000). Public health: The health and wealth of nations. *Science, 287,* 1207–1209.

Bloom, D. E., Canning, D., & Jamison, D. T. (2004). Health, wealth, and welfare. *Finance and Development, 41,* 10–15.

Bourguignon, F., & Morrisson, C. (2002). Inequality among world citizens: 1820–1992. *American Economic Review, 92,* 727–744.

Bromley, D. W., & Paavola, J. (Eds.). (2002). *Economics, ethics, and environmental policy: Contested choices.* Malden, MA: Blackwell.

Canadian Institute for Health Information. (2004). *Improving the health of Canadians: Patterns of health and disease are largely a consequence of how we learn, live and work.* Ottawa, Ontario, Canada: Author.

Cardarelli, K. M., & Aday, L. A. (2002). Health-centered rural policy: Integrating economic and community development. *Texas Journal of Rural Health, 20*(4), 35–43.

Case, A. C. (2001). *Does money protect health status? Evidence from South African pensions* (NBER Working Paper No. 8495). Cambridge, MA: National Bureau of Economic Research.

Dahlgren, G., Nordgren, P., & Whitehead, M. (Eds.). (1996). *Health impact assessment of the EU Common Agricultural Policy.* Stockholm: Swedish National Institute of Public Health.

Deaton, A. (2002). Policy implications of the gradient of health and wealth: An economist asks, would redistributing income improve population health? *Health Affairs, 21*(2), 13–30.

Deaton, A. (2003). Health, inequality, and economic development. *Journal of Economic Literature, 41,* 113–158.

Department of Health. (2001). *From vision to reality.* London: Author.

Evans, R. G. (2002). *Interpreting and addressing inequalities in health: From Black to Acheson to Blair to . . . ? Seventh annual lecture.* London: Office of Health Economics.

Exworthy, M., Stuart, M., Blane, D., & Marmot, M. (2003). *Tackling health inequalities since the Acheson report.* Bristol, United Kingdom: Policy Press.

Floud, R., & Harris, B. (1996). *Health, height and welfare: Britain 1700–1980* (NBER Working Paper No. h0087). Cambridge, MA: National Bureau of Economic Research.

Fogel, R. W. (1991). *New sources and new techniques for the study of secular trends in nutritional status, health, mortality, and the process of aging* (NBER Working Paper No. 0026). Cambridge, MA: National Bureau of Economic Research.

Fogel, R. W. (1997). New findings on secular trends in nutrition and mortality: Some implications for population theory. In M. R. Rosenzweig & O. Stark (Eds.), *Handbook of population and family economics* (pp. 433–481). New York: Elsevier.

Fogel, R. W. (2000). *The fourth great awakening and the future of egalitarianism.* Chicago: University of Chicago Press.

Franzini, L., Ribble, J., & Spears, W. (2001). The effects of income inequality and income level on mortality vary by population size in Texas counties. *Journal of Health and Social Behavior, 42,* 373–387.

Gallup, J. L., & Sachs, J. (2000). *The economic burden of malaria* (CID Working Paper No. 52). Cambridge, MA: Harvard University, Center for International Development.

Gershman, J., Irwin, A., & Shakow, A. (2003). Getting a grip on the global economy: Health outcomes and the decoding of development discourse. In R. Hofrichter (Ed.), *Health and social justice: Politics, ideology, and inequity in the distribution of disease* (pp. 157–194). San Francisco: Jossey-Bass.

Gorman, D., Douglas, M. J., Conway, L., Noble, P., & Hanlon, P. (2003). Transport policy and health inequalities: A health impact assessment of Edinburgh's transport policy. *Public Health, 117,* 15–24.

Grameen Communications. (1998). *A short history of Grameen Bank.* Retrieved August 16, 2004, from http://www.grameen-info.org/bank/hist.html

Gravelle, H. (1998). How much of the relation between population mortality and unequal distribution of income is a statistical artefact? *British Medical Journal, 316,* 382–385.

Gruber, J., & Wise, D. A. (Eds.). (1999). *Social security and retirement around the world.* Chicago: University of Chicago Press.

Heyne, P., Boettke, P. J., & Prychitko, D. L. (2005). *The economic way of thinking* (11th ed.). Upper Saddle River, NJ: Prentice Hall.

Hobdell, M. H. (2001). Economic globalization and oral health. *Oral Diseases, 7,* 137–143.

Huynh, P. (2002). *The emergence of a population perspective within Canada: The influence of a research organization on the public policy process.* Unpublished doctoral dissertation, University of Texas Health Science Center at Houston School of Public Health.

Institute of Medicine, Committee on Assuring the Health of the Public in the 21st Century. (2003). *The future of the public's health in the 21st century.* Washington, DC: National Academies Press.

International Conference on Reducing Social Inequalities in Health. (2002). The Copenhagen declaration on reducing social inequalities in health. *Scandinavian Journal of Public Health, 59*(Suppl.), 78–79.

Jack, W. (1999). *Principles of health economics for developing countries.* Washington, DC: World Bank Institute.

James, W.P.T., Nelson, M., Ralph, A., & Leather, S. (1997). Socioeconomic determinants of health: The contribution of nutrition to inequalities in health. *British Medical Journal, 314,* 1545–1549.

Jamison, D. T., Sachs, J. D., & Wang, J. (2001). *The effect of the AIDS epidemic on economic welfare in sub-Saharan Africa* (CMH Working Paper No. WG1: 13). Geneva: World Health Organization Commission on Macroeconomics and Health.

Johnson, J. V., & Hall, E. M. (1995). Class, work, and health. In B. C. Amick III, S. Levine, A. R. Tarlov, & D. C. Walsh (Eds.), *Society and health* (pp. 247–271). New York: Oxford University Press.

Johnson, T. G. (2001). The rural economy in a new century. *International Regional Science Review, 24*(1), 21–37.

Judge, K. (1995). Income distribution and life expectancy: A critical appraisal. *British Medical Journal, 311,* 1282–1285.

Judge, K., Mulligan, J. A., & Benzeval, M. (1998). Income inequality and population health. *Social Science and Medicine, 46,* 567–579.

Kaplan, G. A., & Lynch, J. W. (2001). Is economic policy health policy? *American Journal of Public Health, 91,* 351–353.

Kaplan, G. A., Pamuk, E. R., Lynch, J. W., Cohen, R. D., & Balfour, J. L. (1996). Inequality in income and mortality in the United States: Analysis of mortality and potential pathways. *British Medical Journal, 312,* 999–1003.

Kawachi, I. (2000). Income inequality and health. In L. F. Berkman & I. Kawachi (Eds.), *Social epidemiology* (pp. 76–94). New York: Oxford University Press.

Kawachi, I., & Kennedy, B. P. (1999). Income inequality and health: Pathways and mechanisms. *Health Services Research, 34,* 215–227.

Kawachi, I., & Kennedy, B. P. (2002). *The health of nations: Why inequality is harmful to your health.* New York: New Press.

Kennedy, B. P., Kawachi, I., Glass, R., & Prothrow-Stith, D. (1998). Income distribution, socioeconomic status, and self-rated health in the United States: Multilevel analysis. *British Medical Journal, 317,* 917–921.

Kennedy, B. P., Kawachi, I., & Prothrow-Stith, D. (1996). Income distribution and mortality: Cross sectional ecological study of the Robin Hood index in the United States. *British Medical Journal, 312,* 1004–1007.

Kitagawa, E. M., & Hauser, P. M. (1973). *Differential mortality in the United States: A study of socioeconomic epidemiology.* Cambridge, MA: Harvard University Press.

Krasnik, A., & Rasmussen, N. K. (2002). Reducing social inequalities in health: Evidence, policy, and practice. *Scandinavian Journal of Public Health, 59*(Suppl.), 1–5.

Krieger, N. (2000). Discrimination and health. In L. F. Berkman & I. Kawachi (Eds.), *Social epidemiology* (pp. 36–75). New York: Oxford University Press.

Krieger, N. (2001). Theories for social epidemiology in the 21st century: An ecosocial perspective. *International Journal of Epidemiology, 30,* 668–677.

Krieger, N., Northridge, M., Gruskin, S., Quinn, M., Kriebel, D., Smith, G. D., et al. (2003). Assessing health impact assessment: Multidisciplinary and international perspectives. *Journal of Epidemiology and Community Health, 57,* 659–662.

Labonte, R. (2003). Globalization, trade, and health: Unpacking the links and defining health public policy options. In R. Hofrichter (Ed.), *Health and social justice: Politics, ideology, and inequity in the distribution of disease* (pp. 469–500). San Francisco: Jossey-Bass.

Lalonde, M. (1974). *A new perspective on the health of Canadians: A working document.* Ottawa, Ontario, Canada: Department of National Health and Welfare.

Lantz, P. M., House, J. S., Lepkowski, J. M., Williams, D. R., Mero, R. P., & Chen, J. M. (1998). Socioeconomic factors, health behaviors, and mortality: Results from a nationally representative prospective study of US adults. *Journal of the American Medical Association, 279,* 1703–1708.

Lavis, J. N., Ross, S. E., Hurley, J. E., Hohenadel, J. M., Stoddart, G. L., Woodward, C. A., et al. (2002). Examining the role of health services research in public policymaking. *Milbank Quarterly, 80,* 125–154.

Lavis, J. N., Ross, S. E., Stoddart, G. L., Hohenadel, J. M., McLeod, C. B., & Evans, R. G. (2003). Do Canadian civil servants care about the health of populations? *American Journal of Public Health, 93,* 658–663.

Leventhal, T., & Brooks-Gunn, J. (2000). The neighborhoods they live in: The effects of neighborhood residence on child and adolescent outcomes. *Psychological Bulletin, 126,* 309–337.

Lock, K., Gabrijelcic-Blenkus, M., Martuzzi, M., Otorepec, P., Wallace, P., Dora, C., et al. (2003). Health impact assessment of agriculture and food policies: Lessons learnt from the Republic of Slovenia. *Bulletin of the World Health Organization, 81,* 391–398.

Lurie, N. (2002). What the federal government can do about the nonmedical determinants of health. *Health Affairs, 21*(2), 94–106.

Lynch, J. W., Kaplan, G. A., Pamuk, E. R., Cohen, R. D., Heck, K. E., Balfour, J. L., et al. (1998). Income inequality and mortality in metropolitan areas of the United States. *American Journal of Public Health, 88,* 1074–1080.

Lynch, J. W., Smith, G. D., Harper, S., Hillemeier, M., Ross, N., Kaplan, G. A., et al. (2004). Is income inequality a determinant of population health? Part 1: A systematic review. *Milbank Quarterly, 82,* 5–99.

Lynch, J. W., Smith, G. D., Hillemeier, M., Shaw, M., Raghunathan, T., & Kaplan, G. (2001). Income inequality, the psychosocial environment, and health: Comparisons of wealthy nations. *Lancet, 358,* 194–200.

Lynch, J. W., Smith, G. D., Kaplan, G. A., & House, J. S. (2000). Income inequality and mortality: Importance to health of individual income, psychosocial environment, or material conditions. *British Medical Journal, 320,* 1200–1204.

Macintyre, S., Chalmers, I., Horton, R., & Smith, R. (2001). Using evidence to inform health policy: Case study. *British Medical Journal, 322,* 222–225.

Macintyre, S., Ellaway, A., & Cummins, S. (2002). Place effects on health: How can we conceptualise, operationalise and measure them? *Social Science and Medicine, 55,* 125–139.

Mackenbach, J. P., Bakker, M. J., & European Network on Interventions and Policies to
Reduce Inequalities in Health (2003). Tackling socioeconomic inequalities in health:
Analysis of European experiences. *Lancet, 362,* 1409–1414.

Manpower Demonstration Research Corporation. (2000a). *MFIP, Reforming welfare and rewarding work: Final report on the Minnesota Family Investment Program: Vol. 1. Effects on Adults.* New
York: Author.

Manpower Demonstration Research Corporation. (2000b). *MFIP, Reforming welfare and rewarding work: Final report on the Minnesota Family Investment Program: Vol. 2. Effects on Children.* New
York: Author.

Manpower Demonstration Research Corporation. (2000c). *Reforming welfare and rewarding
work: A summary of the final report on the Minnesota Family Investment Program.* New York:
Author.

Marmot, M. G. (1986). Social inequalities in mortality: The social environment. In R. G.
Wilkinson (Ed.), *Class and health: Research and longitudinal data* (pp. 21–33). New York:
Tavistock.

Marmot, M. G. (2002). The influence of income on health: Views of an epidemiologist.
Does money really matter? Or is it a marker for something else? *Health Affairs, 21*(2),
31–46.

Marmot, M. G., Shipley, M. J., & Rose, G. (1984). Inequalities in death: Specific explanations
of a general pattern? *Lancet, 1*(8384), 1003–1006.

Marmot, M. G., Smith, G. D., Stansfeld, S., Patel, C., North, F., Head, J., et al. (1991).
Health inequalities among British civil servants: The Whitehall II study. *Lancet, 337,*
1387–1393.

McDonough, P., Duncan, G. J., Williams, D., & House, J. (1997). Income dynamics and adult
mortality in the United States, 1972 through 1989. *American Journal of Public Health, 87,*
1476–1483.

Mercier, J. R. (2003). Health impact assessment in international development assistance: The
World Bank experience. *Bulletin of the World Health Organization, 81,* 461–462.

Minnesota Health Improvement Partnership Social Conditions and Health Action Team.
(2001). *A call to action: Advancing health for all through social and economic change.* St. Paul, MN:
Division of Community Health Services.

Muurinen, J. M., & LeGrand, J. (1985). The economic analysis of inequalities in health.
Social Science and Medicine, 20, 1029–1035.

National Center for Health Statistics. (2003). Deaths: Final data for 2001. *National Vital Statistics Report, 52*(3), 1–115.

Navarro, V. (2000). Health and equity in the world in the era of "globalization." In
V. Navarro (Ed.), *The political economy of social inequalities: Consequences for health and quality
of life* (pp. 109–120). Amityville, NY: Baywood.

Nordhaus, W. D. (2003). The health of nations: The contribution of improved health to
living standards. In K. M. Murphy & R. H. Topel (Eds.), *Measuring the gains from medical
research: An economic approach* (pp. 9–40). Chicago: University of Chicago Press.

Nurturing economic growth through nutrition (2001, November 3). *United Nations Chronicle
Online Edition, 38*(3). Retrieved October 11, 2004, from http://www.un.org/Pubs/
chronicle/2001/issue3/0103p20.html

Porter, R. (1998). *The greatest benefit to mankind: A medical history of humanity.* New York: Norton.

Preston, S. H. (1975). Changing relation between mortality and level of economic development. *Population Studies: A Journal of Demography, 29,* 231–248.

Rao, M. J. (1999). *Openness, poverty, and inequality (Background paper, country and regional study or background note for Human Development Report 1999)*. New York: United Nations Development Programme.

Rodgers, G. B. (1979). Income and inequality as determinants of mortality: International cross-section analysis. *Population Studies, 33,* 343–351.

Rose, G., & Marmot, M. G. (1981). Social class and coronary heart disease. *British Heart Journal, 45,* 13–19.

Ross, N. A., & Wolfson, M. C. (1999). Income inequality and mortality in Canada and the United States: An analysis of provinces/states. *Annals of the New York Academy of Sciences, 896,* 338–340.

Rowentree, B. S. (2001). Poverty: A study of town life—1901. In G. D. Smith, D. Dorling, & M. Shaw (Eds.), *Poverty, inequality and health in Britain, 1800–2000: A reader* (pp. 97–106). Bristol, United Kingdom: Policy Press.

Samuelson, P. A., & Nordhaus, W. D. (2005). *Economics* (18th ed.). Boston: McGraw-Hill.

Sapolsky, R. M. (1998). *Why zebras don't get ulcers: An updated guide to stress, stress-related diseases, and coping.* New York: W. H. Freeman.

Sen, A. (1970). *Collective choice and social welfare.* San Francisco: North-Holland.

Sen, A. (1976). Real national income. *Review of Economic Studies, 43,* 19–39.

Sen, A. (1999). *Development as freedom.* New York: Oxford University Press.

Shively, C. A., Laber-Laird, K., & Anton, R. F. (1997). Behavior and physiology of social stress and depression in female cynomolgus monkeys. *Biological Psychiatry, 41,* 871–882.

Smith, J. P. (1999). Healthy bodies and thick wallets: The dual relation between health and economic status. *Journal of Economic Perspectives, 13,* 145–166.

Social Research and Demonstration Corporation. (2002). *Making work pay: Final report on the self-sufficiency project for long-term welfare recipients.* Ottawa, Ontario, Canada: Author.

Social Research and Demonstration Corporation. (2003). *Can work incentives pay for themselves? Final report on the self-sufficiency project for welfare applicants.* Ottawa, Ontario, Canada: Author.

Sorlie, P. D., Backlund, E., & Keller, J. B. (1995). U.S. mortality by economic, demographic, and social characteristics: The National Longitudinal Mortality Study. *American Journal of Public Health, 85,* 949–956.

Stiglitz, J. E. (2002). *Globalization and its discontents.* New York: Norton.

Subramanian, S. V., Belli, P., & Kawachi, I. (2002). The macroeconomic determinants of health. *Annual Review of Public Health, 23,* 287–302.

Subramanian, S. V., & Kawachi, I. (2003). The association between state income inequality and worse health is not confounded by race. *International Journal of Epidemiology, 32,* 1022–1028.

Subramanian, S. V., & Kawachi, I. (2004). Income inequality and health: What have we learned so far? *Epidemiologic Reviews, 26,* 78–91.

Subramanian, S. V., Kawachi, I., & Kennedy, B. P. (2001). Does the state you live in make a difference? Multilevel analysis of self-rated health in the U.S. *Social Science and Medicine, 53,* 9–19.

Syme, S. L., Lefkowitz, B., & Krimgold, B. K. (2002). Incorporating socioeconomic factors into U.S. health policy: Addressing the barriers: Commissions and special reports can get the ball rolling, but success hinges on getting various sectors into the game. *Health Affairs, 21*(2), 113–118.

Theodore, K. (2001). *HIV AIDS in the Caribbean: Economic issues—impact and investment response, 2000* (CMH Working Paper Series No. WG1: 1). Geneva: World Health Organization Commission on Macroeconomics and Health.

Townsend, P., & Davidson, N. (1992). The Black Report 1982. In P. Townsend, N. Davidson, & M. Whitehead (Eds.), *Inequalities in health: The Black Report* (New, revised, and updated ed., pp. 29–213). New York: Penguin Books.

United Nations Development Programme. (1990). *Human development report 1990: Concept and measurement of human development.* New York: Author.

Uno, H., Tarara, R., Else, J. G., Suleman, M. A., & Sapolsky, R. M. (1989). Hippocampal damage associated with prolonged and fatal stress in primates. *Journal of Neuroscience, 9,* 1705–1711.

U.S. Census Bureau. (2004, July 14). *Current populations survey, annual demographic survey, March supplement: Age and sex of all people, family members and unrelated individuals iterated by income-to-poverty ratio and race, below 100% of poverty—2002.* Retrieved October 13, 2004, from http://ferret.bls.census.gov/macro/032003/pov/new01_100.htm

Usher, D. (1973). An imputation to the measure of economic growth for changes in life expectancy. In M. Moss (Ed.), *The measurement of economic and social performance* (pp. 193–226). New York: Columbia University Press for the National Bureau of Economic Research.

Wallace, L. (2004). Freedom as progress: Linda Wallace interviews Nobel Prize winner Amartya Sen. *Finance and Development, 41,* 4–7.

Whiteis, D. G. (1998). Third world medicine in first world cities: Capital accumulation, uneven development and public health. *Social Science and Medicine, 47,* 795–808.

Whiteis, D. G. (2000). Poverty, policy, and pathogenesis: Economic justice and public health in the U.S. *Critical Public Health, 10,* 257–271.

Wilkinson, R. G. (1992). For debate: Income distribution and life expectancy. *British Medical Journal, 304,* 165–168.

Wilkinson, R. G. (1996). *Unhealthy societies: The afflictions of inequality.* New York: Routledge.

Wilkinson, R. G. (1997). Socioeconomic determinants of health: Health inequalities: Relative or absolute material standards? *British Medical Journal, 314,* 591–595.

Wilkinson, R. G. (2001). *Mind the gap: Hierarchies, health and human evolution.* New Haven, CT: Yale University Press.

Wolfson, M., Kaplan, G., Lynch, J., Ross, N., & Backlund, E. (1999). Relation between income inequality and mortality: Empirical demonstration. *British Medical Journal, 319,* 953–955.

Wolfson, M., Rowe, G., Gentleman, J. F., & Tomiak, M. (1993). Career earnings and death: A longitudinal analysis of older Canadian men. *Journals of Gerontology, 48*(Suppl. 4), 167–179.

World Bank Group. (2004). *About us: What is the World Bank?* Retrieved August 4, 2004, from http://web.worldbank.org/WBSITE/EXTERNAL/EXTABOUTUS/0,,contentMDK:20040558~menuPK:34559~pagePK:34542~piPK:36600,00.html

World Health Organization. (1999). *The world health report 1999: Making a difference.* Geneva: Author.

World Health Organization. (2000). *The world health report 2000: Health systems: Improving performance.* Geneva: Author.

World Health Organization. (2001). *Macroeconomics and health: Investing in health for economic development: Report of the Commission on Macroeconomics and Health.* Geneva: Author.

World Health Organization, Commission on Macroeconomics and Health, Working Group 1. (2002). *Health, economic growth, and poverty reduction: The report of Working Group 1 of the Commission on Macroeconomics and Health.* Geneva: Author.

World Health Organization, Stop TB Partnership Secretariat. (2002). *Stop TB annual report 2001* (Report No. WHO_CDS_STB_2002.17). Geneva: Author.

Yach, D., & Bettcher, D. (1998). The globalization of public health, I: Threats and opportunities. *American Journal of Public Health, 88*, 735–738.

Zollner, H. (2002). National policies for reducing social inequalities in health in Europe. *Scandinavian Journal of Public Health, 59*(Suppl.), 6–11.

Appendix 5.1

The Impact of Globalization on Local Urban and Rural Economies in the United States

Globalization has had a manifest impact on development in both developed and developing countries. The deindustrialization of inner-city economies and large-scale corporatization of agriculture in rural areas of the United States provide compelling examples of the local and regional impact of the rapid and fluid movement of capital into and out of geographic localities and regions.

Inner Cities

The industrial revolution in the late 19th and early 20th centuries led to the growth of industrial cities in the eastern and midwestern United States (such as New York, Detroit, and Chicago). A working-class, increasingly unionized workforce grew adjacent to the factories and sources of production. This growth, however, eventually grew to be self-limiting. As production increased, unemployment was reduced; wages and rents increased; and corporate profits diminished. An important cost-cutting mechanism introduced in the mid-20th century was the relocation of capital into regions where raw materials and labor were less expensive. Following World War II and the growth of highways and communication technologies, this resulted in the growth of exurbia. In the 1970s and 1980s, industry moved into the nonunionized Deep South and the Sun Belt; and since the mid-1980s, with the advent of globalization, it has moved to developing countries. Historical patterns of racism and residential segregation exacerbated by successive loss of jobs, reduction in low-income housing stock, and diminished public support for human services have resulted in a deterioration of the economic and social infrastructure in inner-city areas that has placed the poor and minority urban populations in conditions resembling those of the developing countries, including corollary health and public health consequences (Whiteis, 1998, 2000).

Local Rural Economies

Comparable trends regarding the growth and concentration of corporate capital and its rapid movement to areas in which raw materials and production and labor costs, as well as international trade policies, have also had manifest consequences for the major industries supporting local rural economies and communities—agriculture and mining (oil and gas production, coal mining, etc.). The increasing mechanization of agriculture and U.S. and international trade policies have compelled greater capital-intensive investments, corollary growth in the size of farms, and a shift to large-scale productivist and corporate agriculture. Expanded access to international oil and gas sources has also resulted in the abandonment of less profitable mineral extraction operations within the United States and the movement into countries where development costs are lower and environmental regulations weaker or nonexistent. The industries that may offer promising hopes for reinvestments in rural communities, for example, large-scale corporate hog farming, dairy, or poultry operations, often offer low-wage unskilled jobs without benefits and with increased occupational or environmental health risks. The consequence for the largely rural Great Plains and Appalachian regions of the United States, heavily dependent on agriculture and mining, is the depopulation of the rural landscape, the growing concentration of the elderly and poor, the corollary diminishment of the local tax base, and the shutting down of public institutions such as schools and hospitals that are essential for promoting reinvestment in the community (Cardarelli & Aday, 2002; Johnson, 2001).

CHAPTER SIX

COMMUNITY DEVELOPMENT AND PUBLIC HEALTH

Cynthia Warrick, Dan Culica, Beth E. Quill,
William D. Spears, Rachel Westheimer Vojvodic

Chapter Highlights

- Community development is a process that serves to empower individuals and groups as citizens in collective activities aimed at positive change.
- Economic and political institutions create, enforce, and perpetuate economic and social privilege and inequality that are the root causes of social inequalities of health.
- Community development that incorporates strategies for community empowerment and social change is vital for the development of a healthy republic.
- The equity of social and economic arrangements in a given locality, resulting from the full and effective participation of affected parties in shaping the decisions that affect them, represents the desired outcomes of successful community development.
- Public health practice combined with social support and targeted strategies aimed at community-based issues (racial discrimination, race-based and economically based residential and occupational segregation, toxic and hazardous living conditions, targeted marketing of commodities such as alcohol

237

and fast-food in poor neighborhoods, and inadequate health care) supports community development in the service of creating healthy communities.

- For public health the desired consequences of community development are to achieve the nation's population health goals and objectives and to reduce and/or eliminate health disparities.

Introduction

Community development is a process of engagement in which community members participate voluntarily in efforts aimed at improving their physical, social, and economic conditions (Lindsey, Stajduhar, & McGuinness, 2001). In this chapter we provide an overview of the theoretical foundation for community development, present evidence on the fundamental determinants, and provide examples of models and policies currently in practice.

Our goal is to show how current activities support and/or fall short of the success that could be accomplished through a community development approach to building a healthy (re)public. The chapter points out how the success of public health in achieving its essential mission of *healthy people in healthy communities* can be enhanced by enlarging and strengthening its role in local community development.

Overview

Community development builds on mutual trust and shared expectations among residents to mobilize cooperation and collaboration to solve problems and/or advance community goals through community building and community organizing. These activities produce assets such as reinforced values and reliance that improve neighborhood quality of life (Ferguson & Dickens, 1999; Lindsey et al., 2001; McNeely, 1999). How successful a community is at solving problems and achieving its goals depends on the resources, leadership, trust, communication, cooperation, and networks that make up its social and cultural capital (social ties and community values). Community development is an approach that works from the ground up, using democratic participatory processes to channel political and economic forces to promote change. By incorporating public health goals into community development strategies, sustainable improvements in population health can be achieved.

Why is public health important in community development? The Institute of Medicine's Committee for the Study of the Future of Public Health (1988, p. 43) identified the three major functions of public health as a field:

1. *Assessment*—assessment and monitoring of the health of communities and populations at risk to identify health problems and priorities
2. *Policy development*—formulating public policies, in collaboration with community and government leaders, designed to solve identified local and national health problems and priorities
3. *Assurance*—assuring that all populations have access to appropriate and cost-effective care, including health promotion and disease prevention services, and evaluation of the effectiveness of that care

The role of the field of public health in community development is the facilitation, development, and management of social capital to monitor the health of communities, develop community-based strategies and interventions to address community health problems, and improve population health through disease prevention and greater accessibility to quality and effective health care.

The Healthy People Agenda. Healthy People, the nation's public health promotion and disease prevention agenda, is a framework that recognizes that individual health and community health are interdependent and that community health is affected by the beliefs, attitudes, and behaviors of all members in the community (U.S. Department of Health & Human Services [USDHHS], 2001). Healthy People sets goals and objectives to improve health and reduce mortality. The first Healthy People set of national health targets was released in 1979 and adopted five goals: to reduce mortality among four age groups—infants, children, adolescents and young adults, and adults—and to increase independence among older adults. The first report, *Healthy People 2000*, was released in 1990 and established a more comprehensive agenda organized into 22 priority areas, with 319 supporting objectives. Its three overarching goals were to increase years of healthy life, reduce disparities in health among different population groups, and achieve access to preventive health services (USDHHS, 1991, 2000a).

The public health agenda, *Healthy People 2010*, adopted the vision "Healthy People in Healthy Communities" and proposed a systems approach to community health improvement (Figure 6.1). A *healthy community* is a place in which the community assumes a leadership role in assessing its own resources and needs, where public health and social infrastructure and policies support health, and where essential public health services are available (Wilcox & Knapp, 2000). The two principal goals of *Healthy People 2010* are to "increase quality and years of healthy life" and to "eliminate health disparities" (USDHHS, 2000b).

The *Healthy People 2010* approach to the improvement of health status as portrayed in Figure 6.1 is an interactive process from the development of goals and objectives that support policies and interventions to improve population health

FIGURE 6.1.   HEALTHY PEOPLE IN HEALTHY COMMUNITIES:
A SYSTEMATIC APPROACH TO HEALTH IMPROVEMENT.

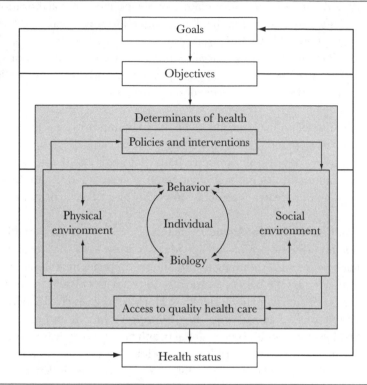

Note. From *Healthy People 2010: Introduction,* by U.S. Department of Health and Human Services, 2000, p. 6, retrieved from http://www.healthypeople.gov/document/html/uih/uih_1.htm

through increased access to quality health care. The Healthy People agenda has made some progress toward improving health in areas, such as firearm-related deaths and syphilis, at the national level. Improvements measured at the national level, however, may not be evidenced at the community level. For example, although infant mortality has decreased from 10.1 deaths per 1,000 live births in 1987 to 7.1 deaths per live births for the nation in 2000, for black infants the 2000 rate was 17.1 deaths per 1,000 live births (USDHHS, 2001). The rates in some minority communities are even higher; the infant mortality rate in 2000 for Ward 8 in Washington, DC, equaled 27.5 deaths per 1,000 live births, exceeding the rates of some developing countries (District of Columbia, State Center for Health Statistics Administration, Department of Health, 2002).

The Healthy People approach has made progress through enhancing community involvement in the national agenda-setting process, but it has not been successful in eliminating health disparities at the community level. Financial (health insurance), structural (facilities and services), and personal (culture and education) barriers to health care have been offered as explanations for the differences in mortality and morbidity between ethnic minority populations and the white (non-Hispanic) majority (USDHHS, 2001). Health disparities, however, are multidimensional, complicated issues that cannot be addressed through the provision of health care alone. As argued and documented in the earlier chapters of this book, "Health disparities are rooted in fundamental social structure inequalities" (Cohen & Northridge, 2000, p. 841). In this chapter we propose that health disparities could be addressed more effectively through public health–based community development.

The Healthy Communities Movement. In 1984 Dr. Leonard Duhl outlined a comprehensive community-based approach to improving public health by addressing the broad range of factors that influence the health and quality of life in cities. In contrast to the Healthy People agenda, Duhl's vision of "Healthy Cities" goes beyond a health care approach to a holistic commitment that directly involves citizens in the decision making and action required for community and social change (Kesler, 2000).

The Healthy Communities movement that resulted adopted eight guiding principles (Norris & Pittman, 2000):

- The use of a broad definition of *health* that encompasses the full range of quality-of-life issues, including behavior, genetics, socioeconomic, cultural, and the physical environment
- The use of a broad definition of *community* to include faith, professional, and geographic perspectives
- A shared vision from community values to identify goals and priorities
- The pursuit of an improved quality of life
- Diverse citizen participation and community empowerment
- A focus on systems change toward community decision making
- The development of local assets and resources to create a community infrastructure that encourages health
- The development of performance measures and community indicators to provide information to the community about their progress

These ideals are integral to our concept of community development and public health. By building on the foundation put forth by Healthy People in Healthy

Communities, also known as *Healthy People 2010,* the Healthy Communities agenda campaign provides evidence for how to put the theories and principles of community development into practice. As part of its goals and objectives, *Healthy People 2010* encourages local and state leaders to develop communitywide and statewide efforts that promote healthy behaviors, create healthy environments, and increase access to high-quality health care (USDHHS, 2001). We will discuss specific initiatives later in this chapter.

The Healthy People and Healthy Communities processes have helped to ground our approach on the role of community development and public health in improving the health of the public. The Healthy People agenda recognizes the disparities in population health and sets goals and objectives that establish policy priorities to address these issues. Some of the policies and programs have been effective in improving the nation's health overall but have been ineffective in addressing the disparities in racial and ethnic minorities. We propose that by taking a community development approach in public health, the policy and program outcomes will be more successful in relieving health disparities and sustaining improvements in population health. The Healthy Communities movement provides an important foundation for understanding how public health may facilitate community development. In discussing the strengths and limitations of current policies later in this chapter, we review a program that resulted from the Healthy Communities movement, California Smoke-Free, that demonstrates how community development activities can stimulate positive change toward health improvement.

Fields of Study

In the following sections, we present the essential components to define and understand community development that include illuminating what is meant by community (or neighborhood), a sense of community, collective efficacy, social capital, community building, and community-based participatory research.

Community. Communities can be defined by their location or geography, values and interests, or by affiliation. Most research in this area focuses on communities formed on the basis of where people live (Mattessich & Monsey, 1997). Community is the social place shared by family, friends, neighbors, clubs, civic groups, churches, ethnic groups, local media, and local government (McKnight, 1995). It is the collective association of groups who share geographic boundaries, sense of membership, culture, norms, language, values, interests, the reality of living or working in the same location, and common health risks and problems (Institute of Medicine, Committee on Assuring the Health of the Public in the 21st Century, 2003). These associations are often interdependent and built on trust. The capacity of the associations is demonstrated through collective effort, informality, stories, celebration, and tragedy. Although researchers tend to define communities on the basis of demographic characteristics, it is important to ask members of the community what they perceive their boundaries, representatives, and concerns to be (Sullivan et al., 2003).

Communities may also be defined as settings when actions are directed to change individual behaviors in certain geographic locations. When changes in the health status of a community as a result of policies and programs are the principal goal, the community is viewed as a target (McLeroy, Norton, Kegler, Burdine, & Sumaya, 2003). As an asset, community places emphasis on ownership and participation to achieve desired outcomes, and interventions may involve external resources as well. Community can also be identified as an agent when interventions do not involve external resources and when the community relies on its own units of solution (practice) for community development (McLeroy et al., 2003). Although communities participate as (potential) resources in government-centered models, they become agents (of change) in community-based models, targeting a population that lives in a setting. Consequently, community as a resource is related to the development of community infrastructure and capacity, whereas community as an agent works to sustain itself as a functioning civil society (McLeroy et al., 2003).

Sense of Community and Collective Efficacy. Community psychologists have defined *sense of community* as a feeling of belonging and a commitment to fulfill the needs of community members (Chipuer & Pretty, 1999). McMillan and Chavis (1986) incorporate these dynamics into a model that consists of four dimensions:

- Membership and identification with the larger collective that produces a sense of belonging
- Influence characterized by reciprocity among individuals and community to affect change in each other
- Fulfillment of needs through cooperative behavior within the community
- Emotional connection characterized by mutual support through the struggles and successes of community living

Similar ideas are expressed in the health promotion literature through terms like *social cohesion* and *collective efficacy*, which equate with developing a sense of community. *Social cohesion* refers to two closely related features of society, the absence of latent conflict and the presence of strong social bonds (Colletta & Cullen, 2002). Latent conflict exists because of income or wealth inequality, racial and ethnic tensions, disparities in political participation, and other forms of polarization. Social bonds are reflected in the levels of trust and norms of reciprocity that produce civil society through institutions of conflict management such as a responsive democracy, an independent judiciary, and an independent media (Colletta & Cullen, 2002).

Collective efficacy, the ability of communities to come together for the common good (Sampson, Raudenbush, & Earls, 1997), provides the foundation for community sustainability, that is, maintaining residents' interest and investment in assuming responsibility for the environmental, economic, and/or equity affairs of the neighborhood over the long term (Hyman, 2002; Innes & Booher, 2000). A theoretical concept more than a community action, collective efficacy is highlighted as the result of trust and social cohesion of community members coming spontaneously together as a mechanism for maintaining public order (Sampson, Morenoff, & Gannon-Rowley, 2002).

A task-oriented construct, collective efficacy emphasizes community members' expectations and ability to act (engage) jointly for a common purpose or against a common threat (Morenoff, Sampson, & Raudenbush, 2001). It was introduced in association with the study of variation in violent crimes, showing a strong association with low rates of violence (Sampson et al., 1997). Collective efficacy operates by capitalizing on the community's ability to gather its own resources (assets).

Social Capital. *Social capital* is defined as the networks, norms, and social trust that facilitate coordination and cooperation for mutual benefit that result from a strong civil society (Putnam, 2000). *Civil society* refers to groups of people who contribute to community change through participation in activities that are not part of the formal political or market system, such as neighborhood associations (Baum & Ziersch, 2003). Social capital is a social good embodied through people's relationships and is created when the structure of these relationships facilitates action, making possible the achievement of certain goals that in its absence would not be possible. Social capital is not within individuals but in the structure of their social organization (Ferguson & Dickens, 1999, p. 255). It is the attitudinal, behavioral, and communal glue that holds society together through relationships among individuals, families, and organizations.

Social capital is measured by the extent of community associations and networks that produce information sharing and mutually beneficial collective action (Grootaert & van Bastelaer, 2002). Social capital and collective efficacy play complementary roles in community development and are interdependently linked for successful community development. Table 6.1 outlines the domains and local policies related to social capital.

TABLE 6.1. THE DOMAINS OF SOCIAL CAPITAL AND APPROPRIATE NEIGHBORHOOD POLICIES TO SUPPORT THEM.

Domain	Description	Local Policies
Empowerment	People feel they have a voice that is listened to, are involved in processes that affect them, can themselves take action to initiate changes.	Providing support to community groups; giving local people "voice," helping to provide solutions to problems, giving local people a role in policy processes
Participation	People take part in social and community activities, local events occur and are well attended.	Establishing and/or supporting local activities and local organizations; publicizing local events
Associational activity	People cooperate with one another through the formation of formal and informal groups to further their interests.	Developing and supporting networks between organizations in the area
Supporting networks and reciprocity	Individuals and organizations cooperate to support one another for either mutual or one-sided gain; they have an expectation that they would give or receive help when needed.	Creating, developing, and/or supporting an ethic of cooperation between individuals and organizations that develop ideas of community support; good neighbor award schemes
Collective norms and values	People share common values and norms of behavior.	Developing and promulgating an ethic that residents recognize and accept, securing harmonious social relations, promoting community interests
Trust	People feel they can trust their neighbors and local organizations responsible for governing or serving their area.	Encouraging trust in residents in their relationships with each other, delivering on policy promises, bringing conflicting groups together
Safety	People feel safe in their neighborhood and are not restricted in their use of public space by fear.	Encouraging a sense of safety in residents, involving them in local crime prevention, providing visible evidence of security measures
Belonging	People feel connected to their neighbors and their community and have a sense of belonging to the place and its people.	Creating, developing, and/or supporting a sense of belonging in residents; boosting the identity of a place through design, street furnishings, naming

Note. From "Social Cohesion, Social Capital and the Neighbourhood," by R. Forrest and A. Kearns, 2001, *Urban Studies, 38,* p. 2140, tab. 5. Used with permission.

Some forms of social capital, however, do not benefit vulnerable communities but provide barriers to the prevention of poverty, racism, and injustice, thus serving to produce and maintain inequality. These social networks assist white advancement through racial discrimination and segregation, "concentrating wealth and whites in suburbs, and poverty and minorities in cities" (Saegert, Thompson, & Warren, 2001, p. 37). "The deeper the inequality, the more exclusive social networks may become" (McClenaghan, 2000, p. 572). Additionally, local communities may exhibit internal cohesiveness, but the quality and resource value of their social networks may be very different. African Americans living in poor urban environments display some of the strongest forms of social capital, having the highest rates of church membership and participation in the nation (Saegert et al., 2001). However, health disparities within and between these communities occur because their social capital is not the type that can mobilize resources for community development, such as organizing to prevent a locally unwanted land use (such as the placement of a waste transfer station in the area). "The problem is not the absence of social capital in poor communities, but the fact that social capital is being asked to compensate for a lack of other resources" (Saegert et al., 2001, p. 274).

Link and Phelan (1995, p. 87) argue that the fundamental causes of disease are related to social conditions (race or ethnicity and socioeconomic status) that prevent access to resources (money, power, prestige, and/or social connectedness) that can be used to avoid risks or to minimize the consequences of disease. Incorporating public health strategies with community-based social capital assets could assist in the development of policies and interventions that successfully empower communities and improve and maintain community health.

Community Building. Local governments have increasingly begun to view their role as that of "convener of the various sectors and citizens rather than the sole entity responsible for making policy" (O'Connor & Gates, 2000, p. 159). Instead of engaging citizens to ratify a plan developed by government officials or staff, citizens are involved as participants in the development and decision making, thus building capacity in the citizenry to partner in problem solving. This activity represents *community building,* a holistic approach designed to strengthen the community, while addressing issues of inequity and poverty (Blackwell & Colmenar, 2000). Community building represents the efforts and activities of communities to develop and/or increase social capacity (the ability to work together). It works by building community and reviving civic life in neighborhoods to establish and reinforce sound values. People learn to develop attitudes of self-reliance, self-confidence, and responsibility to create human and social capital. Community building stresses working through community residents to develop relationships, cohesion, mutual trust, and strong community-owned institutions (McNeely, 1999).

The outcomes of community building are improved capacity to accomplish goals and a heightened sense of community through the strengthening of social and psychological ties within the community (Mattessich & Monsey, 1997). For community building to be effective, social capital, social capacity, economic resources, external investment, and community stability are needed. It requires policies that are sensitive to neighborhood stability and community-informed economic development. Communities with high social capacity can identify problems and needs, achieve consensus on goals and priorities, and cooperate with strategies to achieve goals (Mattessich & Monsey, 1997). These community-building activities are needed for sustainable community development. The following list provides examples of community-building activities (Ferguson & Dickens, 1999, p. 271):

- Establish social order and reduce crime.
- Collective strategies to clean up litter, vandalized cars, broken windows, and drug needles; remove or rehabilitate abandoned housing; stagger bar closing times to control unruly crowds; picket or protest public drinking, drug use, and prostitution; and organize walking groups for adults in public areas.
- Policies to encourage informal social control–organized supervision of leisure-time youth activities, enforcement of truancy and loitering laws, staggered school closing times to reduce thresholds or flash points of peer congregation, parent surveillance and involvement in after-school and nighttime youth programs, and adult-youth mentoring systems.
- Land-use planning to promote community–neighborhood environments that foster social interaction and public activities; limitation of neighborhood size.
- Integrating community with child development policy.
- Promoting housing-based neighborhood stabilization.
- Deconcentration of poverty.
- Maintaining the public service base—maintain fire, sanitation, and other vital municipal services.
- Increasing community power and organizational base—stable interlocking organizations, ability to secure public and private goods and services, promote community empowerment by involvement in local organizations and voluntary associations, tied to neighborhood associations and local institutions.

For community building to influence public health, Ellen, Mijanovich, and Dillman (2001) introduced four pathways: neighborhood institutions and resources, reducing stressors in the physical environment, reducing stressors in the social environment, and using neighborhood-based networks and norms. Community development occurs when democratic processes enable these activities to emerge. When residents are empowered to define their problems and develop their own solutions in the context of a safe and secure environment, trust is produced and motivates communities to organize and network, thus producing social capital and social capacity. Community building helps residents galvanize resources to shift local power toward community and policy development. Greater empowerment of community groups will help achieve changes in the physical environment, but "the very process may be beneficial to health through increasing collective efficacy, building social capital, and enhancing the social environment. The health effects associated with this process might be equal to or even greater than those associated with the outcome" (Institute of Medicine, Roundtable on Environmental Health Sciences Research and Medicine, 2001, p. 34). This is accomplished through governmental and public- and private-sector alliances and support.

Community-Based Participatory Research. Community-based participatory research (CBPR) is a method of bringing together community members with community development researchers for the purpose of "involving all partners in the research process and recognizing the unique strengths that each brings" (Minkler & Wallerstein, 2003, p. 4). The methods come from a variety of epistemological roots and have various names: CBPR, rapid epidemiological appraisal, environmental justice, and empowerment evaluation. All have common principles that involve participants integrally in the research process. CBPR methods emerged from work done with oppressed groups in Third World nations that involved community members in conducting research. CBPR methods involve community members in designing, implementing, evaluating, and reporting results. In this process the academic researcher serves not as an expert but rather as a facilitator and co-learner (Thrall, 2001). CBPR is an indispensable research model for understanding effective community development.

Policy Domains

Community development policy is grounded in an understanding of the principles of deliberative democracy. Freire (1970), Gutmann and Thompson (1996), Habermas (1984, 1996), Minkler and Wallerstein (2003), Young (1990, 2000), and others have identified a set of guiding principles underlying deliberative democracy. These include the discourse principle, as well as the principles of inclusion, political equity, reasonableness, reciprocity, and accountability. These principles in effect provide the theoretical and normative grounding for community development as a field of study and practice.

Deliberative Democracy. Jürgen Habermas is a German philosopher and author best known for developing the theory of communicative action. His belief that communication forms the common ground for solving society's problems is embodied in the concept of the lifeworld (Habermas, 1984). The lifeworld is formed by individuals' historical context and material condition and is the basis for their worldviews. This is relevant to community development because communities are formed by groups of people with shared locations or geography; because of that physical relationship, they also share experiences. When people communicate with each other, they discover shared common life relations (values, respect, and equality) and therefore share a particular worldview that defines their community. To achieve mutual goals and problem solving, Habermas (1996, p. xxvi) argued that communication must be fundamentally grounded in the discourse principle: "Only those norms are valid to which all affected persons could agree as participants in rational discourses."

Recognizing that community members have different goals and values, the discourse principle describes activities that are aimed at reaching consensus about a problem and the possible ways to deal with it that the stakeholders who are most likely to be affected by the outcomes agree on. Rational discourse involves a process of discussing positions in which participants make arguments in order to test whether a proponent's claims are valid (Habermas, 1996). This process of testing involves members developing their reasons for or against collective endeavors and having the opportunity to present their arguments. This process is most successful when it is noncoercive and is based on sound information and reason. The participants must be mutually committed to reaching an agreement in which each member understands that his or her individual needs will most likely be met by aiming for a result that is best for the group (Young, 2000).

Related to Habermas's communicative action and discourse theories, Freire's dialogical theory proposes that revolutionary leaders, who "believe in the potentialities of the people," dialogue with the members (oppressed) and join in "communion with the people" (Freire, 1970, pp. 169, 170) to establish true cooperation to carry out a liberating praxis, thus transforming their unjust reality. Through discourse, leaders and people, mutually identified, create the guidelines for action. Both Habermas and Freire emphasize the importance of engagement by all parties who will be affected by the outcomes of decision making in order to ensure that they agree on the outcomes, that the outcomes will be fair and equitable and will therefore serve the larger good.

Discourse is a type of dialogue. Dialogue is an act of communicating, such as having a conversation, and it is a way for people to learn of each other's perspectives and underlying reasoning. According to Freire (1970), dialogue can establish trust and provide a forum for transforming the community. The manner in which participants dialogue with one another is vital to carrying out democracy and achieving more just outcomes. For example, community development experts may transfer knowledge about procedures for successful community development to community members via a (one-way) monologue; however, a two-way dialogue in which members discuss personal views of the community and what they hope to gain may improve the chance of the community achieving its goals. When people are able to express how they really feel, to speak using words that characterize their perceptions about the world, it is then possible to begin the process of change. Participants who communicate rationally and toward mutual understanding, rather than being purely self-interested or coming to the discussion with preconceived goals and suppositions, are best able to establish the foundations of trust and collaboration that are necessary to solve community problems despite differing points of view (Habermas, 1996).

Deliberation is a discussion process aimed at producing reasonable, well-informed opinions through the uncovering of differing points of view (Chambers, 2003; O'Connor & Gates, 2000). The ideal but not necessarily required outcome of deliberation is consensus. Deliberation is important because people have limited generosity, which means that although most people are not entirely self-interested and selfish, there is a limit to the extent to which any given member will think of the greater good (Gutmann & Thompson, 1996). Deliberation provides a forum for community members to take a broader perspective than they might otherwise take; community members are able to sort out which disagreements are indicative of genuinely moral and potentially incompatible values and which ones might be due to merely a misunderstanding or lack of information. Through deliberation community members "can learn from one another, come to recognize their individual and collective mistakes, and develop new views and policies that are more widely justifiable" (Gutmann & Thompson, 1996, p. 43).

Young (2000) discusses the principle of deliberative democracy as a means of building social justice. According to Young (1990, p. 91), *justice* is

> the institutionalized conditions that make it possible for all to learn and use satisfying skills in socially recognized settings, to participate in decision making, and to express their feelings, experience, and perspective on social life in contexts where others can listen.

Deliberative democracy is a principle for guiding discussions in which differences in perceptions and beliefs may influence the decision-making process.

Five major principles emerge to guide the process of deliberative democracy in the service of social justice: inclusion, political equity and equal opportunity, reasonableness, reciprocity, and accountability (Gutmann & Thompson, 1996; Habermas, 1984, 1996; Young, 1990, 2000).

Inclusion. Essential to the practice of deliberative democracy is the ideal of inclusion. *Inclusion* means that all of those affected by the decision are included in the process of discussion and decision making (Young, 2000). When people become directly connected to the outcomes through participation in the decision-making process, they are more likely to be satisfied with the resulting solutions.

Political Equity. Political equity is achieved when affected parties are included on equal terms and have an effective opportunity to express their interests and concerns, to question one another, and to respond to and to criticize one another's proposals and arguments (Young, 2000). When major changes are occurring in the community, such as gentrification of old neighborhoods, it is important to encourage the participation of those who may be more vulnerable to exclusion from community development activities (such as poor elderly residents on fixed incomes) in order to achieve equal consideration and political equity (Gutmann & Thompson, 1996). Participants can achieve just outcomes when each member has an equal opportunity to make his or her case.

Reasonableness. *Reasonableness* refers to a set of dispositions that discussion participants have that aim to reach agreement, that is, willingness to listen, willingness to compromise, respect for others, and willingness not to judge others too quickly (Young, 2000). It is important for members to accept that each person has a right to be heard and to express an opinion even if it differs from other members' perspectives.

Reciprocity. Reciprocity is also necessary for deliberative democracy in that participating entities (such as researchers or government agencies) take the interests of others (the community) directly into account (Young, 2000). In order to receive a good on terms that one set of participants would consider acceptable, other participants must return a proportionate good in terms acceptable to them (Gutmann & Thompson, 1996). For example, when a local city government decides to locate a new freeway through a particular neighborhood, the freeway provides a good that serves the larger community but at a cost to the community adjacent to the freeway. For reciprocity to occur, government must negotiate with the local community to provide a proportionate good, such as erecting barriers to the freeway noise or investing in new neighborhood amenities, for example, parks and recreational facilities. Reciprocity does not always result in agreement; however, it does require that participants continually cooperate to seek fair terms.

Accountability. Finally, each participant is accountable to the others and therefore should express his or her interests in terms that aim to persuade others rather than to disregard their legitimate interests (Young, 2000). This ability to be accountable and justify decisions to affected parties is essential in a deliberative democracy (Gutmann & Thompson, 1996). In the example of the new freeway construction, the local government is accountable to the community that the freeway will most directly affect, and government would need to be able to justify the location decision and make a proportionate return for a good considered equally or more important to the greater community.

Inclusion, political equity, reasonableness, reciprocity, and accountability are conditions that create an optimum environment for deliberation; and they are the defining elements that support the principles of deliberative democracy (Gutmann & Thompson, 1996; Young, 2000). Just outcomes will result from deliberative democracy when all affected parties are included in the decision-making process (Habermas, 1984, 1996), when members have an equal opportunity to be heard (Gutmann & Thompson, 1996; Young, 2000), and when members are reasonable about how they treat each other during discourse (Young, 2000). Deliberative democracy is an important principle for community development because it can enhance the likelihood of both fairer and more effective outcomes (Young, 2000).

Community Development Model for a Healthy (Re)Public. The following model (Figure 6.2) presents our perspective on how community development and public health improve population health. It is based on theories of deliberative democracy and participative action operating through a public health and social capital context.

A partnering of assets between the public health infrastructure, collective efficacy, and community social capital work together and develop a strategy to solve a problem or achieve a goal through community development. The community development activities (sustainable community building and CBPR) produce a healthy republic, and the product of those activities creates a healthy public. This population health approach to improving community health combines the goal and agenda-setting activities of Healthy People and the grassroots community involvement processes of Healthy Communities.

Evidence Regarding Research on Fundamental Determinants

A large body of evidence indicates that social or societal factors exert a major influence on population health. Researchers studying social capital have used multilevel models that include the influence of community and regional factors along

FIGURE 6.2. COMMUNITY DEVELOPMENT MODEL
FOR A HEALTHY (RE)PUBLIC.

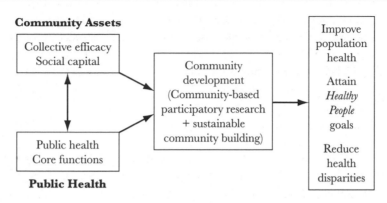

with individual measures to understand the impact of social policy on individual health. In this section we will discuss the process of CBPR in enhancing social capital and present evidence to show how community social capital works through deliberative democracy and CBPR to advance population health.

Social Capital as a Resource for Community Development

The domains of social capital outlined in Table 6.1 (empowerment, participation, associational activity, supporting networks and reciprocity, collective norms and values, trust, safety, and belonging) support the determinants of health in community development. In our community development model (Figure 6.2), we propose that social capital assets be generated in communities in order for community development to occur. Social capital is enhanced by partnering with the public health infrastructure to facilitate the development of policies that protect the community's voice in local decision making.

The concept of social capital has facilitated considerable dialogue among researchers, policymakers, and practitioners throughout various disciplines, including public health. In the previous section, we discussed how the principles of deliberative democracy could serve to facilitate dialogue and involvement among affected members of a community, but whether communication occurs and of what quality depend on the community's social capital.

A community's social capital is composed of a variety of relationships including friendship, workplace ties, membership in voluntary organizations, and neighborly interaction (Kilpatrick, Field, & Falk, 2003). The social capital domains identify the characteristics of communities that allow deliberative democracy to be possible. Veenstra (2001) indicates that social capital exists at multiple levels. Working at the surface or visible level, social capital is active in the daily personal interactions that reflect the connectedness within a community. It is also influenced at a deeper or less noticeable level by the economic system, political system, and civic society that underpin a state or community. The divides of race, social class, power, and deeply held moral values that characterize the deep structure of societies can have manifest consequences for generating and maintaining the connective ties of social capital within communities. Evidence regarding the role of social capital as a fundamental determinant of population health is presented in Chapter Two.

Establishing trust and respect is often a challenge to conducting effective community-based endeavors (Freire, 1970; Israel, Schulz, Parker, & Becker, 1998). Conflict associated with differing perspectives, values, and beliefs may be difficult to overcome and may hinder community development. Measures of social capital include trust in others and trust in institutions, civic engagement (membership or participation in organizations and groups), and social networks (close family, friends, and neighbors who provide support) (Caughy, O'Campo, & Muntaner, 2003).

Sampson et al. (1997) used multilevel modeling to study the influence of social capital on violence in neighborhoods. The researchers collected individual-level information on social cohesion among neighbors (collective efficacy) and violence. They used census data to measure differences in neighborhoods by levels of poverty, race and ethnicity, immigration, the labor market, age composition, family structure, and home ownership. After controlling for individual characteristics, they found that high social capital was negatively associated with rates of violent crime.

The principles that Young (2000) and Habermas (1984, 1996) discussed regarding the optimum conditions for achieving successful community development practices are based on a theoretical democracy in which all people are equal, reasonable, and included. In practice, democracies are riddled with inequalities such as inequalities of wealth, social and economic power, access to knowledge, and status; and people are pressed for time, participate in varying degrees, and have unconscious prejudices that all have an impact even on the most well-intentioned deliberations (Young, 2000). When inequalities of money and power exist, as in economic development and gentrification of old neighborhoods, the voices and issues of less privileged people may be marginalized by powerful outside interests of the more privileged. In such cases political power and material privilege may dominate and override the interests of affected communities.

Building collaborative relationships among community members may not be sufficient to surmount differences because power differentials among members and organizers are often substantial (Minkler & Wallerstein, 2003). For example, "the distribution of information, time, formal education, and income reflects broader social inequalities structured around race/ethnicity, class, and gender" (Israel et al., 1998, p. 183). Community development must focus around specific improvement initiatives that reinforce community values and build social and human capital. If social capital is to be built, success depends on shared power, capable leadership accountable to the community, and the involvement of a substantial proportion of residents (McNeely, 1999).

A community with a community vision, a desire for an improved quality of life, strong social cohesion, trust among neighbors, and high and diverse participation is a healthy community and has a greater potential for improving the health of the people residing within it.

CBPR as a Resource for Community Development

Public health professionals can advance community health through CBPR, one essential component of which is the principle of deliberative democracy. Israel et al. (1998) developed the following principles of CBPR:

- Recognize community as a unit of identity.
- Build on strengths and resources within the community.
- Facilitate collaborative partnerships with all phases of the research.
- Integrate knowledge and action for mutual benefit of all partners.
- Promote a co-learning and empowering process that attends to social inequalities.
- Involve a cyclical and iterative process.
- Address health from both positive and ecological perspectives.

CBPR methods involve community participants in the decision-making process and support and encourage them in continuing their involvement in other community activities. Kahn Rahi, of the Loka Institute in Washington, DC, says, "Community-based participatory research, for us, is conducted by, for, or with lay people. In many instances, lay people's involvement in research has had a profound impact on environmental health issues and social determinants of health" (Agency for Healthcare Research and Quality, 2003, p. 3).

Hindrances to community development are conflict within the community, differing values, beliefs, and perspectives that may be difficult to overcome. Establishing social trust and respect within a community is often a challenge to conducting effective community-based activities (Freire, 1970; Israel et al., 1998). Measures of social trust in others and in institutions, civic engagement (membership or participation in organizations and groups), and the extent to which one turns to close family, friends, and neighbors for support (Caughy et al., 2003) are operational proxies used to measure social capital. CBPR uses a deliberative process to engage the community in a dialogue facilitated by the researcher (community builder) that empowers the community through capacity building for improved health. Working together in this manner, the group builds trust and social cohesion among community members and between the community and the academic community, thus generating social capital.

A critical distinction is the extent to which community-based research emphasizes conducting research in a community as place or setting—in which community members are not actively involved—versus conducting research in the community as a social and cultural entity with the active engagement and influence of community members in all aspects of the research process (Israel et al., 1998). Conducting research in the community may provide useful information about disparities within the community, but it does little or nothing to build community capacity to deal with those disparities.

Communities engaged in community-driven research can strive to develop local assets and resources to assist in empowering the community to attain its vision (Etzi, Lane, & Grimson, 1994). CBPR engages community residents in activities that help them to better understand the strengths and resources of their community and teaches skills that can be beneficial in community building. Methods that CBPR researchers use engage individuals from the ranks of the community to become involved (Thrall, 2001). Hundreds of examples of successful citizen-led community-based projects related to building healthy communities, sustainable communities, and social justice exist across the United States. Most of these projects have implicit or explicit goals of using holistic approaches designed to strengthen community and address issues of inequity and poverty (McCulloch, 2003; Minkler, 2000). The following section will examine two projects, the Healthy Communities agenda campaign and the federal Healthy Start program; both use CBPR principles to put theory into the practice of community development.

Healthy Communities. The Coalition for Healthier Cities and Communities initiated the Healthy Communities agenda campaign, a project that identifies common patterns of a healthy community and provides specific policies and procedures for incorporating these patterns into communities (Adams, 2000). The campaign builds on the *Healthy People* principles by providing a tool for achieving the *Healthy People* strategy for creating a healthy community (see Figure 6.1). The strategy recommends that communities wanting to create a plan to achieve the goal of improving health should use a process to mobilize, assess, plan, implement, and track (MAP-IT) progress (USDHHS, 2001). The MAP-IT approach can help communities to build a structured plan that they tailor to the specific community. The communities mobilize individuals and organizations that care about community; assess the needs and interests of the community as well as the resources and other strengths available; plan the approach, such as the vision of the community and the action steps to meet the vision; implement the plan using action steps that the community can monitor; and track progress over time.

The Healthy Communities agenda recognizes that dialogue plays a key role in building and maintaining healthy communities. During 1999 more than 4,000 people took part in a campaign to develop the Healthy Community Agenda Dialogue Guide (Association for Community Health Improvement, 2005; Public Health Foundation, 2002). Communities can use the dialogue guide as a tool to achieve the objectives of MAP-IT. The dialogue guide attempts to bridge the gap between informal conversations among neighbors and civic governance by helping communities employ their voices and talents in order to get in touch with shared values. The goals of the guide are to establish shared purpose, break stereotypes, build working and trusting relationships, create new ideas, align multiple strategies, and take sustained action. The dual purpose of the guide was to stimulate action at the local level in order to build healthier communities and to provide a national message from communities themselves about the common patterns that were found for what creates health and improves quality of life (Association for Community Health Improvement, 2005; Public Health Foundation, 2002).

The following seven common patterns emerged from the dialogues for what a community can do to create health and improve quality of life for its members:

- Practice ongoing dialogue
- Embrace diversity
- Shape its future
- Know its defining values and identity
- Generate leadership everywhere
- Connect people and resources
- Create a sense of community

By following the process laid out in the guide, communities build consensus for communal action. They begin by asking community members questions such as these (Association for Community Health Improvement, 2005; Public Health Foundation, 2002):

- What are the two to three most important characteristics of a healthy community?
- What makes you most proud of your community?
- What would excite you enough to become involved (or more involved) in improving your community?

The protocol also offers guidelines such as establishing ground rules for the group: listen respectfully; everyone has an opportunity to speak; one person speaks at a time; making dialogue successful is the responsibility of all participants; and be tough on ideas, not on people—no personal attacks (Association for Community Health Improvement, 2005; Public Health Foundation, 2002). Asking participants to follow these ground rules exemplifies a way of including people in decision-making discussions and increasing the likelihood that people will feel their voices are heard. This process initiates a dialogue for finding common ground and shared purpose. The rules for dialogue attempt to create an environment that will facilitate rational discourse.

The Healthy Communities agenda campaign is an example of a community development initiative that incorporates the theories of community development. Applying the MAP-IT approach and the dialogue guide are examples of ways to achieve deliberative democracy because they are inclusive of community members, encourage reasonableness and reciprocity, and establish rules for achieving political equity and holding people accountable. This also creates the kind of legitimate process for rational discourse that Habermas (1984, 1996) describes. He discusses the engagement in rational discourse as an example of a just process that leads to just outcomes. The Healthy Communities agenda campaign exemplifies the concept of deliberative democracy by integrating these theories into its suggested process for community members who are working toward improving health in their communities.

Healthy Start. Another example of a large-scale community development policy initiative that incorporates community participation is the federal Healthy Start program that began in 1991 (Blackwell & Colmenar, 2000). At the program's start, the United States ranked 22nd in the world in infant mortality; and the goal of the program was to reduce infant mortality by 50% in the areas with the highest impact (PolicyLink, 2000). The program mandated that participants, residents, community organizations, and health care providers serve as community members in the planning, implementation, and evaluation process (PolicyLink, 2000).

PolicyLink (2000) initiated a nine-city study of the effects of community involvement in the Healthy Start program. The study found that "Community involvement played a key role in the development and delivery of training of health education, empowering individuals to change behaviors, improve health outcomes and become better parents" (p. 7). For example, caseworkers and outreach workers motivated their clients to become part of the consortium and arranged for their transportation to meetings. These clients motivated others to join Healthy Start, such as pregnant women bringing other pregnant women into the program.

By having program participants as consortium members, the program was more reflective of community concerns and more able to gain the community's trust.

Healthy Start was successful in focusing institutional and organizational attention on the needs and concerns that specific communities identified. For example, community leaders in New Orleans identified food access as a major concern; therefore, the consortium supported the development of a supermarket in a target community that had no food stores (PolicyLink, 2000). All of the Healthy Start programs are designed to meet the program's long-term goal of reducing infant mortality and improving health outcomes; however, specific programs implemented in each community depend on unique community needs and the community's involvement in designing programs to meet the Healthy Start goal.

The Healthy Start program also exemplifies the principles of deliberative democracy. Built on the foundations of successful community development that Gutmann and Thompson (1996), Young (1990, 2000), Habermas (1984, 1996), and Freire (1990) described, Healthy Start uses fair processes such as including community members and pregnant women in the decision-making process and encouraging participants to rationally and reasonably debate a variety of positions. By mandating the involvement of a variety of community members, Healthy Start allows for political equity and encourages reciprocity and accountability in the decision-making process.

Following the principles of deliberative democracy ensures community involvement and enables communities to develop according to what its members most need and desire. Through active engagement in community dialogue, members will enhance the prospect for creating healthy communities. The section that follows views alternative policy models for translating community development principles into practice.

Current Policies That Address Fundamental Determinants

This section reviews the applications of models of government, community, and market-centered decision making to community development and public health. We will focus on community-driven policies and compare different approaches to dealing with communities. Table 6.2 presents a framework to compare these models as they emerge at the government, community, and market level, emphasizing their focus and means for development, as well as particular scientific methods that explain different health policy approaches to community development. Critical analyses will identify the contributions of each model and their associated strengths and limitations in addressing the health of communities.

TABLE 6.2.   MODELS OF COMMUNITY DEVELOPMENT.

	Government	Community	Market
Dimensions	Building	Sustainability	Growth
Focus	Infrastructure	Empowerment	Investment
Means	Needs assessments	Community values and assets assessments	Economic growth
Research base	Scientific studies (positivist science)	Postpositivist methods (social learning, ethnography)	Supply-demand analyses

Government Models

Government-centered policies focus on building community infrastructure with support from technical experts. This model of community development engages a technocratic (expert-dominated) approach (Rosenau, 1994). Highly identified with community health planning and mostly performed by experts in management, planning, and policy analysis, this community-building strategy is the one that those in governing positions prefer (Rohrer, 1999). It is grounded in the positivist paradigm, which argues that an objective reality exists that can be captured and understood, and it relies on the scientific method and related hypothesis testing. The research base for the governmental planning model is typically grounded in needs assessments and performance measurement to identify and monitor community health problems (Denzin & Lincoln, 2000). Proponents of government-centered policies are viewed as pragmatists because they emphasize the necessity of having government and donors involved in identifying needs and outside resources, in order to generate and generalize a program or product (one-size-fits-all approach) once established (Morgan, 2001).

Community Models

Community-centered policies for sustainable community development emphasize the process of involving the local community in decision making about their own health through community empowerment and related CBPR (Morgan, 2001; Rohrer, 1999; Rosenau, 1994). This multidimensional approach of collaboration between population health research and practice communities is rooted in the ecological paradigm, which acknowledges the role of multiple systems (social, economic, and political) on community behavior and access to health (Institute of Medicine, Committee on Assuring, 2003; Israel et al., 1998). Community-centered policies advance the consideration of community values and assets in community development to increase the likelihood of sustainable communities (Campbell & Jovchelovitch, 2000). The development of CBPR created the opportunity to unveil and incorporate community values (context) and culture into policymaking and involve the public in the discourse regarding health improvement. Morgan (2001) demonstrated that government-centered proponents viewed context and culture as barriers to health policy development, whereas community-centered advocates (activists) saw merit in local initiatives related to the community's perspective of public health.

Whereas a deficiency model (needs assessment) is characteristic of government-centered policies, the asset model (assets assessment) supports community-centered policies. The principle is to identify strengths and resources within communities and mobilize community members to act in their own interest (Kretzmann & McKnight, 1993). This alternative model does not exclude external resources or the professional assistance of decision makers for community building, development, and planning; but it includes the community members as experts for identifying the community's needs and assets. Integration of this portfolio of assets represented by local realities, values, knowledge, and other resources enables the dialogue between community members to reach a level of critical awareness. These principles characterize the community model approach in policy development and planning (Campbell & Jovchelovitch, 2000; Freire, 1970; Moser, 1998).

Critical thinking is achieved through the process of social learning, democratic dialogue, and participation producing empowerment. Through empowerment local communities are able to acknowledge their assets and reinforce their identity. Community empowerment, also related to the community's social capital, produces the collective efficacy and social identity needed for health-enhancing behaviors, central to a model for sustainable community development policies (Campbell & Jovchelovitch, 2000).

Market Models

Market-dominated models (discussed in Chapter Three) affecting population health at the community level encompass market-dominated medical care systems, economic development, and community development.

The U.S. health care system is largely dominated by the market, which can have adverse consequences for particularly at-risk populations. Insurance companies are consolidating and integrating providers into larger groups. The costs of medical services are rising dramatically, and health insurers are maintaining profit margins by shifting costs from the employer to the employee. Selective inclusion of members in the risk pools also continues to increase the exclusion of uninsured individuals and implicitly reduces community participation (Whiteis, 2000).

From an economic development perspective, market models, with their emphasis on growth, have dominated community development strategies as well. Investments such as bringing new businesses and creating tax benefits for investors produced economic growth in local areas. The market paradigm underlying local economic and community development initiatives has not necessarily adhered to community values nor contributed to sustaining community well-being (Aday, 1997). Failures and critiques of market-dominated economic strategies are presented in Chapters Three and Five.

The impact of market growth on populations at the community level has led to economic and social discrepancies that ultimately account for poor health and community underdevelopment. This is especially true among poor and minority socioeconomic groups due to inequality (Whiteis, 2000). These socioeconomically vulnerable communities predominantly located in inner-city areas bear the brunt of the gentrification process of rediscovery, redevelopment, and reinvestment of capital that displaces the areas' long-time residents. The result is that community development strategies may largely fail in terms of both empowering communities and enlarging their access to economic opportunity.

Promising New Models. Neither the government policies nor market-dominated community and economic development strategies have succeeded in directing policies and programs toward population health and sustainable community perspectives (Rohrer, 1999). In the discussion that follows, we review recommended strategies for public health interventions that involve the market or corporate model in improving the health of populations based on the report *The Future of the Public's Health in the 21st Century* (Institute of Medicine, Committee on Assuring, 2003).

Public and private employers can influence population health by providing health insurance coverage as an employee benefit. However, the challenges of a fluctuating economy with increased health care and prescription costs create additional burdens on employees who must pay higher insurance premiums and cover larger parts of their health expenses (co-insurance, deductibles) out of pocket, especially if they are employees of smaller firms. Policy analysts criticize this market domination, questioning the role and the ability of the employer to regulate the insurance market, and they support the idea that decisions regarding insurance options should reside with the employee or consumer of health care.

Moreover, it is in the interest of the employer to maintain the health and well-being of its workforce because this leads to a reduction in the employees' overall use of health insurance benefits. Illness is correlated with exposure to lifestyle risk factors, and many of these behaviors are associated with and influenced by work stress. The corporate world faces low productivity and reduced profits due to employee illness or injury. Employers could improve health by adopting health promotion and disease prevention strategies in the workplace to modify behavioral risk factors.

Another important role of business in influencing the health of the public is its impact on environmental health and mass behavior. Corporate industry in general has had a long-lasting impact on the physical environment through contamination and occupational health hazards. When problems arise (e.g., severe pollution, child obesity), the government will intervene to regulate the business or market in the absence of market forces (through the actions of the Environmental Protection Agency, for example).

Efforts have been made in recent years to redirect the market and business community approach to improving population health (referred to in Chapter Three). Investment by a corporation in community health is not only a corporate social responsibility but also an avenue to increase the profits of the corporation itself (Institute of Medicine, Committee on Assuring, 2003, p. 292). Investment in education, health promotion, and disease prevention programs can improve medical care delivery and enhance the perception of corporate industry as a good citizen. These investments motivate and attract a healthier and better-educated community toward local business.

Schlesinger et al. (1998) recommended a Healthy Communities perspective oriented toward community benefit in the organization and provision of health care. Borrowing elements of social justice theory, this multidimensional model places emphasis on health policymaking, allocating more resources to other essential determinants of health rather than exclusively to medical care, on limiting environmental hazards, and on transferring some responsibility for disease prevention to the managed care system. A collective effort between the medical care system (managed care in particular), public health, and other sectors is needed in order to make a positive impact on the community (Schlesinger & Gray, 1998). Suggested avenues to achieve this effort are developing minimum standards for public participation in community development, designing performance indicators to show community health improvement, and creating an incentive system to encourage collaboration between health plans, public hospitals, and community clinics.

To advance the vision of healthy people in healthy communities, the Institute of Medicine reports (Committee on Assuring, 2003; Committee on Using Performance Monitoring to Improve Community Health, 1997) make recommendations that support enlarging the role of public health in community development. Major directions include strengthening the public health infrastructure, generating intersectoral collaboration (including community participation), improving communication within and across sectors, creating accountability systems for public health services, and basing decisions on evidence, within a population health approach, to account for multiple determinants of health. Government, communities, and industry can all help to actualize these recommendations.

Summary

Government-centered policies can strengthen the public health infrastructure through reform of public health laws. Policies can assure competence in the public health workforce, including communication skills; development of information networks; continuous assessment of the public health infrastructure; increased access to public health services; improved flexibility of funding; development of accreditation and quality assurance systems; initiation of research to provide evidence for decisions, policies, and practice; and increased collaboration among elements of the public health system, including all levels of government (Institute of Medicine, Committee on Assuring, 2003). The role of governmental public health is more fully discussed in Chapter Seven.

Based on their resources and assets, communities are playing an increasing role in improving local population health. Community-centered initiatives require assistance in assessing their capacity, developing programs, and evaluating population outcomes to lead to reduction of local disparities in health.

The various contributions of market forces and businesses and employers need to evolve in a new direction with changed roles and new methods of engagement. Market-centered policies can assist community development to accomplish the nation's public health agenda through partnerships with local governments and communities. Through intersectoral collaboration with government agencies, industry can become actively involved in promoting healthy behavior and preventing illness and injury through health improvement programs at the work site, environmentally responsible corporate management practices, and related activities that promote community health and well-being.

Strengths and Limitations of Current Policies

Public policies present examples of community development and define actions in achieving population health outcomes along the behavioral, biological, environmental, and social dimensions (see Figure 6.1). Specific policies provide a means for illustrating various community development strategies. The models described in Table 6.2 illustrate that these policies to develop health and well-being can be manifested in government, community, and market approaches.

McKnight (1994) suggests that two critical tools for building community well-being are a system and a community. He describes the system as a tool composed of a few participants who desire to control and standardize outputs based on diverse inputs. Consumers and clients represent the major participants in government- and market-dominated systems, respectively. Community, he posits, represents social associations and active, self-generating groups of citizens. Community operates through a process of consent and citizen power. Complex systems that health professionals design without community involvement often grow and expand at the expense of the community social associations. In considering the formulation of community development policies designed to achieve healthy community policies, one must acknowledge both system and community influences.

Acosta (2003) makes a further distinction in policy, noting that the two sources of policy are the private sector (internal) or the public sector (external). Private policymakers include community-based organizations, corporate employers, faith-based organizations, hospitals, and local businesses. Public policymakers include state legislatures, county commissioners and boards of supervisors, city councils, county and city health departments, and local school boards, for example. Both private and public policymakers contribute to the development of communities.

Partnerships often provide a framework to link the multiple sectors and bridge the gaps between systems and the community, public, and private sectors. Mitchell and Shortell (2000) describe the performance of community health partnerships (CHPs) as an example of collaboration. CHPs are the voluntary collaboration of diverse community organizations, which have joined forces in order to pursue a shared interest in improving community health. CHP presents a community-organizing or -building example that reflects action on the institutional level. Many studies of CHP, however, have revealed that the partnerships often fail to achieve measurable outcomes. Nonetheless, the CHPs have a contribution to make. Molinari, Ahern, and Hendryx (1998) underscore the benefits of public-private collaborations in a 1995 survey elucidating the relationship of community quality of life and health status. Tarlov (1999) extends the argument for multiple sectors in policy development, integrating several conceptual models of public policymaking to specifically address the determinants of health and civic will.

As the previous discussion suggests, the interaction of government, community, and market models determines the success of efforts to improve population health. Further, these policies will be successful to the extent that they operationalize the principles of equity, efficiency, and effectiveness in attaining *Healthy People 2010* objectives and reducing disparities (see Figures 6.1 and 6.2). Thus, critically examining selected models through the lenses of equity, efficiency, and effectiveness provides insight regarding the process and outcome of community development policies.

Assessing Community Development Policies

We will analyze the strengths and limitations of community development policies in two ways. First, we will select six policies and present them in a typology of community development policies (see Table 6.3). Policies are organized by model of community development: government, community, and market. The values listed illuminate the underlying constructs that frame each community development policy (Aday, 1997). These policies create impacts at the individual, institutional, and community level. Central to the analysis is the extent to which citizens have participated in the decision-making process and in what form the participation is evident.

The second test of community development policies is an assessment of their strengths and weaknesses and their responsiveness to the criteria of efficiency, effectiveness, and equity (see Table 6.4). We will measure effectiveness by answering the question: Do current policies serve to improve population health and health disparities? We will measure efficiency by addressing the question: Do current policies invest in the most efficient mix of inputs to produce health improvements? And we will measure equity, expressed in terms of intergenerational justice, distributive justice, deliberative justice, and social justice, by the question: Do current policies satisfactorily address some or all of the equity criteria? In the following sections, we will designate the policies as meeting the respective criteria fully, partially, or not at all based on a qualitative assessment of the strength and consistency of evidence regarding these outcomes.

Selected Policies

The review of specific policies highlights the dimensions of the major types of community development models.

Policy Descriptions. We have selected six policies, two for each model (government, community, and market). These models notably are not mutually exclusive and may share characteristics to maximize the assets of each model. However, we have used the predominant characteristics for this analysis. We designed the review of policies to elicit a broad view of the types of policies inherent in the examination of community development. This perspective includes recognition of the international initiatives that inform the understanding of community development policies. Several studies in Europe, England, Sweden, Germany, Canada, and Australia examine the status of community development, health status, and policy development (Glouberman & Millar, 2003; Jan, 1998; Krasnik & Rasmussen, 2002; McCarthy, 2000; Morgan, 2001; Poland, Boutilier, Tobin, & Badgley, 2000;

TABLE 6.3. TYPOLOGY OF SELECTED COMMUNITY DEVELOPMENT POLICIES.

	Government		Community		Market	
Values	• Beneficence • Dependence • Public good		• Reciprocity • Interdependence • Mutual benefit		• Autonomy • Independence • Private interest	
Specific policy	**Community Services Block Grant**	**California Smoke-Free**	**Turning Point Land Use**	**Boston Community Policing**	**Enterprise Zone**	**Health Care Access**
Policy intent	Poverty reduction	Healthier air in buildings	Community planning	Reduced youth homicides	Economic vitality	Care for uninsured women
Domains of influence (determinants)	Economic, human, and community development	Community and human development	Community development	Human and community development	Economic development	Human and community development
Level of participation and decision making	*Moderate* Participation in governance and programs	*High* Organized community groups Advocacy for new policies	*High* Citizen planning and voting	*High* Citizens plan and operate community programs.	*Low* Business and government develop plans.	*Moderate to low* Professionals with some citizen participation

TABLE 6.4. EVALUATION OF SELECTED COMMUNITY DEVELOPMENT POLICIES BASED ON EFFECTIVENESS, EFFICIENCY, AND EQUITY CRITERIA.

	Government		*Community*		*Market*	
	Community Services Block Grant	California Smoke-Free	Turning Point Land Use	Boston Community Policing	Enterprise Zone	Health Care Access
Effectiveness: Do current policies serve to improve population health and reduce health disparities?	Partially met	Fully met	Partially met	Fully met	Not met	Partially met
Efficiency: Do current policies invest in the most efficient mix of inputs to produce health improvements?	Partially met	Partially met	Partially met	Partially met	Not met	Not met
Equity: Do current policies satisfactorily address some or all of the equity criteria?	Partially met	Fully met	Partially to fully met	Fully met	Not met	Partially met

Note. Fully met = strong evidence; partially met = mixed evidence; not met = little or no evidence.

Wismar & Busse, 2002). These studies underscore the need for community-specific research; and many countries, especially Canada, have well-developed community models. However, the international examples posed major challenges in comparability at the level of analysis and availability of outcome information.

Therefore, we provide only U.S. examples as a first step in exploring the relevance of the typology and constructs discussed in this chapter. Selection was further influenced by the amount of information regarding the policy, the significance of the policy, and the relevance to community development. The classifications serve to illustrate key elements of community development that are most prevalent and representative.

Government Policies. Government policies provide insight into the relationship of governmental imperatives to community development outcomes.

Community Services Block Grant. Community action has a long history initially marked by the Economic Opportunity Act of 1964 (Garson, n.d.). This statute was designed to eliminate the causes and consequences of poverty. It established community action agencies with a governance structure designed to promote maximum participation by low-income people; the agencies hired low-income persons and appointed them to the board. The premise was to involve impoverished citizens in identifying and promoting solutions to problems in their local community. Early programs included Head Start, Legal Services, the Community Food and Nutrition Program, Foster Grandparents, and National Youth Sports (National Association for State Community Services Programs, 2003a, 2003b).

In 1981 President Reagan consolidated many domestic social programs into the Community Services Block Grant (CSBG). Formerly, funds had gone directly to local communities, but under the CSBG, funds went to states for awards to local entities (usually community action agencies). New initiatives, under the CSBG in the 1980s and 1990s, included developing services for the homeless, child care, and assistance in natural disasters. In 1997 Congress increased the allocation for CSBG by 25%. This was noted to be a supportive gesture to states as they implemented the Personal Responsibility and Work Opportunity Reconciliation Act of 1996 (Welfare Reform Act). This legislation affected communities through individual income, employment opportunities, labor market shifts, and health care access for vulnerable community members.

CSBGs illustrate approaches to strengthen the community. The $672 million that Congress appropriated to the states in 2001 provided services to the poorest of the poor (National Association for State Community Services Programs, 2003b). The intent of this long-standing public policy is specifically to reduce poverty through local services. CSBGs provide nutrition, education, and employment to individuals.

Their domains of influence include economic development (employment and training), human development (Head Start), and community development (participation in and development of services). The level of participation and decision-making process is apparent in three basic tenets of the program: the community identifies the needs; participants are part of agency governance; and CSBGs created opportunities in the community for participants to improve their health and social circumstances. Participation was moderate in terms of visible input to agency governance and the development of agency programs.

Analysis of CSBGs yields evidence that the program only partially met all the criteria. The impacts of CSBG on the fundamental determinants of health show success in effectiveness. The familiar Head Start program suggests effectiveness in influencing human development. Success in changing the economic circumstances and contributing to the labor pool through education and training programs suggests success in terms of economic impact. Efficiency is difficult to determine. CSBG expenditures have not been successful in reducing the national poverty rate. Rather, real income of the poorest dropped, and the national poverty rate increased. A plausible explanation is that the resources may have been used efficiently and even leveraged nongovernmental resources to support the program but that the scope of the problem is large and allocated resources are insufficient to alter the national rates of poverty. We found evidence of equity in the CSBG policies in the fair distribution of services for those in need and the inclusion of citizens in the determination of programs. Fundamentally, this policy was designed to give a voice to the very poor through participation in agencies and program development. Little evidence is available to document the extent and level of participation. But researchers have documented the receipt of housing, education, and employment services (Claeson et al., 2002; Culyer & Wagstaff, 1993; Wagstaff & Van Doorslaer, 1993).

California Smoke-Free. Healthy Cities and Healthy Communities established principles of community development that stimulated many local and state policy initiatives. The California Smoke-Free Cities in 1990, using funds generated by the tobacco tax, engaged in developing policies to regulate secondhand smoke. Adhering to the principles of citizen participation, an extensive education campaign of the public and public officials began. The wave of local ordinances from 1990 to 1993 resulted in a state law in 1994 that banned smoking in all workplaces, including bars (Adams, 2000). This success reinforced the opportunity for citizens to participate and develop a positive outcome. Regulation of the environment through control of secondhand smoke is a policy that emerged in other states and communities with attendant community participation.

The intent of the policies was to improve the air quality in California buildings and communities. The principal domains of influence were community development and human development. Human development was enhanced by the elimination of the consequences of secondhand smoke and community development by noteworthy civic engagement. The level of participation and decision making is notably high, with organized groups of citizens developing, advocating, and successfully disseminating their policies.

This policy ranks high in effectiveness (improving health) and equity (fairness and distribution of benefits). Reducing smoking as well as secondhand smoke is quite likely to lead to lower health care costs and related reductions in absences from work due to illness, but the efficiency of this policy is likely to vary depending on the level of community and workplace enforcement. Efficiency was partially met through the allocation of tax dollars for this effort and the deliberate partnership of government and business. We were not able to discover the specific amounts of funds to quantify the analysis, however.

Community Policies. Community policies reveal the relationship of community cultures and values to community development.

Turning Point. The W. K. Kellogg and Robert Wood Johnson foundations were concerned about the capacity of the public health system to respond to emerging challenges in public health, specifically collaboration in explaining the health status of the U.S. population (Nicola, Berkowitz, & Lafronze, 2002). Initiated in 1996, Turning Point's goal "is to transform and strengthen the current public health infrastructure so that states, tribes, communities and their public health agencies may respond to the challenge to protect and improve the public's health in the 21st century" (National Association of County and City Health Officials, 2001, p. 9). Initially, Turning Point funded 41 communities in 14 states ($60,000 for a three-year period); later, it funded an additional seven states.

Turning Point health improvement experiments have three primary themes: "(a) a broader vision of what public health activity is, (b) a sharing of responsibilities for public health across the community, and (c) a drive to put the public voice back in public health activity" (National Association of County and City Health Officials, 2001, p. 49). Turning Point's public and private partnerships have focused on but are not limited to eliminating health disparities, increasing access to quality health care, preventing infectious disease, promoting healthier lifestyles, and protecting the population from hazards and toxins in the environment (Nicola et al., 2002). As a consequence, this national initiative spawned many local community-level policies. Many of the sites focused on assessment of the community. The following example illustrates an advancement to establish policies to promote community development, and it therefore characterizes the early actions of a community development approach.

The Turning Point project in Texas County, City of Guymon, Oklahoma, engaged citizens in planning and deciding on land use in their community. Developers seeking to develop a 700-unit mobile-home park wanted to build outside the city limits in order to avoid regulations of water, sewer, paved streets, and restrictions on lot size. Citizens assessed the benefits to the city from such construction and voted down the request; they subsequently approved the building of 150 subsidized homes within the city. Planning and land-use regulations are a common way that citizens participate in policy development to control their environment. Further, planned land use promotes optimal air and water quality and environmentally safe waste disposal practices to ensure healthier communities.

Turning Point programs, similar to the Healthy Cities and Healthy Community approaches, engage citizens in individual and collective action to improve the quality of their lives in their communities. The intent of Turning Point is to conduct community assessment and planning efforts with an emphasis on collaboration, multisector partnerships, and implementation of strategies. Community development is the fundamental focus through creating a collaborative process and structure to improve health. The means for doing so include assessing community health needs and assets and developing and targeting programs. Many Turning Point sites experienced growth in the number and types of institutional partners (National Association of County and City Health Officials, 2001). The level of participation and decision-making process, although varying from project to project, include structures at the national, state, and local level. A primary emphasis is on citizen participation, as evidenced by the land-use policy in the Texas County example.

Turning Point overall and with specific local examples is effective in developing and documenting partnerships to improve health. Health outcomes to support this success may not be realized or evidenced yet. The Turning Point initiatives can be presumed to be efficient because of the modest foundation and community investment and the subsequent results. The modest investment and scope of activities, however, may be inadequate to achieve the objectives. Lack of evidence on the scope of resources related to outputs limits definitive conclusions. Equity measures reveal that Turning Point has garnered success in including citizens and developing structures and processes that promise fairness. Its various sites either partially or fully met this criterion.

Ten Point Coalition. Concerned over gang-related killings, citizens and clergy in Boston initiated the Ten Point Coalition in 1995 to develop a citywide strategic plan. A key component of the neighborhood-specific plan was to retain a local neighborhood police presence to work with community members on prevention and youth development. Youth leadership and summer job programs with responsible adults were initiated to support the neighborhood youth. Further collaboration with the judicial system resulted in court advocacy and mentoring programs for youth. The Ten Point Coalition acts as a referral system for youth in trouble with the law. The policies resulting from this coalition have shown visible effects in the crime and health statistics. In 1994, prior to the program, six juveniles had been murdered; from July 1995 to December 1997, not one juvenile under the age of 16 was murdered by a firearm in the city of Boston. During the latter half of 1996, gun-related murders of those under age 25 dropped by 65%. Overall, the murder rate dropped to its lowest in three decades (Blackwell & Colmenar, 2000).

This policy illustrates community safety issues. The specific intent of the Ten Point Coalition policy was to reduce youth homicides in Boston neighborhoods. The domains of influence are human development and community development. Individuals benefited from the programs designed to prevent crimes. The community benefits from a safe environment in which youth can expect to advance and thrive. The Boston community policing effort ranks high in community participation because citizens volunteer in the programs as well as work with community partners to maintain community safety.

This policy is an example of effectiveness in a community development policy. The documented health statistics are evidence of the policy's positive outcomes. Reducing the rates of violent crime and related costs of incarceration and prosecution are likely to have benefits in terms of efficiency, but the costs and related benefits may vary across communities. Equity in this policy was fully met through broad participation and efforts to sustain the community policing.

Market Policies. Market policies focus on the role that private corporations and industry play in the economic revitalization of communities.

Enterprise Zones. Enterprise zones, originally a British concept, were designed to stimulate economic activity in industrial areas largely devoid of residents (Vidal, 1995). The U.S. derivation has included revitalizing adjacent residential neighborhoods as a complementary objective (Butler, 1991). The policy expressed the premise of employment as a benefit for the unemployed, but specific programs largely emphasized benefits for business. The primary focus of the state enterprise zones was economic development. Although the supporters of the enterprise zones shared the view that disadvantaged neighborhoods contained untapped human resources and capital, state programs did not design programs to achieve this objective. Studies of state programs reveal broad variability in employment opportunities. Empirical evidence suggests that communities of color and urban poor communities experienced limited employment opportunities. When new opportunities became available, the match between skills required and the local workforce often precluded local residents from participating in employment opportunities that the enterprise zones generated. In a review of the 36 state programs, Erickson and Freidman (1991) noted that all the programs consider levels of unemployment and household well-being but that the incentives to firms (tax credits and wage credits for employers who hire local residents) primarily stimulate business investment.

The enterprise zones are an example of a policy with an intent to address issues of poverty and with a primary focus on economic development. The economic investment and stimulation of economic resources is viewed as a mechanism to highlight the economic domain of influence. The predominant beneficiaries are the institutions (businesses). Limited community benefits from community employment opportunities are evident. Enterprise zones by design have a low level of participation and decision making. Government and business are the parties largely determining programs and policies.

In terms of effectiveness, the enterprise zones may contribute to population health and health disparities, but this appears to be a secondary outcome when compared to the primary goal of economic vitality. Likewise, investments in businesses may not be the most efficient means to produce population health improvements. Further, the policy is directed at supporting industrial vitality and not fairness or equity per se.

Health Care Access. Access to health care is a common concern of communities and a manifestation of the market-dominated medical system that often precipitates exclusion of specific populations that do not have insurance. In 1995, following the principles of Turning Point, Wyandotte County Community Health Partners in Wyandotte, Kansas, convened citizens, public officials, health care providers, and social service organizations to address two specific issues: access to care and maternal-child health services. Central to these issues was the concern about the level of services, access to care, and uninsured women. Community efforts resulted in two task forces: Access to Care and Healthy Pregnancy. Further, the mayor established the Access to Health Care Commission and provided local resources to support improved capacity of the local health department to monitor health and provide services. This is an example of partnerships that include public and private collaboration to influence the system and market imperatives (National Association of County and City Health Officials, 2001).

This county initiative had a particular intent to eliminate the risks to pregnant women and, through system changes, produce a more favorable market condition for at-risk women. Two determinants of health can be identified in the domains of influence: human development and community development. Most of the participation was on the part of health professionals and governmental representatives. Thus, citizen input was low.

The initiative partially met the effectiveness criterion because it established concrete efforts to reduce the risks specific to a health problem. With little data that directly link program costs to outcomes, it is very difficult to adequately assess the efficiency of the program. Individuals benefit from services, and the community benefits from system changes, though citizen input was low, resulting in an assessment that the initiative only partially met the equity criterion.

Summary. Our assessment of six selected community development policies provides a profile of some of the strengths and weaknesses of such policies. A major strength of the policies is that all the policies purported to have community objectives and participation as an objective or subobjective. Secondly, many of the policies influenced more than one health determinant and had impacts at multiple levels. This argues for multilevel analysis that captures the effectiveness, efficiency, and equity outcomes. Third, many policies resulted in secondary benefits (social cohesion, collective advocacy, etc.) that, if sustained, could be a framework for further advancing policies. In addition, community development policies provide support and actualization of the democratic process. The Boston community policing policy, which met most of the evaluation criteria, illustrates a series of activities from community participatory planning, implementation, and evaluation that present a model for data collection and analysis to assess community health benefits.

We noted several limitations of this analysis. First, data to substantiate the extent to which policies achieve their objectives and result in benefits to the community was frequently missing or of variable quality. It is apparent that government and market policies are most likely to have documented evaluations and quantifiable information to measure performance. Thus, the criterion for judging the effectiveness, efficiency, and equity of policies becomes subjective in many cases because the information across the types of policies varies. In addition, it is difficult to document the health outcomes and their link to these policies. Second, the description of the policies often emphasizes community participation but details little about the ways in which civic involvement is manifest. Third, policies vary widely in their scope and may not be mutually exclusive, influencing several domains. Selection of the policies was arbitrary, although we attempted to include several types and topical areas. Specifically, the effectiveness and efficiency of community development initiatives are not yet well documented, and the evidence with respect to equity is quite variable across programs.

Mechanic (2002) points out, as argued in Chapter One (see Table 1.3) as well, that improving population health and reducing disparities are often different objectives that sometimes conflict. Sen (1992, p. 136) further advances this notion: "A conflict can arise between aggregate considerations (generally enhanced individual advantages, no matter how distributed) and distributive ones (reducing the disparities in the distribution of advantages)." Practitioners, researchers, and citizens concerned with examining the policies related to community development and health disparities face the challenge of distinguishing the contribution of the policies to the eventual outcome. This critical linkage determines the extent to which evidence supports the policy's success. Many outcomes of the policies are not apparent for long periods of time. Thus, the impact of these community development policies requires longitudinal evaluation to ensure that investigators consider evidence of all aspects of policy development, implementation, and evaluation. Researchers, practitioners, and citizens must ensure that appropriate data collection is part of the policy design and implementation and evaluation phases.

In summary, the application of the effectiveness, efficiency, and equity criteria will prove increasingly valuable as investigators extend them to other policies and the programs meet the standard of evidence. Community development policies require ongoing evaluation to provide the best insight into these policies' contributions to improved population health.

Recommendations

Community development to improve public health is produced when community social capital assets (i.e., empowerment, participation, networks, reciprocity, and trust) link with the major functions of public health (assessment, assurance, and policy development) to achieve population health goals (increase years of healthy life, reduce racial and ethnic health disparities, and achieve access to preventive health services), as depicted in Figure 6.2.

In this chapter we have compared current approaches and presented a rationale for participatory approaches toward healthy communities. Our core philosophy of community development and public health practice is that local residents must be empowered to join together, define their goals, and create networks within the public health infrastructure; further, public health facilitators or community builders must engender trust and a commitment to community goals through policy and program development with input from the affected populations. We make the following recommendations to assist the transdisciplinary development of approaches for community development to enhance public health.

Evaluate Existing Models

In order for public health to facilitate successful community development, practitioners must understand what the various community development models are, how they have succeeded and failed, and what their community health impact is likely to be. Because public health has not fully succeeded in the past in engaging communities and improving community health, the field will need to incorporate the principles of participatory communication; build information networks; conduct continuous assessment of public health system performance; enhance the accessibility of public health services; improve the flexibility of funding; conduct research for evidence-based decisions, policies, and practice; and strengthen collaboration among elements of the public health system.

The government model dominates the field of public health. We recommend that public health professionals begin to step outside of traditional structures and consider how the public health system could operate more effectively with communities through CBPR approaches. Through matched funding and collaborations with public health agencies, such as the Centers for Disease Control and Prevention, change that promotes real partnerships between local government and communities will support community development and reduce disparities. The design of an intersectoral public health system and alternative models of collaborative decision making will be more fully discussed in Chapter Seven.

Strengthen the Role of Public Health in Community Development

Examination of community development policies, initiatives, and projects reveals several approaches that strengthen the linkages between community development activities and public health. The field of public health, which is primarily concerned with health outcomes and specific disease-prevention actions, can learn valuable lessons from community development examples and provide leadership in advancing community health.

Three recommendations may be particularly beneficial. First, the public health community must expand beyond the traditional participants to include professionals in urban planning, economists, developmental specialists, ecologists, architects, educators, anthropologists, and historians, for example, to forge transdisciplinary frameworks and methods for innovatively addressing persistent population health problems and disparities. Second, the infrastructure of public health provides a framework for measuring the progress in community development and community health. Expanding the capacity and capability of public health surveillance systems to include social determinant indicators will advance the evaluation of more comprehensive community impacts including population health and yield best practices in community health. Third, policies that derive from government, business, and market domains must reflect citizen participation to achieve community development objectives. Public health resources and practice that are more fully grounded in principles of deliberative democracy can help to strengthen community development efforts through convening multiple stakeholders to develop policies and programs.

Support Workforce Development and Training

The public health workforce should be trained to facilitate community development efforts directed toward the public health mission of healthy people in healthy communities. Challenging questions to address in preparing the workforce include, for example, the following:

- How can we apply community organizing models around issues like civil rights and social justice to population health and public health consequences such as health disparities?
- How can we define the public health perspective in these issues?

Because communities differ, one application will not be sufficient. However, training community leaders to collaborate with the public health infrastructure can help to support social movements toward improving public health. These types of partnerships, such as MAP-IT, will tailor the policies and programs to fit the goals of the particular community. Schools of public health should produce MPH graduates with community-building skills to commandeer the political environment that controls the power to make the changes required for healthy communities. This may involve building social capital in communities to encourage active participation in communities toward community goals.

Recognize the Need for Political Action

Oppressive political and economic barriers (segregation, voting rights, etc.) have resulted historically in major social movements to alter these arrangements. Public health practitioners in community development must be able to maneuver the political environment. Knowledgeable leaders take advantage of the political climate and opportunities, such as during election years, to move community concerns onto the political agenda. Governmental policy and investment operate on short-term intervals such as political office terms of two to four years. Community development requires long-term time frames. Political expectations from community development need to identify short-term benefits for political support but look for the production of healthier communities in the long term. The promise of community development is shifting to local leadership, power, and control; and this will require building relationships. However, trust and reciprocity take time and require a redefining of the social relationships; the elitist dimension, in which outside interests dominate the distribution of power in communities, must shift to a grassroots dimension that listens and acts on community concerns.

Respect Community Interests and Values

Members of the public health community must acknowledge that the community's interests may not fully overlap with their interests. The lifeworld of a community centers on shared lived experiences around things that matter to the community's members. Sustainable community development will occur when the foundation is rooted in the lifeworlds and related local cultural values and goals. Programs disregarding this reality will fail. When experts drive the model, the program may fail because of a lack of community buy-in. When government, nongovernmental organizations, and academics disregard this reality, they disrespect the community's time and energy.

Government models of leadership often operate within a hierarchical framework. Public health must come into communities ready to listen to community members about their needs, values, and interests; moreover, public health must be ready to compromise in order to facilitate programs that will achieve success. Promising models that use democratic principles (such as MAP-IT) will tailor the policies and programs to fit the goals of the particular community.

Public health practitioners and researchers must demonstrate respect for the goals and values of community members, because it is the community that will remain after the funding is gone. A reinvigorated commitment to healthy communities would be evidenced by public health programs and policies that entail the full and effective participation of community members and that are planned to assure long-term sustainability as well as short-term success.

Chapter Seven, the final chapter of the book, provides a blueprint for how the field of public health might better accomplish its defining mission of assuring healthy people in healthy communities.

References

Acosta, C. M. (2003, April). Improving public health through policy advocacy. *Community-Based Public Health Policy and Practice*, pp. 1–8.

Adams, C. F. (2000). Healthy communities and public policy: Four success stories. *Public Health Reports, 115,* 212–215.

Aday, L. A. (1997). Vulnerable populations: A community-oriented perspective. *Family and Community Health, 19*(4), 1–18.

Agency for Healthcare Research and Quality. (2003). *Creating partnerships, improving health: The role of community-based participatory research* (AHRQ Publication No. 03-0037). Washington, DC: Author.

Association for Community Health Improvement. (2005). *Association for Community Health Improvement: Planning, outcomes and evaluation resources.* Retrieved May 25, 2005, from http://www.communityhlth.org/communityhlth/resources/planning.html

Baum, F. E., & Ziersch, A. M. (2003). Social capital. *Journal of Epidemiology and Community Health, 57,* 320–323.

Blackwell, A. G., & Colmenar, R. (2000). Community-building: From local wisdom to public policy. *Public Health Reports, 115,* 161–166.

Butler, S. M. (1991). The conceptual evolution of enterprise zones. In R. E. Green (Ed.), *Enterprise zones: New directions in economic development* (pp. 27–40). Newbury Park, CA: Sage.

Campbell, C., & Jovchelovitch, S. (2000). Health, community and development: Towards a social psychology of participation. *Journal of Community and Applied Social Psychology, 10,* 255–270.

Caughy, M. O., O'Campo, P. J., & Muntaner, C. (2003). When being alone might be better: Neighborhood poverty, social capital, and child mental health. *Social Science and Medicine, 57,* 227–237.

Chambers, S. (2003). Deliberative democratic theory. *Annual Review of Political Science, 6,* 307–326.

Chipuer, H. M., & Pretty, G.M.H. (1999). A review of the sense of community index: Current uses, factor structure, reliability, and further development. *Journal of Community Psychology, 27,* 643–658.

Claeson, M., Griffin, C. C., Johnston, T. A., McLachlan, M., Soucat, A.L.B., Wagstaff, A., and Yazbeck, A.S. (2002). Health, nutrition, and population. In J. Klugman (Ed.), *A sourcebook for poverty reduction strategies: Vol. 2. Macroeconomic and sectoral approaches* (pp. 201–230). Washington, DC: World Bank.

Cohen, H. W., & Northridge, M. E. (2000). Getting political: Racism and urban health. *American Journal of Public Health, 90,* 841–842.

Colletta, N. J., & Cullen, M. L. (2002). Social capital and social cohesion: Case studies from Cambodia and Rwanda. In C. Grootaert & T. van Bastelaer (Eds.), *The role of social capital in development: An empirical assessment* (pp. 279–309). New York: Cambridge University Press.

Culyer, A. J., & Wagstaff, A. (1993). Equity and equality in health and health care. *Journal of Health Economics, 12,* 431–457.

Denzin, N. K., & Lincoln, Y. S. (Eds.). (2000). *Handbook of qualitative research* (2nd ed.). Thousand Oaks, CA: Sage.

District of Columbia, State Center for Health Statistics Administration, Department of Health. (2002, February 22). *Draft briefing paper on the 2000 infant mortality rate for the District of Columbia.* Retrieved July 27, 2004, from http://www.doh.dc.gov/services/administration_offices/schs/pdf/infantmortality00.pdf

Ellen, I. G., Mijanovich, T., & Dillman, K. N. (2001). Neighborhood effects on health: Exploring the links and assessing the evidence. *Journal of Urban Affairs, 23,* 391–408.

Erickson, R. A., & Freidman, S. W. (1991). Comparative dimensions of state enterprise zones policies. In R. E. Green (Ed.), *Enterprise zones: New directions in economic development* (pp. 155–176). Newbury Park, CA: Sage.

Etzi, S., Lane, D. S., & Grimson, R. (1994). The use of mammography vans by low-income women: The accuracy of self-reports. *American Journal of Public Health, 84,* 107–109.

Ferguson, R. F., & Dickens, W. T. (Eds.). (1999). *Urban problems and community development.* Washington, DC: Brookings Institution Press.

Forrest, R., & Kearns, A. (2001). Social cohesion, social capital and the neighbourhood. *Urban Studies, 38,* 2125–2143.

Freire, P. (1970). *Pedagogy of the oppressed* (M. B. Ramos, Trans.). New York: Continuum.

Garson, G. D. (n.d.). Economic Opportunity Act of 1964. Retrieved June 5, 2005, from http://cwx.prenhall.com/bookbind/pubbooks/burns4/medialib/docs/eoa1964.htm

Glouberman, S., & Millar, J. (2003). Evolution of the determinants of health, health policy, and health information systems in Canada. *American Journal of Public Health, 93,* 388–392.

Grootaert, C., & van Bastelaer, T. (Eds.). (2002). *The role of social capital in development: An empirical assessment.* New York: Cambridge University Press.

Gutmann, A., & Thompson, D. F. (1996). *Democracy and disagreement.* Cambridge, MA: Harvard University Press.

Habermas, J. (1984). *The theory of communicative action: Vol. 1. Reason and the rationalization of society* (T. McCarthy, Trans.). Boston: Beacon Press.

Habermas, J. (1996). *Between facts and norms: Contributions to a discourse theory of law and democracy* (W. Rehg, Trans.). Cambridge, MA: MIT Press.

Hyman, J. B. (2002). Exploring social capital and civic engagement to create a framework for community building. *Applied Developmental Science, 6,* 196–202.

Innes, J., & Booher, D. (2000). Indicators for sustainable communities: A strategy building on complexity theory and distributed intelligence. *Planning Theory and Practice, 1,* 173–186.

Institute of Medicine, Committee for the Study of the Future of Public Health. (1988). *The future of public health.* Washington, DC: National Academies Press.

Institute of Medicine, Committee on Assuring the Health of the Public in the 21st Century. (2003). *The future of the public's health in the 21st century.* Washington, DC: National Academies Press.

Institute of Medicine, Committee on Using Performance Monitoring to Improve Community Health. (1997). *Improving health in the community: A role for performance monitoring.* Washington, DC: National Academies Press.

Institute of Medicine, Roundtable on Environmental Health Sciences Research and Medicine. (2001). *Rebuilding the unity of health and the environment: A new vision of environmental health for the 21st century.* Washington, DC: National Academies Press.

Israel, B. A., Schulz, A. J., Parker, E. A., & Becker, A. B. (1998). Review of community-based research: Assessing partnership approaches to improve public health. *Annual Review of Public Health, 19,* 173–202.

Jan, S. (1998). A holistic approach to the economic evaluation of health programs using institutionalist methodology. *Social Science and Medicine, 47,* 1565–1572.

Kesler, J. T. (2000). The healthy community movement: Seven counterintuitive next steps. *National Civic Review, 89,* 271–284.

Kilpatrick, S., Field, J., & Falk, I. (2003). Social capital: An analytical tool for exploring lifelong learning and community development. *British Educational Research Journal, 29,* 417–433.

Krasnik, A., & Rasmussen, N. K. (2002). Reducing social inequalities in health: Evidence, policy, and practice. *Scandinavian Journal of Public Health, 59*(Suppl.), 1–5.

Kretzmann, J. P., & McKnight, J. (1993). *Building communities from the inside out: A path toward finding and mobilizing a community's assets.* Evanston, IL: Institute for Policy Research, Northwestern University.

Lindsey, E., Stajduhar, K., & McGuinness, L. (2001). Examining the process of community development. *Journal of Advanced Nursing, 33,* 828–835.

Link, B. G., & Phelan, J. (1995). Social conditions as fundamental causes of disease. *Journal of Health and Social Behavior* [Special issue], 80–94.

Mattessich, P., & Monsey, B. (1997). *Community building: What makes it work: A review of factors influencing successful community building.* St. Paul, MN: Amherst H. Widler Foundation.

McCarthy, M. (2000). Social determinants and inequalities in urban health. *Reviews on Environmental Health, 15,* 97–108.

McClenaghan, P. (2000). Social capital: Exploring the theoretical foundations of community development education. *British Educational Research Journal, 26,* 565–582.

McCulloch, A. (2003). An examination of social capital and social disorganisation in neighbourhoods in the British household panel study. *Social Science and Medicine, 56,* 1425–1438.

McKnight, J. (1995). *The careless society: Community and its counterfeits.* New York: Basic Books.

McKnight, J. L. (1994). Two tools for well-being: Health systems and communities. *American Journal of Preventive Medicine, 10,* 23–25.

McLeroy, K. R., Norton, B. L., Kegler, M. C., Burdine, J. N., & Sumaya, C. V. (2003). Community-based interventions. *American Journal of Public Health, 93,* 529–533.

McMillan, D. W., & Chavis, D. M. (1986). Sense of community: A definition and theory. *Journal of Community Psychology, 14,* 6–23.

McNeely, J. (1999). Community building. *Journal of Community Psychology, 27,* 741–750.

Mechanic, D. (2002). Disadvantage, inequality, and social policy: Major initiatives intended to improve population health may also increase health disparities. *Health Affairs, 21*(2), 48–59.

Minkler, M. (2000). Using participatory action research to build healthy communities. *Public Health Reports, 115,* 191–197.

Minkler, M., & Wallerstein, N. (Eds.). (2003). *Community based participatory research for health.* San Francisco: Jossey-Bass.

Mitchell, S. M., & Shortell, S. M. (2000). The governance and management of effective community health partnerships: A typology for research, policy, and practice. *Milbank Quarterly, 78,* 241–289.

Molinari, C., Ahern, M., & Hendryx, M. (1998). Gains from public-private collaborations to improve community health. *Journal of Healthcare Management, 43,* 498–510.

Morenoff, J. D., Sampson, R. J., & Raudenbush, S. W. (2001). Neighborhood inequality, collective efficacy, and the spatial dynamics of urban violence. *Criminology, 39,* 517–559.

Morgan, L. M. (2001). Community participation in health: Perpetual allure, persistent challenge. *Health Policy and Planning, 16,* 221–230.

Moser, C.O.N. (1998). The asset vulnerability framework: Reassessing urban poverty reduction strategies. *World Development, 26,* 1–19.

National Association for State Community Services Programs. (2003a). *Community services block grant statistical report, FY 2001.* Washington, DC: Author.

National Association for State Community Services Programs. (2003b). *Community services network: The community services block grant in action fiscal year 2001.* Washington, DC: Author.

National Association of County and City Health Officials. (2001). *Advancing community public health systems in the 21st century: Emerging strategies and innovations from the Turning Point experience.* Washington, DC: Author.

Nicola, R. M., Berkowitz, B., & Lafronze, V. (2002). A turning point for public health. *Journal of Public Health Management and Practice, 8*(1), iv–vii.

Norris, T., & Pittman, M. (2000). The healthy communities movement and the coalition for healthier cities and communities. *Public Health Reports, 115,* 118–124.

O'Connor, D., & Gates, C. T. (2000). Toward a healthy democracy. *Public Health Reports, 115,* 157–160.

Personal Responsibility and Work Opportunity Reconciliation Act of 1996 (Welfare Reform Act) (PL 104-193). Retrieved June 5, 2005, from http://frwebgate.access.gpo.gov/cgi-bin/getdoc.cgi?dbname=104_cong_public_laws&docid=f:publ193.104.pdf

Poland, B., Boutilier, M., Tobin, S., & Badgley, R. (2000). The policy context for community development practice in public health: A Canadian case study. *Journal of Public Health Policy, 21,* 5–19.

PolicyLink. (2000). *Community involvement in the federal Healthy Start program: Summary document.* Oakland, CA: Author.

Public Health Foundation (2002). *Healthy people 2010 toolkit: A field guide to health planning.* Washington, DC: Author.

Putnam, R. (2000). *Bowling alone: The collapse and revival of American community.* New York: Simon & Schuster.

Rohrer, J. E. (1999). *Planning for community-oriented health systems* (2nd ed.). Washington, DC: American Public Health Association.

Rosenau, R. V. (1994). Health politics meets postmodernism: Its meaning and implications for community health organizing. *Journal of Health Politics, Policy and Law, 19,* 303–333.

Saegert, S., Thompson, J. P., & Warren, M. R. (Eds.). (2001). *Social capital and poor communities.* New York: Russell Sage Foundation.

Sampson, R. J., Morenoff, J. D., & Gannon-Rowley, T. (2002). Assessing "neighborhood effects": Social processes and new directions in research. *Annual Review of Sociology, 28,* 443–478.

Sampson, R. J., Raudenbush, S. W., & Earls, F. (1997, August 15). Neighborhoods and violent crime: A multilevel study of collective efficacy. *Science, 277,* 918–924.

Schlesinger, M., & Gray, B. (1998). A broader vision for managed care, part 1: Measuring the benefit to communities. *Health Affairs, 17*(3), 152–168.

Schlesinger, M., Gray, B., Carrino, G., Duncan, M., Gusmano, M., Antonelli, V., et al. (1998). A broader vision for managed care, part 2: A typology of community benefits. *Health Affairs, 17*(5), 26–49.

Sen, A. (1992). *Inequality reexamined.* Cambridge, MA: Harvard University Press.

Sullivan, M., Chao, S. S., Allen, C. A., Koné, A., Pierre-Louis, M., & Krieger, J. (2003). Community-researcher partnerships: Perspectives from the field. In M. Minkler & N. Wallerstein (Eds.), *Community based participatory research for health* (pp. 113–130). San Francisco: Jossey-Bass.

Tarlov, A. R. (1999). Public policy frameworks for improving population health. *Annals of the New York Academy of Sciences, 896,* 281–293.

Thrall, T. H. (2001). Coverage & access: Communities take charge. *Hospitals and Health Networks, 75,* 52–54.

U.S. Department of Health and Human Services. (1991). *Healthy people 2000: National health promotion and disease prevention objectives: Full report, with commentary* (DHHS Publication No. PHS 91-50212). Washington, DC: Author.

U.S. Department of Health and Human Services. (2000a, November 30). *Healthy people 2000 fact sheet*. Retrieved November 14, 2004, from http://www.odphp.osophs.dhhs.gov/pubs/HP2000/hp2kfact.htm

U.S. Department of Health and Human Services. (2000b, November). *Healthy people 2010: Introduction*. Retrieved November 24, 2003, from http://www.healthypeople.gov/document/html/uih/uih_1.htm

U.S. Department of Health and Human Services. (2001). *Healthy people 2000 final review* (DHHS Publication No. PHS 2001-0256). Hyattsville, MD: Public Health Service.

Veenstra, G. (2001). Social capital and health. *ISUMA: Canadian Journal of Policy Research, 2*(1), 72–81.

Vidal, A. C. (1995). Reintegrating disadvantaged communities into the fabric of urban life: The role of community development. *Housing Policy Debate, 6,* 169–230.

Wagstaff, A., & van Doorslaer, E. (1993). Equity in the finance and delivery of health care: Concepts and definitions. In E.K.A. van Doorslaer, A. Wagstaff, & F.F.H. Rutten (Eds.), *Equity in the finance and delivery of healthcare: An international perspective* (pp. 7–19). New York: Oxford University Press.

Whiteis, D. G. (2000). Poverty, policy, and pathogenesis: Economic justice and public health in the U.S. *Critical Public Health, 10,* 257–271.

Wilcox, R., & Knapp, A. (2000). Building communities that create health. *Public Health Reports, 115,* 139–143.

Wismar, M., & Busse, R. (2002). Outcome-related health targets: Political strategies for better health outcomes: A conceptual and comparative study (part 2). *Health Policy, 59,* 223–241.

Young, I. M. (1990). *Justice and the politics of difference.* Princeton, NJ: Princeton University Press.

Young, I. M. (2000). *Inclusion and democracy.* New York: Oxford University Press.

CHAPTER SEVEN

TOWARD A HEALTHY (RE)PUBLIC

Lu Ann Aday, Beth E. Quill, Hardy D. Loe Jr.,
Charles E. Begley

Chapter Highlights

- Population health–centered policy is concerned with the direct and indirect impacts of policies and programs in health sectors (medical care, public health) and nonhealth sectors (sustainable, human, economic, and community development, as well as other sectors) on the fundamental determinants of health and health disparities within defined populations.
- Population health–centered practice requires that governmental public health agencies and professionals reorient and expand core public health functions and essential services.
- The public health system dictated by more population health–centered policy would be intersectoral in design and practice.
- A healthy republic forges effective collaborations across traditional disciplinary, institutional, professional, and political divides to enhance the health of the public.
- To achieve a healthy republic, the field of public health must envision a systems approach, assume leadership, measure

performance, and train for the future while remaining grounded in the lessons of the past.

This book is intended to provide a road map and guidelines for developing an expanded public health system and partnerships, grounded in a broad ecological and transdisciplinary framework for designing and evaluating policies to address the fundamental determinants of population health.

The final chapter highlights the implications of the framework that the preceding chapters introduced and elaborated for enlarging the vision and role of public health in addressing the fundamental social, economic, and ecological determinants of poor health and health disparities and the design of more population health–centered policies and practice in addressing these fundamental causes at the international, national, state, and local levels.

Population Health–Centered Policies—Issues and Examples

As indicated in Chapter One, a central thesis underlying the book is that the prospects for improving the health of individuals and communities are enhanced by interventions addressing the fundamental social, economic, and ecological determinants of health in policy domains that lie outside the conventional public health infrastructure. This broader policy vision has not yet been fully operationalized in practice.

This section of the final chapter highlights examples of policies for improving population health and health disparities, based on evidence, analyses, and examples presented in the preceding chapters (see Table 7.1); and it reviews the major issues related to the effectiveness, efficiency, and equity of current policies (see Table 7.2). The preceding chapters have amply documented the evidence regarding the fundamental determinants of population health outlined in the framework for the book (see Table 1.1). They have also illuminated the role of the major policy domains in influencing these determinants and ultimately population health and health disparities (see Table 1.4).

Examples

Table 7.1 summarizes key examples of policies for addressing the fundamental determinants of population health in the respective policy domains. The recommended policies encompass a range of options that assume and require leadership on the part of governments, the market, and communities. Many of these

TABLE 7.1. SELECTED POLICIES AFFECTING POPULATION HEALTH AND HEALTH DISPARITIES.

Government	←→	Community	←→	Market
Economic development: national and international monetary, fiscal, income, and trade policies	*Human development:* early childhood development and education policies			*Sustainable development:* environmentally responsive vs. conventional corporate policies
Community development: government-oriented community infrastructure–building programs and policies		*Community development:* community-oriented local empowerment programs and policies		*Community development:* market-oriented local economic growth pro-grams and policies

policies lie outside what some deem to be the conventional province of public health. They are, however, essential to consider because policies in these areas have major impacts on the fundamental determinants of human health.

- National and international monetary, fiscal, income, and trade policies play a central role in the distribution of income and related health inequalities in developed and developing countries (Chapter Five).
- Public and community investments in early childhood development and education contribute to developing and sustaining health and human capital throughout the life course (Chapter Four).
- Socially responsible and environmentally responsive corporate decision making is essential to minimize the consequences of practices in conventional business—and increasingly international business—in producing environmental stressors and related population health impacts (Chapter Three).
- Community development policies supported through either government-, community-, or market-centered strategies focus on contrasting but potentially complementary community development goals—building community infrastructure, empowering community residents, and promoting economic growth—to facilitate and sustain healthy communities (Chapter Six).

TABLE 7.2.   MAJOR ISSUES OF POLICY EFFECTIVENESS, EFFICIENCY, AND EQUITY.

| Policy Domain | *Summary of Issues* | | |
	Effectiveness	Efficiency	Equity
Sustainable development	*Ecological effectiveness:* minimize the impact of the economic system on ecological determinants of population health	*Economic efficiency:* maximize profits	*Intergenerational justice:* balance the benefits and burdens across generations *Environmental justice:* minimize differences in environmental risks between groups and neighborhoods
Human development	*Life-course epidemiology:* positively influence the determinants of developmental health at all stages of the life course	*Allocative efficiency:* to maximize developmental health over the life course, given limited resources, invest in early childhood interventions	*Social justice:* allocate resources to the most at-risk groups to ameliorate developmental health differentials over the life course between groups
Economic development	*Welfare economics:* maximize aggregate utility (including population health)	*Technical efficiency:* invest in policies that maximize the generation of economic resources (e.g., jobs, income) at the least cost	*Distributive justice:* distribute the benefits and burdens fairly across countries, communities, population subgroups, and individuals
Community development	*Community benefit:* facilitate positive change in the community through collective action	*Dynamic efficiency:* invest in the generation of social capital within communities to sustain community benefits over time	*Deliberative justice:* maximize the full and effective participation of affected communities and populations in decision making

Evaluation

Table 7.2 highlights the principal effectiveness, efficiency, and equity criteria for evaluating the success of policies in the respective policy domains.

Sustainable development initiatives focus on minimizing the impact of the economic system—and specifically the corporate business sector—on the ecological determinants of population health. As Chapter Three argued, however, a framework for socially responsible corporate practices must be constrained by the realistic acknowledgement that the defining goal of the business economy is to maximize profits. *Economic efficiency* refers to the allocation of the corporation's resources that results in the maximization of net benefits or profits. The corporate social responsibility framework presented argues that environmental consequences are quite likely to transpire if business practices fail to take the environment into account, thereby ultimately resulting in significant costs to corporations and to society. The equity consequences of corporate business practices are judged cross-sectionally in terms of the extent to which environmental risks and consequences result in differing burdens for different groups and neighborhoods, and over time in terms of the balance of burdens and benefits that are passed on to future generations.

Human development research identifies the essential indicators and determinants of healthy human development at all stages of the life course (see Chapter Four). Education is a fundamental determinant of human productive potential and has ramifications for social and economic opportunities, resources for coping with stressors, and health throughout an individual's life. Investing in early childhood interventions is a much more allocatively efficient strategy than are the investments required later in remediating educational or development delays and deficiencies. Some groups, especially poor and minority children, are particularly at risk. From a social justice point of view, early childhood intervention programs for high-risk children are especially important for maximizing the human productive potential and capacities for these children and ameliorating developmental health differentials over the life course between groups of children.

Economic development has tended to focus on economic growth. But as Chapter Five pointed out, growth can have costly human and environmental consequences. A critical review of economic policies and their consequences acknowledges the impact and effectiveness of these policies in contributing to income and related health disparities in developed and developing nations. The concept of *capacity* directly incorporates considerations of the human impact of economic policies in terms of gains in the quality and value of life years for populations directly or indirectly affected by these policies. The technical efficiency criterion attempts to identify those policies that generate economic resources, such as jobs and income, at the least cost. Small investments in very poor people or nations, through microcredit or microfinance initiatives, for example, may yield substantial economic and health benefits. The growth and expansion of multinational corporations and their dominance in the global economy have had dramatic consequences for increasing the concentrations of wealth among a very small proportion of the population in many countries and widening the gap between those at the lowest and highest ends of the wealth and income distributions. This raises serious equity considerations in terms of the distribution of material resources as well as the consequences for exacerbating the health gap and gradient between those with the most versus the fewest resources.

Community development initiatives seek to facilitate positive change in the community through collective action. As indicated earlier, the precise goals of different community development initiatives may differ in the changes they seek: building community infrastructure, empowering community residents, and/or promoting economic growth. Community development at its best takes a long-term view of the dynamic efficiency of community benefits through investing in the generation of social capital within the community to sustain community benefits over time. As Chapter Six documents, community development efforts have varied widely and been more or less successful in identifying and achieving community goals. Due to differentials in status, power, expertise, and/or resources between outside agencies and researchers who initiate or advise regarding community development projects and community representatives and leaders, the priorities of community members may not be effectively heard or addressed. A defining equity benchmark for evaluating community development initiatives is the norm of deliberative justice, which demands the full and effective participation of affected communities and populations in the decision-making process.

The discussion that follows views the profile of current public health policies, systems, and practice in order to set the context for exploring how to expand the mission and operation of the field to encompass the role of sustainable development and related human, economic, and community development programs and policies in influencing the fundamental determinants of population health.

Public Health Policies, Systems, and Practice— Present Realities

The report *The Future of Public Health* (Institute of Medicine, Committee for the Study of the Future of Public Health, 1988) set out an assessment and vision for the future of the field grounded in three defining core functions: assessment, policy development, and assurance. In addition, the report described a predominantly governmental mission and model of public health. A major premise of this work was to articulate the tenet that effective service delivery is contingent on the quality and capacity of the infrastructure. Critiques of the assessment noted major shortcomings in the governmental public health system and made recommendations for improvement to achieve the national public health objectives. Researchers and practitioners further advanced the understanding of the public health system through the *Public Health in America* statement (U.S. Department of Health and Human Services [USDHHS], 1994), which extended the three core functions to an array of ten essential services:

Assessment Function

1. Monitor health status to identify community health problems
2. Diagnose and investigate health problems and health hazards in the community

Policy Development Function

3. Inform, educate, and empower people about health issues
4. Mobilize community partnerships and action to identify and solve health problems
5. Develop policies and plans that support individual and community health efforts

Assurance Function

6. Enforce laws and regulations that protect health and ensure safety
7. Link people to needed personal health care services and assure the provision of health care when otherwise unavailable
8. Assure a competent public health and personal and population-based health workforce (i.e., a workforce that is well trained in the delivery of personal health care services as well as the management and administration of population health-oriented services for entire populations or communities)
9. Evaluate effectiveness, accessibility, and quality of personal and population-based health services

Serving All Functions

10. Research for new insights and innovative solutions to health problems

The defining mission and objectives of the U.S. public health system detailed in the *Healthy People 2010* agenda (USDHHS, 2000) profiles the promise of a revised and more effective public health system. For the first time, the report included a chapter (Chapter 23) titled "Public Health Infrastructure." This chapter identifies five fundamental components of public health infrastructure: data and information systems, workforce, public health organizations, resources, and prevention research. A companion Centers for Disease Control document, *Public Health's Infrastructure* (USDHHS, 2001, p. iii), puts forth recommendations in three areas to achieve the objective of "[e]very health department fully prepared; every community better protected." These areas are a skilled public health workforce, robust information and data systems, and effective health departments and laboratories.

Several initiatives illustrate efforts to remediate weaknesses in the public health infrastructure. Data and information systems have been strengthened by the development of the Centers for Disease Control and Prevention's (CDC) Public Health Information Network, HealthAlert, and Disease Surveillance systems.

National efforts to expedite the collection, analysis, and dissemination of key public health and safety information have proven critical to protecting the national health and welfare (Baker & Koplan, 2002). Federal support of Health Resources and Services Administration Public Health Training and CDC Emergency Preparedness Centers emphasizes the importance of enumerating, educating, and training the public health workforce to manage emerging public health challenges. Leadership training and development at the national, regional, and state levels (Public Health Leadership Institutes), funded by CDC, provide an example of the advanced expertise necessary to meet these challenges and move successfully toward population-centered objectives. Public health organizations have been buttressed by the allocation of funds to state and local health departments specifically to strengthen the capabilities of the departments and the scope of laboratory activities. Further, funds specifically designed to support emergency preparedness have necessitated the development of strong community alliances to achieve system effectiveness.

In a climate of fiscal restraint with challenges to document and analyze expenditures, agencies allocate resources to priority health issues in the name of efficiency and effectiveness. The development of the National Public Health Performance Standards in 1997 reflects the imperative to measure the performance of these initiatives, in terms of their effectiveness, efficiency, and eventual outcomes. Prevention research through Prevention Research Centers has received renewed attention from federal agencies that now recognize the role of preventive interventions in improving health status. The National Institutes of Health road map further endorses and challenges researchers to translate their findings into practical applications and programs to improve health and well-being (Zerhouni, 2003).

Evolving concepts of the public health system, however, move beyond considerations of the formal governmental public health infrastructure per se. The concept of a public health system "includes the complement of public and private organizations that contribute to the delivery of public health services for a given population, including governmental public health agencies as well as private and voluntary organizations" (Mays, Halverson, & Scutchfield, 2003, p. 180). The public health system infrastructure as developed by the National Association of County and City Health Officials (2004, p. 4) represents "the capacities and resources that make the provision of the essential services possible within a community." Handler, Issel, and Turnock (2001, p. 1237) emphasize the "structural capacity" or "cumulative resources *and relationships* necessary to carry out the important processes of public health," including information resources, organizational resources, physical resources, and human and fiscal resources. This concept of a public health system goes beyond governmentally supported public health programs and services per se to encompass building partnerships within communities and between and among public and private organizations (e.g., school systems, the business sector, and private philanthropies), in the service of promoting and protecting the health of the public.

Two recent reports (Institute of Medicine, Committee on Assuring the Health of the Public in the 21st Century, 2003; Institute of Medicine, Committee on Educating Public Health Professionals for the 21st Century, 2003) assay the strengths and limitations of the current U.S. public health system and suggest fruitful new directions for better achieving U.S. public health policy objectives in the 21st century. The reports argue for a promising future through grounding innovations in the design and implementation of public health policies and programs in an ecological and transdisciplinary model of population health, based on research on the multifactorial determinants of health.

This book builds on but goes beyond these reports on the future of public health in providing guidance for creating a healthy (re)public in the following ways (review Table 1.1):

- Transdisciplinary: *Reinventing Public Health* draws on a very broad array of fields of study including ecology, managerial economics, corporate social responsibility, human capital and development theory, life-course epidemiology, macroeconomic theory, deliberative democracy, social capital theory, community development theory, and participatory action research, as well as ecosocial theory, public health research, health services research, and policy analysis.
- Population health–centered: This book identifies a number of units of analysis and related levels of intervention that must be considered in ultimately and effectively improving population health (including individuals; populations; communities; corporations; international, national, regional, state, and/or local economies; and the ecosystem).
- Grounded in the fundamental social and economic determinants of health: It directly links research on the fundamental determinants of health to specific policy options that lie outside the conventional public health and health care policy domain, including sustainable development, human development, economic development, and community development policy.
- Participatory and inclusive: This book explicitly identifies and applies benchmarks of fairness for evaluating the performance and outcomes of policies and programs, including deliberative justice, social justice, distributive justice, and intergenerational justice.
- Intersectoral in design: It provides concrete guidance regarding the components and design of an intersectoral public health system as well as the specific implications for more population health–centered public health practice (discussed later in this chapter).

- Critical and evaluative: It delineates and critically applies effectiveness, efficiency, and equity criteria for evaluating existing policies and programs.

Toward a Healthy (Re)Public

As Chapter One documented, the health of the (re)public reflects the inextricable link between the health of populations and policies related to the fundamental determinants of health. The *public* refers to populations that are the focus of public policy decisions. A *republic* refers essentially to a form of government in which power ultimately resides in a body of citizens entitled to vote and in which elected officers and representatives responsible to them exercise power and govern according to law. A *healthy republic* is one in which public decision making takes into account the impacts of policies related to fundamental determinants on the health of the populations that these policies target. The specific dimensions and criteria characterizing a healthy (re)public are highlighted in Table 7.3.

TABLE 7.3. DIMENSIONS AND CRITERIA FOR A HEALTHY (RE)PUBLIC.

Dimensions	Criteria
A Healthy Republic	
Structure	
Policy	Intersectoral population health–centered policy
• Health sectors: Medical care, public health	
• Nonhealth sectors: Sustainable, human, economic, and community development; other sectors	
System	Intersectoral public health system
Process	
Partnerships	Participatory public-private decision-making process
Practice	Population health–centered public health practice
A Healthy Public	
Outcomes	
Health levels	Improved population health
Health disparities	Reduced health disparities

Overview

A healthy republic may be characterized in terms of structure and process dimensions. The principal structure criteria include the formulation of intersectoral population health–centered policies and an intersectoral public health system, encompassing both health and nonhealth sectors. The process through which these policies and systems emerge requires building a participatory public-private decision-making process and related intersectoral partnerships, as well as more explicitly population health–centered public health practice arrangements.

A healthy public focuses on population health outcomes and related population health levels and disparities. Measures of achieving a healthy public encompass improvements in population health and reduced health disparities relative to desired benchmarks, such as those incorporated in the U.S. Healthy People and World Health Organization (WHO) 2010 Health Objectives (U.S. Department of Health and Human Services, 2000; World Health Organization, 2000).

The central thesis underlying this book is that to effectively improve population health and reduce health disparities, policymaking in a variety of policy domains must take into account the fundamental social, economic, and ecological determinants of health. The discussion that follows elaborates how this might be achieved.

Structure

The principal structural issues to address include the formulation of more population health–centered public policies and the development of an intersectoral public health system.

Formulate a Population Health–Centered Policy. Steps for formulating population health–centered policies include broadening the scope of health policy, defining population health objectives and criteria, and highlighting the need for population health policy research.

Broadening the Scope of Health Policy. Health policy agendas in the United States and throughout most of the world continue to focus on issues and strategies for improving the performance of health care services and systems. U.S. reform debates have remained essentially the same for the past two decades, focusing on how to address the problem of the large and growing number of uninsured and slow the growth in health care costs while maintaining a voluntary employer-based private insurance system (Evans, 1998). At one extreme are those who desire to move the health care system to a more publicly controlled, nonmarket, compulsorily financed model that has proven to be relatively successful in other developed countries. At the other extreme are constituents who support limiting the role of government and moving the health care system further in its promarket direction, with greater consumer choice, more out-of-pocket financing, and further minimization of government regulation (Anderson, 1989).

The first major U.S. effort to look at the policy implications of the broader determinants of health focus was *Healthy People: The Surgeon General's Report on Health Promotion and Disease Prevention* (U.S. Department of Health Education and Welfare, 1979). Its publication led to Healthy People reports setting goals for 1990, 2000, and 2010. Later reports focusing on *Healthy People 2010* emphasized the social determinants of health, particularly the goals of eliminating racial and socioeconomic disparities in health (National Center for Health Statistics, 1998; USDHHS, 2000).

While defining a broad set of health objectives, neither the Healthy People reports nor subsequent federal government efforts have defined on a national scale the population health–centered policies needed to address these objectives. Rather, the health policy community continues to struggle with alleviating major inequalities in access to health care and rising costs of care. A reflection of the lack of emphasis on population health policy in the United States is the fact that 93% to 95% of public health expenditures made by federal, state, and local governments are still directed at financing or directly providing personal health care services, whereas only 5% to 7% is spent on health protection, promotion, and prevention activities aimed at the determinants of health (Cowan, Catlin, Smith, & Sensenig, 2004).

As earlier chapters described, the broader view of population health–centered policy is receiving more attention in international organizations such as the Organisation for Economic Co-operation and Development (OECD) and the WHO (Exworthy, Stuart, Blane, & Marmot, 2003). The population health–centered framework that the WHO is using to assess health systems throughout the world considers maximizing population health and minimizing health disparities as major social goals (WHO, 2000). Improved population health and reduced health disparities, measured respectively as the level of and variation in disability-adjusted life expectancy (DALE), are the objectives of health policy aimed at influencing the basic determinants of health (Institute of Medicine, Committee on Summary Measures of Population Health, 1998; Murray & Evans, 2003).

The WHO framework defines health policies to include government activities with the primary purpose of promoting, restoring, or maintaining health and intersectoral policy developed primarily to influence broader socioeconomic conditions that have a large influence on population health (Murray & Frenk, 2000). Policies and programs aimed at the provision, financing, or regulation of personal health services are clearly within these boundaries, as are policies and programs aimed at providing traditional public health services such as health education and disease prevention programs and vehicle and environmental safety regulations. Intersectoral policy related to economic development, human development, and environmental sustainability is increasingly being emphasized to address the complex determinants of health that lie outside the reach of health care and public health.

Examples of individual countries stressing the role of medical and nonmedical determinants of health and the need for joining health care, public health, and intersectoral policies to address population health include the United Kingdom, Canada, and Sweden, among others. (See Chapter Two for a review of the role and history of population health policies in these and other countries.)

The United Kingdom has made a major commitment to monitor inequalities in health and develop interventions to reduce them. This includes specific initiatives in early education, child care, health, and family support for children; a national strategy for improving housing and increasing other social infrastructure in poor neighborhoods; and initiatives to reduce behavioral risk factors related to tobacco use, obesity, and injuries (Acheson, 1998; Black, 1980; Exworthy, 2003; Exworthy, Blane, & Marmot, 2003; Exworthy, Stuart, Blane, & Marmot, 2003). Table 7.4 lists specific policy initiatives in the United Kingdom by their health care, public health, or development focus and identifies the principal population health determinants being targeted. The initiatives rely on forging intersectoral collaborations and policies. The United Kingdom is ahead of most other developed countries in implementing nonhealth care, especially economic, policies with the intent to influence health. However, some have criticized the policies for being vague and lacking a well-articulated focus on health (Evans, 2002). Recent reform initiatives tend to focus more on the National Health Service, shifting policy away from economics to health care.

The official endorsement of population health in Canada builds on a long-standing tradition of public health, community health, and health promotion research and activities in that country (Epp, 1986; Federal, Provincial and Territorial Advisory Committee on Population Health [Canada], 1994, 1996, 1999; Lalonde, 1974). Canada has been successful in incorporating nonmedical determinants of health in federal policymaking. The creation of population health divisions of government, dealing with nonmedical determinants of health, provides an institutional base to ensure the broad acceptance of the population health perspective. Still, the growing acceptance of population health ideas has largely been limited to the health sector and not influenced policy agendas outside the health sector, particularly the economic and finance sectors, where much of the potential lies (Lavis et al., 2003).

**TABLE 7.4.   SPECIFIC POLICIES ADDRESSING POPULATION HEALTH
DETERMINANTS IN THE UNITED KINGDOM.**

Population Health Determinants	Population Health Policy Initiatives
Human development: life-course approach, early childhood development	Sure Start program offering early education, child care, health, and family support to reduce the consequences of child poverty
Community development: area-based initiatives focusing on disadvantaged communities	Health action zones to improve housing and other environmental factors in poor neighborhoods
Economic development: redistribution of income through welfare to work	Child tax credits for low-income families Increases in the minimum wage and minimum income employment policies Employment policies for disabled people
Health care services: availability of services	Organizational reform in the National Health Service to improve availability of services in poor neighborhoods
Community education: targets and performance culture	Public service agreements Health inequality reductions specified for the nation

Among developed countries, Sweden has created perhaps the most comprehensive and integrated set of policy objectives and specific strategies aimed at population health. A set of national objectives addresses important determinants of health, including strengthening public participation and influence in the policy development process, promoting economic security through antipoverty measures, providing secure and favorable conditions during childhood and adolescence, facilitating healthy workplaces, creating healthy environments, protecting food products through import barriers and farm subsidies, providing preventative health services, and promoting healthy behavior (Ågren, 2003). A major national program addressing socioeconomic inequalities in health includes strong employment protection and active labor market policies for chronically ill citizens. Sweden has been most successful in obtaining the involvement of policymakers throughout government in developing and implementing its population health ideas.

The development of a specific population health policy agenda in the United States is beginning to be adopted on an experimental basis at the state and local levels of government. The leaders of the National Policy Association and the Academy for Health Services Research have proposed an agenda addressing social determinants of health (Auerbach, Krimgold, & Lefkowitz, 2000). The agenda urges that policy be developed to address social factors in five specific areas, which encompass many of the policy domains that are the focus of this book:

- Investing in children through policies that explicitly recognize the importance of early development throughout the life span
- Providing services and opportunities to those at the lower end of the socio-economic scale
- Improving the work environment, including policies aimed at increasing opportunities for development, worker protections, a greater variety of work, and improved leave
- Strengthening support at the community level through policies that build social networks and encourage economic development and reduce the effects of economic and racial segregation
- Creating a more equal economic environment through tax, transfer, and employment policies

Another example of local population health–centered policy development in the United States is the Turning Point initiative, an effort begun in 1997 by the Robert Wood Johnson Foundation and W. K. Kellogg Foundation (see Chapter Six; Hassmiller, 2002; Turning Point, 2005). The goal of this project was to broaden public health policies and programs at the state and local level to better address population health. Working with 41 communities in 14 states, the two foundations helped build the capacity for public and private policy development that addressed the determinants of health and had broad-based support.

A related example is the Minnesota Health Department's plan to address racial or ethnic health disparities focusing on nonmedical determinants, including housing and increasing civic engagement, as ways to improve health (Minnesota Health Improvement Partnership Social Conditions and Health Action Team, 2001). Produced as part of the Minnesota Health Improvement Project, the plan calls for policies and programs to:

- Help people move out of poverty and meet their basic needs
- Promote optimal early childhood development and attachment
- Assure opportunities for quality education and lifelong learning
- Link economic development, community development, and health improvement
- Elevate the standard of living and prospects for future generations

A comprehensive approach at the national level to address the determinants of health does not appear likely for the United States in the near future. However,

Lurie (2002) has identified several steps that the federal government could undertake to advance a population health–centered policy agenda:

- Provide leadership and education on economic and social determinants of health
- Develop mechanisms for interdepartmental policy development aimed at nonmedical determinants
- Enhance monitoring and reporting of nonmedical determinants
- Strengthen the science base by funding research in population health
- Expand the scope and definition of health policy to include nonmedical determinants as health objectives

Lurie's analysis (2002) is, however, limited to the role of the federal government and specific governmental agencies and departments in addressing the nonmedical determinants of health. The pursuit of a broader population health–centered agenda must take into account the role of diverse sectors (including corporations, community organizations, the media, and academia) in contributing to the health of communities and populations. It also requires collaborations across sectors and at the federal, state, and local levels in order to enhance intersectoral collaboration and coordination. The usual mechanisms for funding personal health care programs through block, program, formula, and categorical grants from the federal government to states and nongovernmental entities must be modified to allow mixing of funds. Public health protection policy must include integration of federal standards and regulations with those of health and health-related agencies of state and local government. The federal government's vast amount of information collection and dissemination activity must also shift from focusing on health care delivery to other factors that affect health (Milbank Memorial Fund, 2001).

Defining Population Health Objectives and Criteria. The population health framework proposes to shift policy objectives and reform agendas from the performance of the health care system to the more fundamental question of how to improve population health and reduce health disparities (Figure 7.1). The shift is based on the recognition that health services, be they preventive, curative, or rehabilitative, play a relatively small role in determining individual and population health and that trade-offs need to be made between investments in health care services and other determinants of health (Evans, Barer, & Marmor, 1994; McGinnis & Foege, 1993). Although the United States is the acknowledged world leader in investments in medical technology, it continues to lag behind other developed countries in population health levels achieved (WHO, 2000; also see Chapter Five). Some of the gap reflects inequities in access to health care services among the poor and the uninsured, but the difference may also be due to the lack of policy initiatives stressing behavioral and environmental factors, as well as the broader economic, social, and human development conditions that influence health.

A population health–centered policy approach would consider communitywide health improvement at all stages of the policy development cycle: in the choice of problems or opportunities to work on; in the choice of strategies or alternatives to develop and apply; in the decision of how to implement past actions; and in the decision to continue, modify, or repeal a policy. Related to the choice of strategies to improve health, a population health approach analyzes the available evidence on which policies or combinations of policies are the most effective in modifying specific types of health outcomes, decreasing health inequities, improving the health of the population as a whole, or achieving change in the determinants of health. It poses the central question: Will we make the population healthier by spending more on health care or by investing in other programs that affect health? (Health Canada, Population Strategic Policy Directorate of the Population and Public Health Branch, 2001).

Policies aimed at influencing upstream determinants of health are a central focus, including broad socioeconomic determinants as well as environmental and behavioral factors. The key is to identify what combination of health care services, health promotion programs aimed at groups and individuals, and health promotion and protection strategies aimed at communitywide socioeconomic and environmental factors will have the greatest impact on aggregate levels of health.

The objective of effectiveness in a population health policy agenda focuses on the relative impact of and the interactions among intersectoral health promotion and protection services, population-based and individual behavior change programs, and treatment-oriented acute and long-term health care service programs. Interventions that have the greatest upstream impacts, such as early childhood development, poverty and labor market policies, and socially responsible corporate business practices, as well as prevention-oriented public health interventions, would be the central goal within this paradigm. Similarly, efficiency objectives relate to choosing the mix of policy strategies that produces the greatest upstream health impacts given limited resources. One must judge the existing allocation of resources and whether it requires altering to obtain greater health for a society given a limited budget. Population equity objectives are concerned with health disparities produced by the unequal distribution of the social, economic, and environmental determinants of health. Analyses of inequalities in population health focus on the social structural and environmental factors that influence health—a much broader concern than an unequal distribution of health care services alone (Aday, Begley, Lairson, & Balkrishnan, 2004).

A population health approach must balance short-, medium-, and long-term goals. Long-, medium-, and short-term investments broadly correspond to addressing the fundamental, intermediate, and proximate determinants of health respectively (see Figure 1.3). Health problems have to be treated immediately, but at the same time immediate treatment has short-lived returns. Examples of short-term initiatives include responding to citizen concerns about the quality and accessibility of health care, food and drug safety, and emergency response procedures. Upstream investments in ameliorating socioeconomic and environmental risk factors require sustained support, and their impacts will be realized in the medium and long term. Medium-term initiatives include programs to change lifestyle in young adults in order to prevent heart disease and diabetes in middle age.

Examples of long-term upstream initiatives include investment in programs that favor equity, such as redistributing resources and programs that invest in children. An environmental example is investment in alternative energy sources and other technologies that reduce stress on the physical environment. Currently, most countries' health investment portfolios are weighted heavily toward short-term downstream returns. Population health policy strives to strike a more appropriate balance between policies aimed at health services with short-term benefit and those upstream interventions addressing broader and deeper fundamental determinants of health with long-term benefit (Health Canada, 2001).

Highlighting the Need for Population Health Policy Research. Relevant research for population health policy links the major health problems of groups, communities, and populations to their fundamental determinants and clarifies the dynamics by which the various determinants combine to cause health and illness (Kindig & Stoddart, 2003). Valid scientific information is needed on the robustness of the relationship between risk factors and health outcomes and the role of the social, economic, and environmental factors that contribute to the risk factors. As previous chapters reported, various formulations of environmental, human, and economic factors have been empirically linked to a range of public health outcomes. However, significant ongoing disputes over the interpretation of these relationships and the implications for health policy exist (Szreter & Woolcock, 2004). Evidence based on more robust methods, such as multilevel modeling, causal modeling, and controlled experiments, is needed to better understand the mechanisms by which these broad determinants influence health outcomes.

Population health research is also needed to identify a more balanced agenda of medical, public health, and intersectoral health policies to improve health and overcome constraints on intersectoral and intergovernmental population health strategies that existing bureaucratic and political structures pose. Although the volume and diversity of evidence makes clear that these factors are significant determinants of health, we cannot design specific policy interventions without a better understanding of the causes of good health and the relative effects of multiple determinants of health. For example, as Chapters Two and Five discussed, the research on the role of the social environment on health has centered on the influence of socioeconomic position (SEP), but the mechanisms through which SEP is associated with morbidity and mortality are not clear. Likewise, as Chapters Two and Three indicated, abundant evidence exists of an association between environmental conditions and health outcomes independent of SEP, but scholars do not fully understand how the environmental characteristics of communities affect population health. In Chapter Five we learned that the relationship between income and health may be explained by a combination of health risk behaviors, a number of factors associated with poor material conditions, and psychosocial factors that induce health-damaging biological and behavioral consequences. Also, health may be viewed as both a cause and consequence of socioeconomic circumstance.

What the previous chapters abundantly document, however, is that the fundamental determinants of population health have fundamental consequences for health. U.S. health policy has largely focused on downstream, short-term, medical care–oriented interventions. An enlarged and expanded population health–centered policy would encompass upstream, long-term, fundamental investments for improving health and reducing health disparities.

Table 7.5 summarizes the research emphases in the pursuit of an evidence-based approach to defining the problem and assessing solutions in an agenda driven by a population health policy. In order to determine what problems to address to improve population health, we need specific data on the health care and nonmedical factors that create risks for populations and subpopulations, the costs and benefits of various health care and nonhealth care strategies for improving health, the magnitude and predictors of health disparities, and the ways that policymakers can use this new information to make efficient health care, public health, and intersectoral investments.

Currently, evidence-based assessments of the question of what works in health policy is largely restricted to policies aimed at enhancing the effectiveness, efficiency, and equity of health care delivery (Aday et al., 2004). There is a paucity of high-quality studies of policies and strategies aimed at the more upstream social, economic, and environmental factors that determine population health. Such research requires a rich mix of interdisciplinary skills that spans the full spectrum of issues that affect health and well-being.

A population health approach supports research that covers that full spectrum of issues, including health services, biomedical, health promotion, social, economic, and environmental health issues. A rich mix of interdisciplinary skills is also required to span the full range of paradigms, including randomized trials,

**TABLE 7.5.   CATEGORIES OF POLICY QUESTIONS AND RELATED RESEARCH
FOR A POPULATION HEALTH–CENTERED POLICY.**

	Policy Question	Research
Problem analysis	Effectiveness	Identify the health care, behavioral, socioeconomic, and environmental factors that create risks to population health.
	Efficiency	Identify the health care, behavioral change interventions, and socioeconomic and environmental investments that are and are not cost-beneficial or cost-effective.
	Equity	Identify the health care, behavioral, socioeconomic, and environmental inequities that contribute to disparities in population health.
Solution analysis	Effectiveness	Identify health care and nonhealth care–related structures and processes that improve population health.
	Efficiency	Identify cost-beneficial and cost-effective health care, public health, and intersectoral investments that improve population health.
	Equity	Identify health care, public health, and intersectoral investments that reduce inequities in population health.

meta-analysis, case studies, surveys, economic evaluations, and so on. A wide range of data types, both qualitative and quantitative, is also relevant, including environmental, behavioral, social, economic, epidemiological, and health systems data, for example. To improve decision making, a population health research agenda includes producing and analyzing relevant information about which interventions or combinations of interventions are the most effective and efficient in modifying specific types of health outcomes, decreasing health inequities, improving the health of the population as a whole, and intervening to influence the fundamental determinants of health.

Design an Intersectoral Public Health System. As indicated earlier in the chapter, there is a growing interest in conceptualizing and implementing a public health system that encompasses a leadership role for conventional governmental public health but also moves beyond it in terms of aligning with other entities and organizations that affect the health of populations.

A *public health system,* as defined by Mays, Halverson, and Scutchfield (2004, p. 183), represents "the collection of organizations, individuals, and communities that contribute to activities that promote health and prevent disease and injury at the population level." Such a system is inherently intersectoral and requires leadership from multiple sectors to attain excellence.

Table 7.6 highlights the potential building blocks for the design of an intersectoral public health system. Considerations in developing such a system include the policy sectors and related interventions to be encompassed. Relevant policies and interventions could be identified within federal, state, or local governments; communities; programs; and organizations, including international agencies and institutions.

This book has argued for the central role that social and economic policies play in influencing the fundamental determinants of population health and in particular the importance of policies dealing with sustainable, human, economic, and/or community development. The business, education, government, and nongovernmental sectors are all potentially central players in the design of an intersectoral public system attuned to these policy areas.

TABLE 7.6. BUILDING BLOCKS FOR AN INTERSECTORAL PUBLIC HEALTH SYSTEM.

Policy Domains	
Sectors	**Selected Interventions**
Social and economic	
Business	Sustainable development
Education	Human development
Government	Economic development
Nongovernmental	Community development
Other (e.g., media, academia)	Varied
Public health	
	Assessment
	Policy development
	Assurance
Health care	
	Financing
	Availability
	Organization

Note. These domains could also be identified and operate within federal, state, or local governments; communities; programs; and organizations, including international agencies and institutions.

The Institute of Medicine report on the future of the public's health in the 21st century (Committee on Assuring, 2003) also argued for the role of media and academia in contributing to the design of an effective intersectoral public health system. The news, entertainment, and advertising media play a major role in shaping public opinion and consumer activities and preferences. The report calls for public health officials and media leadership to forge more effective approaches for communicating information regarding health issues and risks to the public. Academic public health and health professions training programs, as well as related academic programs (such as urban planning, public administration, social work, and business management, among others), provide significant expertise and opportunities for training practitioners in a variety of disciplines to take into account the population health consequences of their decision making. The report calls for the provision of incentives to universities, faculty members, and students to pursue interdisciplinary and transdisciplinary courses of study and research.

As demonstrated in Table 7.6, collaborations across these various policy sectors can exist in a variety of decision-making domains, including within or across various levels of government (federal, state, or local), communities, programs, and organizations. The table purposely leaves open specific examples of policies and related interventions in each of the domains to signal the flexibility and variability that must exist in the design of such a system within and across policy and decision-making contexts. The table acknowledges the importance of interventions at a variety of levels (e.g., government, communities, programs, and organizations) within a given policy domain (e.g., early childhood development) to effectively influence desired health or development outcomes. Input and engagement are also required across sectors to develop transdisciplinary paradigms for identifying and addressing the multipronged determinants of population health.

Governmental public health would maintain a key leadership role in the development of such a system and would center even more directly on its essential assessment, policy development, and assurance functions in promoting and protecting population health. The health care sector, which consumes the lion's share of public and private resources directed to personal health care services, would also be an important partner in addressing more proximate behavioral risks (e.g., smoking, obesity), providing primary prevention clinical services, and curing and caring for those who are ill. The financing, availability, and organization of personal health care services have been the major engines driving the design and operation of the health care delivery system. Representatives from the social and economic sectors round out the inclusion of fundamental entities that influence the fundamental determinants of health.

The system would be focused on specific target populations within identified jurisdictions (federal, state, local, and international). Collaborations among an array of both public- and private-sector entities would be integral to planning, implementing, and evaluating programs to address the fundamental determinants of population health within a jurisdiction. The collaborative would derive its authority from an appointment procedure originating from elected or appointed officials who are themselves authorized and responsible to the population of the jurisdiction or its government. This procedure is essential to legitimate the collaborative and justify financial support from the public officials and the level of government that they represent.

A blueprint for the design of an intersectoral local public health agency in support of such a system is provided in Exhibit 7.1. (The blueprint is based on the work of the Texas Model Public Health Practice Subcommittee of the House Concurrent Resolution 44 . . .Workgroup, *State of Public Health: Local and State Government Issues in Texas: Report Resulting from House Concurrent Resolution 44 of the 75th Legislature,* 1998.) The design reflects the legal requirements of public health practice and modifies and builds on the experience with traditional public health systems but differs substantially in policies, structures, and functions that promote its intersectoral nature. One important rationale for this approach is that a critical element of effectiveness in achieving public health benefits for populations is the constitutional and statutory authority to (a) spend publicly generated funds (taxes) and resources for public health purposes and (b) manage the trade-off between individual and group rights and freedoms and community benefit. A second reason is to formalize the commitment of multiple partners to a community enterprise as members of an agency rather than proceed with an essentially voluntary arrangement.

The design of an intersectoral public health system may be structured and operate at three levels in the community:

1. The first level conceptualizes and supports the concept of intersectoral policy and decision making essential to defining and bringing to bear the multiple sectors that influence health status as well as the interventions to improve or maintain health status in the community. These are the building blocks of the intersectoral system (see Table 7.6).

2. At the second level, a concrete intersectoral agency organizes, deploys, and evaluates the resources of the intersectoral system. The agency supports the implementation of the traditional enforcement and governmental responsibilities of public health agencies while allowing the formal addition and inclusion of entities and organizations that represent the broader determinants of health. This level is described in the outline of components necessary for the structure and function of an intersectoral local public health agency (see Exhibit 7.1).

3. The third level includes a large number of issue-specific coalitions, partnerships, and/or communities of practice that come together to address particular

EXHIBIT 7.1.   BLUEPRINT FOR THE DESIGN OF
AN INTERSECTORAL LOCAL PUBLIC HEALTH AGENCY.

Auspices
- Constitutional and statutory provisions require that government assume the responsibility for public health.
- Optimal achievement of health status for communities requires official inclusion
  of public- and private-sector organizations whose work is essential to achievement
  of improved health outcomes.
- The intersectoral public health system should define and agree on the appropriate
  role, function, and relationships of federal, state, and local public health jurisdictions. A description, for reference, is included in Chapter One of the Institute of
  Medicine's 1988 report *The Future of Public Health.*
- Effective health departments must have structures that generate and mediate
  community support and assure accountability to local community representatives
  and local commitment of financial support to public health.

Vision and Mission
- A vision lays out the expectations of what a healthy society would be like; it
  serves as the inspiration for the mission and work of the intersectoral public
  health system.
- A mission defines the purpose, major thrusts, and qualities of the health department with regard to how the vision will be satisfied; it shapes specific strategies,
  goals, and programs that focus the public health enterprise and reflect the societal values that determine it. It allows members, stakeholders, and proponents of
  the intersectoral public health system to align and join in a common focus and
  purpose.

Public Policy
- Defined policies authorize and drive the work and priorities of the intersectoral
  public health system, both collectively and for individual members.
- The sources of policy derive from each policy domain and each sector; the system
  members have the obligation to agree on policies that are collective across the
  sectors.
- Legal policies provide authorization to establish the intersectoral system, authority
  to contract between public- and private-sector members of the system, and protection of prerogatives for nongovernmental participants in the system.
- Oversight policies define and promote boards of health or other community
  structures for the intersectoral system.

Geographic Jurisdiction
- The agency defines the boundaries of populations in which the distribution and
  impact of determinants of health, disease occurrence and transmission, accessibility and availability of interventions, are determined. Geographic variations in such
  boundaries will be defined by the missions and functions of individual members
  of the intersectoral system.
- The agency allows the quantification, analysis (interpretation), and findings
  of surveillance, monitoring, and evaluation activities for differing populations
  and geographic areas. It addresses the flexibility required to cover differences
  in urban and rural population distributions as well as differing populations
  according to the service mission of participating members in the intersectoral
  system.

Structure
- The organizational structure of an intersectoral public health system defines the policymaking mechanism and denotes paths of decision making, resource allocation, supervisory responsibility, and action.
- The organizational structure defines the responsibilities and relationships of the various members of the intersectoral system.

Functions and Programs
- The essence of a department of health is what it does to carry out its vision and mission. The choice of core functions, programs, and essential services is the most pragmatic part of the model. A new, expanded set will be required that addresses key determinants and identifies institutional roles and functions of the members of the intersectoral public health system.

---

issues. They may either arise independent of the influence of the intersectoral agency or be commissioned and promoted directly by the agency's decisions (see Table 7.7).

The third level of the intersectoral public health system encompasses the many coalitions, partnerships, and communities of service that are established to address specific health issues and then dissolved as their work is completed. In the recommended model of the intersectoral public health system, these groups may arise independent of the intersectoral agency or be commissioned by them. A supportive relationship with the agency is expected in terms of the provision of data about a community, technical assistance, or other resources. The agency, through its liaison with these groups, could improve its surveillance of community health and has the opportunity to assist in maintaining communications across these diverse sectors.

The proposed multilevel intersectoral design maintains the collective governmental responsibility of the traditional public health system while opening up options to include both policy and service inputs from the many other sectors of society that provide the primary resources in realizing improved health status apart from the traditional public health arenas. Indeed, leadership may emerge from traditional and nontraditional sectors to facilitate the attainment of public health system goals.

The resulting system would not be a static, fixed model that takes on a singular form and design. Because of the social and cultural complexities and diversity in the postmodern globalized society and economy in which public health and other major social institutions must now operate (see Chapter One), different models may be needed for specific political and social contexts.

The Turning Point initiative offers other models of intersectoral collaboration. Its central mission and goal was "to transform and strengthen the public

TABLE 7.7.   MODELS FOR COLLABORATIVE DECISION MAKING.

Government	◄───►	Community	◄───►	Market
Advisory boards	Coalitions	Communities of practice	Public-private partnerships	Socially responsive corporate management

health system in the United States to make the system more effective, more community-based, and more collaborative" (Turning Point, 2005). A variety of models emerged and substantial variability existed in each project's actual operation and impact across states and communities. The Turning Point experience does, however, represent an experiment and an opportunity to learn how to develop and implement intersectoral collaborations across varied political and social contexts. The mandate for future research in this area would be to rigorously evaluate which specific models have succeeded in improving population health, determine why, and research whether the models are transferable (Berkowitz & Nicola, 2003).

Process

Progress in moving toward a healthy republic would be characterized by the evolution of participatory public-private decision-making partnerships and population health–centered public health practice arrangements.

Forge New Collaborative Decision-Making Arrangements. Table 7.7 presents an array of collaborative decision-making arrangements that have been employed in public health, as well as other fields (Berkowitz & Wolff, 2000; Bruce & McKane, 2000; Wenger, McDermott, & Snyder, 2002). Arnstein (1969) conceptualized a ladder of citizen participation, with the ascending rungs representing a gradient ranging from nonparticipation to tokenism to increased levels of citizen power and control. Based on the steps in Arnstein's ladder, the advisory and consultative role characterizing membership in institutional or community advisory boards represents the lowest rung of mutually participatory engagement. Political coalitions represent another point along the continuum of collaborative decision making. Coalitions may emerge from bottom-up grassroots interests in carrying a common cause forward or from a top-down legislative mandate or bureaucratic condition of funding.

Communities of practice and related learning communities represent an innovative but largely unevaluated model for ensuring the authentic interest and engagement of participants in sharing information to improve the quality or outcomes of their work. Communities of practice are "groups of people who share a concern, a set of problems, or a passion about a topic, and who deepen their knowledge and expertise in this area by interacting on an ongoing basis" (Wenger et al., 2002, p. 4). And finally, models of socially responsive corporate governance may represent either a virtual or actual partnership between business, public health, and environmental interests to assure corporate profitability while minimizing the environmental consequences of corporate actions.

The promotion of partnerships as a way of doing business has become almost a prerequisite to success in public health. These partnerships are based on the notion that public health can most effectively achieve its objectives by mobilizing other stakeholders in the community. More recently, these partnerships have included health care providers, community-based organizations, and organizations not directly related to health. As Linder, Quill, and Aday (2001, p. 522) point out, "much of the writing on partnering, however, conveys the impression that partnerships of this kind are new to government. . . . We are led to believe that partnering as a management practice, deserves wide emulation both inside government and out." Partnership is not new and can be traced to the Middle Ages, with a more familiar model rooted in business law. Central to the premise of partnerships is the sense of fairness, with each partner bearing some of the risk, cost, and outcome. The assets of partnerships are well documented, but two aspects key to the new (re)public bear examination.

The first is the symmetry of the partnership formulation (Linder et al., 2001). In the context of the health outcomes and fundamental determinants, the following questions need to be addressed:

- Who are the partners, and have the partners been involved in developing the partnership?
- Do all of the partners share in the design and control over the partnership decisions and actions?

The second aspect of the partnership is symmetry of function (Linder et al., 2001):

- Are the partners appropriately matched to the task by their expertise?
- How will they contribute to community health?
- Do all of the partners share in costs and responsibilities?

Partnerships that meet these conditions have satisfied the central element of successful partnerships: trust.

A look at current partnerships leads to three observations regarding their performance. The first observation is that the public health partnership organizations do not frequently partner with an array of nonhealth care entities. Daft (2004) identifies 10 sectors that need to be considered in collaborations and partnership development: the economic conditions sector, the technology sector, the market sector, the financial resources sector, the human resources sector, the raw materials sector, the industry sector, the international sector, the sociocultural sector, and the government sector. These illustrate the broad scope of potential intersectoral work. Irrespective of recent imperatives to maximize intersectoral capital to ensure the health and protection of the population, many sectors have not been fully tapped in public health alliances. Intersectoral and new collaborations with business, philanthropy, or technology are infrequent; and there are only limited examples of partnerships with other sectors. In addition, the partnerships are often asymmetrical, with one or more partners bearing an unequal share of the funding or resources and subsequently the expectation of more control and decision making. A simple example is when a government agency or foundation funds a local public health project. Although the parties involved use the term *partner*, the terms, functions, and responsibilities are often unequal. Finally, the current partnerships specifically designed to engage citizens often reflect a lack of skill in community and civic engagement.

Reformulation and reformation will be required to advance partnerships capable of meeting future challenges. This reconstitution must include intersectoral collaboration and the exploration of new models such as communities of practice. The benefits of these approaches are largely unmeasured but remain a key to understanding how to secure future success.

Symmetry and trust within and across partnerships in both their formulation and function are evidence of progress toward a healthy republic in the service of improving the health of the public. Their de facto success in doing so can be evaluated by applying the benchmarks of effectiveness, efficiency, and equity criteria.

As reviewed in Chapter Six, a variety of failures have been documented in forging and maintaining collaborative models of decision making within and across communities and sectors. The principles most often violated in the operation and impact of such models may be broadly characterized according to the major criteria of equity:

- Intergenerational justice: maintenance of resources and benefits across generations
- Distributive justice: fair distribution of benefits and burdens across individuals and communities

- Deliberative justice: full and effective participation of affected parties in decision making
- Social justice: minimization of health disparities between groups

The record of the sustainability of such interventions, that is, their being maintained to provide benefits to future generations, is often quite limited. There is also often substantial asymmetry in the distributions of economic and/or political power and benefits of such initiatives across individuals and communities. The defining norm of deliberative justice, which mandates the full and effective participation of affected parties in decision making, is more often honored in the breach. And finally, evidence regarding the success of such initiatives in achieving the social justice goal of minimizing health disparities between groups is scant. Further, little rigorous quantitative evidence is available on the effectiveness and efficiency of collaborative models of decision making in improving population health and reducing health disparities.

As with the design of the intersectoral public health system, no one size fits all in the design of collaborative decision-making arrangements in support of such a system. To fully understand which arrangements might work best, public health and health services researchers need to more explicitly characterize and distinguish the extent to which the arrangements differ in form, function, and impact.

Engage in Population Health–Centered Public Health Practice. A defining parameter in the design of a population health–centered intersectoral public health system is that it focuses on enlivening its essential population health–oriented focus around the core public health functions and essential services. Table 7.8 highlights the shifts that would take place in moving to more population health–centered public health practice.

Assessment Function
Assessment entails monitoring the health of communities and populations at risk to identify health problems and priorities.

Monitor Health Status. A population heath–centered focus would extend beyond the focus on disease surveillance and program client and services that has defined conventional public health information systems to a focus on the design and implementation of population health information systems (Keller, Schaffer, Lia-Hoagberg, & Strohschein, 2002; Roos et al., 1996). Such information systems would have a broader denominator of the target population that the public health system served, regardless of whether the individuals had a reportable disease or received services through the system. The systems would also link data from a

TABLE 7.8. POPULATION HEALTH–CENTERED PUBLIC HEALTH PRACTICE.

Core Public Health Functions	Essential Services	Current Practice	Population Health–Centered Practice
Assessment function	*Monitor* health status to identify community health problems.	Develop and employ disease surveillance systems.	Develop and employ population health information systems.
	Diagnose and investigate health problems and hazards in the community.	Conduct disease outbreak investigations in the community.	Apply ecosocial models to identify the fundamental determinants of population health in the community.
Policy development function	*Inform, educate, and empower* people about health issues.	Inform, educate, and empower individuals and communities to promote their health and well-being.	Inform, educate, and empower various sectors (business, education, community organizations, media, academia, government, public health, health care) to promote population health.
	Mobilize community partnerships and action to identify and solve health problems.	Build local, statewide, or national partnerships to address public health problems.	Build an intersectoral public health system to address population health problems.
	Develop policies and plans that support individual and community health efforts.	Formulate and strengthen public health and health care policy.	Formulate and strengthen population health–centered public policy.

Assurance function	*Enforce* laws and regulations that protect health and ensure safety.	Regulate environmental and occupational hazards and disaster preparedness.	Design model legislation to promote population health–centered programs within and across sectors.
	Link people to needed personal health care services and assure the provision of health care when otherwise unavailable.	Organize and manage the delivery of safety-net health care services in the community.	Collaborate to develop and finance an integrated continuum of primary prevention, treatment, and long-term care programs and services in the community.
	Assure a competent public health and personal and population-based health workforce.	Train and evaluate public health professionals in terms of core public health competencies.	Train public health, planning, and development professionals in the population health approach.
	Evaluate the effectiveness, accessibility, and quality of personal and population-based health services.	Evaluate public health agencies and communities in terms of model and performance-based standards.	Evaluate public health and inter-sectoral initiatives in terms of their population health impact.
Serving all functions	*Research* for new insights and innovative solutions to health problems.	Design and conduct multi-disciplinary and interdisciplinary research to address public health issues.	Design and conduct transdisciplinary research to address fundamental determinants of population health.

variety of providers and sources (other than the governmental public health sector) in the service of calibrating health risks, overall rates and patterns of health services use, as well as communitywide health impacts of broader public health–system interventions. Public health informatics represents "the systematic application of information and computer science and technology to public health practice, research, and learning" (Yasnoff, O'Carroll, Koo, Linkins, & Kilbourne, 2000, p. 68). The evolution of the field of public health informatics and the related emergence of informatics training programs for public health students and practitioners support the development of electronic highways for mapping the design of population health information systems.

Diagnose and Investigate Health Problems. Current public health surveillance systems detect and investigate disease outbreaks in the community and attempt to identify and ameliorate the immediate and proximate causes of such outbreaks. The ecosocial paradigm broadens the scope and deepens the levels at which population health risks and consequences are examined. The ecosocial perspective encompasses a broad array of fundamental (distal) as well as intermediate and proximate causes of health and illness. It also argues for a look at the variety of levels of intervention and impact at which these factors may operate (e.g., individual, family, neighborhood, etc.). The advent of geographic information system and related mapping technologies, multilevel modeling of the predictive importance of determinants at various levels, and the evolution of both quantitative and qualitative methods for analyzing the influence of being embedded in a particular social or economic context on health provide helpful tools for translating the broader ecosocial perspective into practice (Krieger, Chen, Waterman, Rehkopf, & Subramanian, 2003; Richards, Croner, & Novick, 1999).

Policy Development Function
Policy development encompasses the formulation of public policies to address identified local and national health problems and priorities in collaboration with community and government leaders.

Inform, Educate, and Empower People. Engaging affected communities in identifying health needs and assets is an important tenet of current public health practice. The blueprint for an intersectoral public health system (see Table 7.6) shifts the focus not only to affected individuals and communities but to other sectors and institutions that might play a role in developing a population health–oriented system (e.g., business, education, community organizations, media, academia, government, public health agencies, health care providers). Learning and innovation are required on the part of all the sectors involved. Public health agencies must identify the role that the other sectors could play in realizing their essential mission. Other sectors must gain a fuller understanding of the essential impact that their policies and actions have on the distal and proximate determinants of health and illness. Governmental public health agencies can assume leadership in encouraging these collaborations, but the success of such collaborations requires the full engagement of all relevant governmental and nongovernmental sectors (Kimbrell, 2000; Nicola & Hatcher, 2000).

Mobilize Community Partnerships. As discussed earlier, effective collaborative relationships are key for building an effective intersectoral public health system. Public health–planning tools offer a means to forge such relationships in practice. A variety of public health–planning models have been applied to facilitate community participation around health issues, including the Assessment Protocol for Excellence in Public Health (APEX/PH), Planned Approach to Community Health (PATCH), Healthy Communities, and Mobilizing for Action through Planning and Partnerships (MAPP). The MAPP model, for example, provides a systematic approach for organizing and developing partnerships; developing a shared vision; and carrying out assessments of community themes and strengths, community health status, local public health system performance, and likely forces for change. The benchmarks of success against which to evaluate the MAPP and other planning models include, among others, those embodied in the equity criteria reviewed earlier: creating collaborations that are sustainable (intergenerational justice), balancing the benefits and costs to various participants (distributive justice), ensuring that the voices of all those affected are heard (deliberative justice), and resulting in improving population health and reducing health disparities (social justice) (National Association of County and City Health Officials & CDC, n.d.; Scutchfield, Ireson, & Hall, 2004).

Develop Policies. Public health–related policies have typically focused on strengthening or supporting the governmental public health infrastructure or related health care reforms to assure that vulnerable and uninsured populations have access to needed preventive or clinical care services. The population health–centered policy vision articulated earlier in the chapter points to health outcomes as the benchmark of success. Standards of accountability in terms of the structure and process of public health system performance shift to what types of intersectoral arrangements are most effective, efficient, and equitable in achieving benchmarks of success for population health improvements (Aday et al., 2004; Handler et al., 2001).

Assurance Function

The assurance function is concerned with ensuring that all populations have access to appropriate and cost-effective care, including health promotion and disease prevention services, as well as the evaluation of the effectiveness of that care.

Enforce Laws and Regulations. Current public health law reflects a historical accretion of legislation and regulations that have been put into place to deal (often in ad hoc and unsystematic ways) with existent or emergent threats to the health of the public (Gostin, 2001). An assessment of current practice reveals that the corpus of public health law in many states does not provide a strong and coherent legal platform for governmental public health in carrying out its core assessment, policy development, and assurance functions (Gebbie, 2000). The Turning Point project has catalyzed an initiative to develop model legislation that would be supportive of governmental public health in carrying out these core functions and related essential services, as well as provide the blueprint and legislative undergirding for the design of a broader intersectoral public health system (Erickson, 2002).

Link People to Needed Services. The current public health and health care systems in many communities are essentially nonsystems; the array of providers, programs, and services often are not able or do not choose to coordinate services and referrals. The funding streams for programs are often discrete and categorical. *Public health finance* is defined as "a field of science and practice that deals with the acquisition, management, and use of financial resources to advance the health of populations through prevention and health promotion" (Moulton, Halverson, Honoré, & Berkowitz, 2004, p. 377). Though in a largely developmental stage at present, public health finance offers a practical means for funding and fueling a public health vision that centers on population health. Integrating discrete streams of funding for programs in mental health, substance abuse, HIV/AIDS, and homelessness, for example, would offer a promising way to fuel the development of a more coordinated and integrated continuum of care. The Robert Wood Johnson Foundation Child Health Initiative funded demonstration projects in several states to see if it could be done. An evaluation of the project documented that the barriers to doing so were great and the successes—in the short run at least—were few in most of the states (Newacheck, Hughes, Brindis, & Halfon, 1995). The public health community could assume leadership by getting its own accounts in order through developing a conceptual framework and procedures for public health finance to more effectively carry out its mission to improve the health of populations.

Assure a Competent Workforce. Scholars have devoted a significant amount of attention to identifying the number, distribution, training, and leadership development needs of the public health workforce (Gebbie, Merrill, Hwang, Gebbie, & Gupta, 2003). Specific competencies have been developed for readying the workforce to carry out the core public health functions (Lichtveld & Cioffi, 2003). Formal testing and credentialing of public health practitioners in terms of their demonstrated capacity for performing these functions and delivering essential public health services are on the drawing board (Cioffi, Lichtveld, Thielen, & Miner, 2003). But new challenges are introduced in infusing a population health vision and identifying relevant professional capacities for carrying it out in a workforce that has been guided more by program process and performance than by the end point of improved population health (Clark & Weist, 2000). The mandate for an intersectoral public health system also raises the question of what training and development non–public health professionals in other sectors (e.g., business, education, and community organizations) need in order to jointly and effectively realize a shared population health vision (Institute of Medicine, Committee on Educating, 2003).

Evaluate Services. The field of public health has developed model standards and related performance-based standards for evaluating the performance of public health agencies (Corso, Wiesner, Halverson, & Brown, 2000; Suen & Magruder, 2004). The evolution of an intersectoral public health system directed explicitly to population health improvements presents important accountability challenges to public health agencies and their partners (Scutchfield, Knight, Kelly, Bhandari, & Vasilescu, 2004). Health impact assessment methods and strategies represent an approach to assay the extent to which agencies achieve the desired objective of improving population health (Krieger et al., 2003; Mindell, Ison, & Joffe, 2003). Identifying the lines of accountability in a system that engages multiple agencies and sectors raises significant methodological and political issues. Further, agencies or entities that are responsible for the health of the public must often take action even when the evidence regarding likely risks is probabilistic at its best and controversial at worst (such as ordering an industrial plant in a neighborhood in which it is a primary source of employment to investigate what appear to be major health consequences for area residents resulting from plant emissions). The precautionary principle may, however, provide guidance for the prudent balancing of mission-driven responsibility and externally mandated accountability. Kriebel and Tickner (2001, p. 1351) articulate the precautionary principle this way: "When an activity raises threat of harm to human health or the environment, precautionary measures should be taken even if some cause and effect relationships are not fully established scientifically."

Serving All Functions: Research for New Insights and Innovations
The information revolution has dramatically shaped economic and social life in our time, much as the industrial revolution defined the character of the late 19th and

early 20th centuries. The generation, dissemination, and mutual exchange of knowledge that will help in achieving professional and organizational goals is also a means for creating innovative forms of organization (learning organizations) and practice (learning communities) (Senge, 1994; Wenger et al., 2002). The fusion of insights and evidence from across the disciplines has guided the corresponding use of approaches that identify and link the complex array of determinants of population health in the context of transdisciplinary research paradigms and programs (Albrecht, Freeman, & Higginbotham, 1998).

Complex and multidimensional problems, such as those that research on the fundamental determinants of health has identified, require new lenses for revealing previously unexamined complexity. The ecosocial paradigm (see Figure 1.2) and the framework for identifying the role of successive fundamental, intermediate, and proximate determinants in accounting for the ways that racial segregation contributes to racial disparities in health (see Figure 1.3) represent some promising new lenses. The central questions to address are "How will we know we are successful?" and "How do we sustain progress?" What is evident is that new definitions and measures of success will be required to develop and sustain effects.

McDowell, Spasoff, and Kristjansson (2004, p. 391) advocate for an extended population health–measurement approach:

> A measurement protocol for population health must include a broad set of measures that includes aggregate measures of healthy outcomes used for descriptive purposes, plus environmental and global health measures of dynamic population characteristics used for predictive, analytical and explanatory purposes.

Broader population health information systems would, for example, capture measures of social and economic as well as physical health and well-being (Miringoff & Miringoff, 1999).

Public health training and practice will require major renovation and leadership development in order to achieve and assess the success of an intersectoral public health system. The defining principles and focus of a public health university grounded in a population health–centered agenda for the 21st century must be broad and energetic: focused on a clear population health–centered vision, grounded in an understanding of the past and the potential for the future of the public health field, guided by core public health principles, centered on learning throughout all levels of the institution, and motivated by balanced and high standards of excellence in scholarship. Exhibit 7.2 provides some details.

EXHIBIT 7.2. A MODEL PUBLIC HEALTH UNIVERSITY FOR THE 21ST CENTURY.

Focused on a Clear Population Health–Centered Vision
A defining vision for a model public health university would center on the core mission of the field of public health—to improve the health of populations, recognize that public health science and scholarship in the service of this goal must be inherently interdisciplinary and transdisciplinary, and acknowledge that effective public health interventions compel the design of innovative and integrative policy and program strategies that cut across conventionally distinct decision-making domains (Health Canada, Population Strategic Policy Directorate of the Population and Public Health Branch, 2001).

Grounded in an Understanding of the Past and the Potential for the Future of the Public Health Field
The architecture for a model public health university would be characterized by a solid foundation of knowledge and understanding of the past history of public health as a field of study and practice, as well as a forward-looking blueprint for strengthening the academic, research, and practice programs that undergird its core population health–centered mission in the light of future challenges (Institute of Medicine, Committee on Assuring the Health of the Public in the 21st Century, 2003; Institute of Medicine, Committee on Educating Public Health Professionals for the 21st Century, 2003).

Guided by Core Public Health Principles
The internal operations as well as the external interfaces of a model public health university must be guided by core public health principles and ethical and principled leadership in forging problem-centered, participatory partnerships across fields of study, institutions, communities, and individuals, in the service of improving the health of the public (Etienne, McDermott, & Snyder, 2002; Public Health Leadership Society, 2002; Wenger, McDermott, & Snyder, 2002).

Centered on Learning Throughout All Levels of the Institution
To achieve excellence in scholarship, a model public health university would create an atmosphere and opportunities to inspire innovation and lifetime learning on the part of all of those who study and work within it—faculty, students, alumni, staff, and administration (Senge, 1994; Senge, Kleiner, Roberts, Ross, & Smith, 1994).

Motivated by Balanced and High Standards of Excellence in Scholarship
The core institutional missions of research, teaching, and service and the hiring, development, retention, promotion, and tenure of faculty would be motivated by benchmarking and balancing excellence in the scholarships of discovery (the generation of new knowledge), integration (the synthesis and application of existing knowledge in new ways), teaching (transmitting knowledge), and application (translating what is known and learned into practice) (Boyer, 1990; Quill & Aday, 2000).

Outcomes

Two tenets, grounded in research and policy on the fundamental determinants, may be helpful to remember in guiding the development and evaluation of population health–centered policy:

• Think and act globally and locally.
• Levels are not the same as differences.

The first tenet is a variant of the oft-cited admonition to "Think globally, act locally." The revised tenet acknowledges the tightly knit connection and interdependence of opportunities and policies at both the local and global levels. Economically impoverished neighborhoods can emerge in very wealthy countries (such as the United States), often as a consequence of the forces of globalization. And the economic and political elite of developing countries may enjoy wealth and privileges that are similar to those of many people in developed nations. Globalization has multiplied and intensified the intrusions of international markets into local economies. On the other hand, local action in governmental, community, or market sectors may catalyze powerful forces for change globally (Bourdieu, 1998; Hardt & Negri, 2000).

As this chapter argued earlier and as Table 7.6 reflects, building an intersectoral public health system requires policy and program interventions at a variety of levels. An approach to addressing the impact of the social and economic deterioration of inner-city areas in the United States, for example, is a call from within the public health community to rebuild a historical connection between urban planning and public health (Corburn, 2004; Northridge & Sclar, 2003). At the same time, the WHO is calling for a broad global health agenda to address the complex, interrelated, international actions and influences that ultimately shape the health of specific nation-states and localities (Kickbusch, 2000).

The second tenet is that levels are not the same as differences. *Levels* refer to the overall levels of health in a society, and *differences* refer to gaps in health between groups within a society (see Table 1.3). Graham (2004b) has insightfully argued that the specific policy devices and corollary political support may differ, depending on whether the focus is on reducing or narrowing the social disadvantage gap as opposed to improving the social and economic well-being of all members of society. Due to the health gradient associated with improvements in economic well-being, the latter policy strategy would result in health improvements for everyone in general, but if the rate of improvement were similar across groups, any existing gaps between groups would still persist. (Distinctions between the health gap and health gradient perspectives and related policy implications were elaborated in Table 1.3.)

The strategy of diminishing gaps between groups, Graham (2004b) argues, runs the risk of having less political support than an approach to trying to improve population health overall, when the predominant political forces oppose categorical programs for the poor and socially disadvantaged. The general population health improvement strategy may be more politically feasible but may leave unremediated gaps between groups. In a related work, Graham (2004a) convincingly argues for a clear conceptual distinction in the explanatory frameworks for examining the social determinants of population health as opposed to the social determinants of health disparities. The latter framework explicitly compels an examination of the fundamental structural inequalities in a society or community to effectively account for and ameliorate differences in population health outcomes across groups.

The transdisciplinary paradigms emerging from research on the social determinants of health provide mental models for identifying the fundamental determinants of population health. These determinants apply across nations and societies, though the magnitude or relative importance of each may differ. Policy interventions for improving population health and reducing health disparities may differ in specifics across political contexts and social-cultural settings. The common assumption underlying their success, however, is that addressing the fundamental determinants of population health is required in order to ultimately influence either levels or differences in population health.

A framework for evaluating the impact of population health–centered policy and practice on population health and health disparities is highlighted in Figure 7.1.

As described in the earlier discussion and more fully documented in Health Canada's population health template (2001), population health–centered policies require multiple strategies, intersectoral collaboration, and public involvement.

A population health–centered system emerging from such policies must encompass a fuller awareness on the part of a variety of sectors (for example, business, education, and others) of the impacts of their actions and initiatives on the health of populations, as well as the forming of effective working partnerships within and across sectors to successfully address the fundamental determinants of population health.

Two streams of impact on population health and health disparities are formulated to acknowledge that both the pathways for intervention as well as the political possibilities for success are grounded in one of the essential tenets of population health–centered policy design offered earlier: "Levels are not the same as differences," that is, focusing on population health improvements overall will not necessarily reduce the disparities between groups within a population (Graham, 2004a, 2004b). Improvements in overall population health and reductions in health disparities may compel somewhat different policy strategies. Stakeholders must clearly understand and delineate the predictors and indicators for each outcome.

FIGURE 7.1.   FRAMEWORK FOR DESIGNING AND EVALUATING THE IMPACT OF POPULATION HEALTH–CENTERED POLICY.

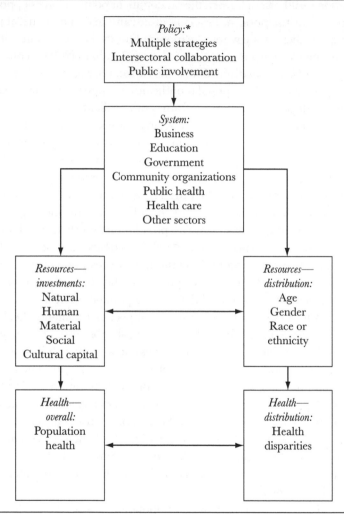

*From *Population Health Template: Key Elements and Actions That Define Population Health,* by Health Canada, Population Strategic Policy Directorate of the Population and Public Health Branch, 2001.

As documented in Figure 1.4, policies in a given area, such as human development and educational policy, may affect population health and health disparities either indirectly through influencing the fundamental determinants of population health (school achievement, level of education, and related skills of individuals and groups) or directly through programs that explicitly target the health needs of selected populations (child nutrition, health education, and school health services, for example). Further, interventions may take place over the long, medium, and short term, broadly corresponding to the fundamental, intermediate, and proximate determinants of health, respectively (delineated sequentially in Figure 1.3).

Health disparities often are visible across age, gender, and (in the United States especially) race or ethnicity. The differential availability of resources essential to promoting and sustaining health across these or other strata (population subgroups) provides a basis for understanding variant health levels and disparities across subgroups.

As the preceding chapters have indicated, a growing body of research has documented the importance of fundamental nonmedical determinants in influencing population health and disparities. The emerging research and policy agenda will need to evaluate the success of policies and programs in a variety of sectors in directly influencing the essential resources that these fundamental determinants represent (renewable and nonrenewable resources, levels of education and skills, distribution of wealth and income, quantity and quality of social ties, and community values) as well as indirectly influencing the health of populations for which disparities in these resources exist. A focal point of the book has been on the indirect impact of policies in conventionally nonhealth sectors on resources that act as fundamental determinants of population health. These resources, highlighted in Table 1.1, include natural, human, material, social, and cultural capital.

Recommendations

The book concludes with specific observations and recommendations for designing and implementing more population health–centered public policy based on the evidence and analyses presented in this and the preceding chapters (see Figure 7.1).

General (Chapters One, Two, and Seven)

- Public health is essentially concerned with improving the health of populations—not just patients.
- The health of populations is influenced by environmental, social, and economic factors that lie outside the conventional province of governmental public health.

- Population health policy encompasses both health and nonhealth policies and programs.
- Population health–centered practice requires that governmental public health agencies and professionals reorient and expand core public health functions and essential services.
- A healthy republic forges effective collaborations across traditional disciplinary, institutional, professional, and political divides to enhance the health of the public.

Sustainable Development (Chapter Three)

- Forge a new strategy for public health that shifts the perspective from a hazard to a habitat dimension—one that focuses on ecosystem stressors rather than individual risk factors and that generates business actions for protecting community health and reducing community health risks.
- Forge a new strategy for socially responsible corporate business practice that sets ecological principles as the foundation for profitable and sustainable business practices.

Human Development (Chapter Four)

- Develop a policy that education starts at birth, explicitly linking child care with formal education for very young children (infancy to 3 years of age, 4 or 5 years of age).
- Develop intersectoral policies that link child care, family support, and education in a seamless and integrated continuum for kindergarten through high school education.

Economic Development (Chapter Five)

- Develop a process for full participation by local and national policymakers, researchers, and affected communities (especially those that are often excluded because of illiteracy, poor health, or poverty) in shaping the policies that affect them.
- Support economic policies that reduce poverty, increase labor market participation, and improve the balance of trade benefits for developing relative to developed countries, as well as policies that directly improve population health.

Community Development (Chapter Six)

- To facilitate successful community development, public health practitioners must understand and evaluate alternative community development models, strengthen the role of public health in community development, and support workforce development and training in this area.

- In particular, public health practitioners need to be trained in promoting deliberative democracy, developing local leadership, respecting community interests and values, and motivating political action in order to facilitate positive change in communities.

Steps to Move the Agenda Forward

Following are a number of steps that are required in order to move this broader public health agenda forward.

Envision a Systems Approach. Systems of public health practice will be successful depending on how well they identify and forecast new intersectoral arrangements that are responsive to emerging public health problems. Success will be determined by how the systems are defined, how they operate, and what effects they generate. Developing, monitoring, and reconstructing effective systems will require risk taking, innovation, and persistence.

Assume Leadership. Public health practice success will require leadership in the following areas: understanding and design of the systems, innovative intersectoral collaboration, and visioning of desirable population-based futures. Leadership approaches that emphasize shared leadership, accountability, ethics, and the inclusion of citizens in decision making offer the promise of realizing the goal of healthy citizens in healthy communities.

Measure Performance. New approaches and methods will be required in order to measure the system effects and population-specific determinants. Partnerships and their influence must also be included in the measurement of system effects. Not only will researchers need to measure different indicators, but they will also perhaps need to develop and apply different methodological approaches. The new applications will challenge existing assumptions regarding public health practice as well as the definition of what success might mean in a practice focused on population health.

Train for the Future, but Stay Grounded in the Past. A new and expanded vision is required for preparing public health professionals to realize the broad practice and policy agenda presented in this book. Such a vision must clearly encompass but move beyond the confines of governmental public health to the design of an integrated public-private system that employs innovative methods and means to respond to existing political and economic realities.

This book provides a compass and a road map for those who work within the field of public health or in collaboration with it for effectively meeting this challenge. Let the journey begin!

References

Acheson, D. (1998). *Independent inquiry into inequalities in health report.* London: Stationery Office.

Aday, L. A., Begley, C. E., Lairson, D. R., & Balkrishnan, R. (2004). *Evaluating the healthcare system: Effectiveness, efficiency, and equity* (3rd ed.). Chicago: Health Administration Press.

Ågren, G. (2003). *Sweden's new public health policy: National public health objectives for Sweden.* Stockholm: Swedish National Institute of Public Health.

Albrecht, G., Freeman, S., & Higginbotham, N. (1998). Complexity and human health: The case for a transdisciplinary paradigm. *Culture, Medicine and Psychiatry, 22,* 55–92.

Anderson, O. W. (1989). *The health services continuum in democratic states: An inquiry into solvable problems.* Chicago: Health Administration Press.

Arnstein, S. (1969). A ladder of citizen participation. *Journal of the American Institute of Planners, 35,* 216–224.

Auerbach, J. A., Krimgold, B. K., & Lefkowitz, B. (2000). *Improving health: It doesn't take a revolution.* Washington, DC: National Policy Association/Academy for Health Services Research and Health Policy.

Baker, E. L., Jr., & Koplan, J. P. (2002). Strengthening the nation's public health infrastructure: Historic challenge, unprecedented opportunity. *Health Affairs, 21*(6), 15–27.

Berkowitz, B., & Nicola, R. M. (2003). Public health infrastructure system change: Outcomes from the Turning Point Initiative. *Journal of Public Health Management and Practice, 9*(3), 224–227.

Berkowitz, W. R., & Wolff, T. (Eds.). (2000). *The spirit of the coalition.* Washington, DC: American Public Health Association.

Black, D. (1980). *Inequalities in health: Report of a research working group.* London: Department of Health and Social Security.

Bourdieu, P. (1998). *Acts of resistance: Against the tyranny of the market* (R. Nice, Trans.). New York: New Press.

Boyer, E. L. (1990). *Scholarship reconsidered: Priorities of the professoriate.* Princeton, NJ: Carnegie Foundation for the Advancement of Teaching.

Bruce, T. A., & McKane, S. U. (Eds.). (2000). *Community-based public health: A partnership model.* Washington, DC: American Public Health Association.

Cioffi, J. P., Lichtveld, M. Y., Thielen, L., & Miner, K. (2003). Credentialing the public health workforce: An idea whose time has come. *Journal of Public Health Management and Practice, 9*(6), 451–458.

Clark, N. M., & Weist, E. (2000). Mastering the new public health. *American Journal of Public Health, 90,* 1208–1211.

Corburn, J. (2004). Confronting the challenges in reconnecting urban planning and public health. *American Journal of Public Health, 94,* 541–546.

Corso, L. C., Wiesner, P. J., Halverson, P. K., & Brown, C. K. (2000). Using the essential services as a foundation for performance measurement and assessment of local public health systems. *Journal of Public Health Management and Practice, 6*(5), 1–18.

Cowan, C., Catlin, A., Smith, C., & Sensenig, A. (2004). National health expenditure, 2002. *Health Care Financing Review, 25,* 143–166.

Daft, R. L. (2004). *Organization theory and design* (8th ed.). Cincinnati, OH: South-Western College.

Epp, J. (1986). *Achieving health for all: A framework for health promotion.* Ottawa, Ontario: Health and Welfare Canada.

Erickson, D. L. (2002). The Public Health Statute Modernization National Collaborative: Developing a model state public health law. *Journal of Public Health Management and Practice, 8*(1), 39–46.

Etienne, W., McDermott, R. A., & Snyder, W. (2002). *Cultivating communities of practice: A guide to managing knowledge.* Boston: Harvard Business School Press.

Evans, R. G. (1998). Going for the gold: The redistributive agenda behind market-based health care reform. In M. A. Peterson (Ed.), *Healthy markets? The new competition in medical care* (pp. 66–103). Durham, NC: Duke University Press.

Evans, R. G. (2002). *Interpreting and addressing inequalities in health: From Black to Acheson to Blair to . . . ?: Seventh annual lecture.* London: Office of Health Economics.

Evans, R. G., Barer, M. L., & Marmor, T. R. (Eds.). (1994). *Why are some people healthy and others not? The determinants of health of populations.* New York: Aldine de Gruyter.

Exworthy, M. (2003). The second Black Report? The Acheson Report as another opportunity to tackle health inequalities. In V. Berridge and S. Blume (Eds.), *Poor health* (pp. 175–197). London: Cass.

Exworthy, M., Blane, D., & Marmot, M. (2003). Tackling health inequalities in the United Kingdom: The progress and pitfalls of policy. *Health Services Research 38*(6), pt. 2, 1905–1921.

Exworthy, M., Stuart, M., Blane, D., & Marmot, M. (2003). *Tackling health inequalities since the Acheson inquiry.* Bristol, England: Policy Press.

Federal, Provincial and Territorial Advisory Committee on Population Health (Canada). (1994). *Strategies for population health: Investing in the health of Canadians.* Ottawa, Ontario: Health Canada.

Federal, Provincial and Territorial Advisory Committee on Population Health (Canada). (1996). *Report on the health of Canadians.* Ottawa, Ontario: Health Canada.

Federal, Provincial and Territorial Advisory Committee on Population Health (Canada). (1999). *Toward a healthy future: Second report on the health of Canadians.* Ottawa, Ontario: Health Canada.

Gebbie, K. M. (2000). State public health laws: An expression of constituency expectations. *Journal of Public Health Management and Practice, 6*(2), 46–54.

Gebbie, K. M., Merrill, J., Hwang, I., Gebbie, E. N., & Gupta, M. (2003). The public health workforce in the year 2000. *Journal of Public Health Management and Practice, 9*(1), 79–86.

Gostin, L. O. (2001). Public health law reform. *American Journal of Public Health, 91,* 1365–1368.

Graham, H. (2004a). Social determinants and their unequal distribution: Clarifying policy understandings. *Milbank Quarterly, 82,* 101–124.

Graham, H. (2004b). Tackling inequalities in health in England: Remedying health disadvantages, narrowing health gaps or reducing health gradients? *Journal of Social Policy, 33,* 115–131.

Handler, A., Issel, M., & Turnock, B. (2001). A conceptual framework to measure performance of the public health system. *American Journal of Public Health, 91,* 1235–1239.

Hardt, M., & Negri, A. (2000). *Empire.* Cambridge, MA: Harvard University Press.

Hassmiller, S. (2002). Turning Point: The Robert Wood Johnson Foundation's effort to revitalize public health at the state level. *Journal of Public Health Management and Practice, 8*(1), 1–5.

Health Canada, Population Strategic Policy Directorate of the Population and Public Health Branch. (2001). *Population health template: Key elements and actions that define population health.* Ottawa, Ontario: Author.

Institute of Medicine, Committee for the Study of the Future of Public Health. (1988). *The future of public health.* Washington, DC: National Academies Press.

Institute of Medicine, Committee on Assuring the Health of the Public in the 21st Century. (2003). *The future of the public's health in the 21st century.* Washington, DC: National Academies Press.

Institute of Medicine, Committee on Educating Public Health Professionals for the 21st Century. (2003). *Who will keep the public healthy? Educating public health professionals for the 21st century.* Washington, DC: National Academies Press.

Institute of Medicine, Committee on Summary Measures of Population Health. (1998). *Summarizing population health: Directions for the development and application of population metrics.* Washington, DC: National Academies Press.

Keller, L. O., Schaffer, M. A., Lia-Hoagberg, B., & Strohschein, S. (2002). Assessment, program planning, and evaluation in population-based public health practice. *Journal of Public Health Management and Practice, 8*(5), 30–43.

Kickbusch, I. (2000). The development of international health policies: Accountability intact? *Social Science and Medicine, 51,* 979–989.

Kimbrell, J. D. (2000). Coalition, partnership, and constituency building by a state public health agency: A retrospective. *Journal of Public Health Management and Practice, 6*(2), 55–61.

Kindig, D., & Stoddart, G. (2003). What is population health? *American Journal of Public Health, 93,* 380–383.

Kriebel, D., & Tickner, J. (2001). Reenergizing public health through precaution. *American Journal of Public Health, 91,* 1351–1355.

Krieger, N., Chen, J. T., Waterman, P. D., Rehkopf, D. H., & Subramanian, S. V. (2003). Race/ethnicity, gender, and monitoring socioeconomic gradients in health: A comparison of area-based socioeconomic measures—The public health disparities geocoding project. *American Journal of Public Health, 93,* 1655–1671.

Lalonde, M. (1974). *A new perspective on the health of Canadians: A working document.* Ottawa, Ontario, Canada: Department of National Health and Welfare.

Lavis, J. N., Ross, S. E., Stoddart, G. L., Hohenadel, J. M., McLeod, C. B., & Evans, R. G. (2003). Do Canadian civil servants care about the health of populations? *American Journal of Public Health, 93,* 658–663.

Lichtveld, M. Y., & Cioffi, J. P. (2003). Public health workforce development: Progress, challenges, and opportunities. *Journal of Public Health Management and Practice, 9*(6), 443–450.

Linder, L. H., Quill, B. E., & Aday, L. A. (2001). Academic partnerships in public health practice. In L. F. Novick & G. P. Mays (Eds.), *Public health administration: Principles for population-based management* (pp. 521–538). Gaithersburg, MD: Aspen.

Lurie, N. (2002). What the federal government can do about the nonmedical determinants of health. *Health Affairs, 21*(2), 94–106.

Mays, G. P., Halverson, P. K., & Scutchfield, F. D. (2003). Behind the curve? What we know and need to learn from public health systems research. *Journal of Public Health Management and Practice, 9,* 179–182.

Mays, G. P., Halverson, P. K., & Scutchfield, F. D. (2004). Making public health improvement real: The vital role of systems research. *Journal of Public Health Management and Practice, 10*(3), 183–185.

McDowell, I., Spasoff, R. A., & Kristjansson, B. (2004). On the classification of population health measurements. *American Journal of Public Health, 94,* 388–393.

McGinnis, J. M., & Foege, W. H. (1993). Actual causes of death in the United States. *Journal of the American Medical Association, 270,* 2207–2212.

Milbank Memorial Fund. (2001). *Health policies for the 21st century: Challenges and recommendations for the U.S. Department of Health and Human Services.* New York: Author.

Mindell, J., Ison, E., & Joffe, M. (2003). A glossary for health impact assessment. *Journal of Epidemiology and Community Health, 57,* 647–651.

Minnesota Health Improvement Partnership Social Conditions and Health Action Team. (2001). *A call to action: Advancing health for all through social and economic change.* St. Paul, MN: Division of Community Health Services.

Miringoff, M., & Miringoff, M.-L. (1999). *The social health of the nation: How America is really doing.* New York: Oxford University Press.

Moulton, A. D., Halverson, P. K., Honoré, P. A., & Berkowitz, B. (2004). Public health finance: A conceptual framework. *Journal of Public Health Management and Practice, 10*(5), 377–382.

Murray, C.J.L., & Evans, D. B. (Eds.) (2003). *Health systems performance assessment: Debates, methods and empiricism.* Geneva: World Health Organization.

Murray, C.J.L., & Frenk, J. (2000). A framework for assessing the performance of health systems. *Bulletin of the World Health Organization, 78,* 717–731.

National Association of County and City Health Officials. (2004). *Local public health agency infrastructure: A chartbook.* Washington, DC: Author.

National Association of County and City Health Officials & Centers for Disease Control and Prevention. (n.d.). *A strategic approach to community health improvement: Mobilizing for action through planning and partnerships (MAPP).* Retrieved September 17, 2004, from http://mapp.naccho.org/MAPP_Home.asp

National Center for Health Statistics. (1998). *Health, United States, 1998, with socioeconomic status and health chartbook* (DHHS Publication No. PHS 98-1232). Hyattsville, MD: Public Health Service.

Newacheck, P. W., Hughes, D. C., Brindis, C., & Halfon, N. (1995). Decategorizing health services: Interim findings from the Robert Wood Johnson Foundation Child Health Initiative. *Health Affairs, 14*(3), 232–242.

Nicola, R. M., & Hatcher, M. T. (2000). A framework for building effective public health constituencies. *Journal of Public Health Management and Practice, 6*(2), 1–10.

Northridge, M. E., & Sclar, E. (2003). A joint urban planning and public health framework: Contributions to health impact assessment. *American Journal of Public Health, 93,* 118–121.

Public Health Leadership Society. (2002). *Principles of the ethical practice of public health* (vers. 2.2). New Orleans: Author.

Quill, B. E., & Aday, L. A. (Eds.). (2000). Practice-academic partnerships in public health. *Journal of Public Health Management and Practice* [Special issue], *6*(1).

Richards, T. B., Croner, C. M., & Novick, L. F. (1999). Geographic information systems (GIS) for state and local public health practitioners, part 2. *Journal of Public Health Management and Practice, 5*(4), 1–6.

Roos, N. P., Black, C., Frohlich, N., DeCoster, C., Cohen, M., et al. (1996). Population health and health care use: An information system for policy makers. *Milbank Quarterly, 74,* 3–31.

Scutchfield, F. D., Ireson, C., & Hall, L. (2004). The voice of the public in public health policy and planning: The role of public judgment. *Journal of Public Health Policy, 25,* 197–205.

Scutchfield, F. D., Knight, E. A., Kelly, A. V., Bhandari, M. W., & Vasilescu, I. P. (2004). Local public health agency capacity and its relationship to public health system performance. *Journal of Public Health Management and Practice, 10*(3), 204–215.

Senge, P. M. (1994). *The fifth discipline: The art and practice of the learning organization.* New York: Currency Doubleday.

Senge, P. M., Kleiner, A., Roberts, C., Ross, R., & Smith, B. (1994). *The fifth discipline fieldbook: Strategies and tools for building a learning organization.* New York: Currency Doubleday.

State of public health: Local and state government issues in Texas: Report resulting from House Concurrent Resolution 44 of the 75th Legislature. (1998). Austin: Texas Legislature.

Suen, J., & Magruder, C. (2004). National profile: Overview of capabilities and core functions of local public health jurisdictions in 47 states, the District of Columbia, and 3 U.S. territories, 2000–2002. *Journal of Public Health Management and Practice, 10*(1), 2–12.

Szreter, S., & Woolcock, M. (2004). Health by association? Social capital, social theory, and the political economy of public health. *International Journal of Epidemiology, 33,* 650–667.

Turning Point. (2005, January 19). *Turning Point: Collaborating for a new century in public health.* Retrieved February 1, 2005, from http://www.turningpointprogram.org

U.S. Department of Health and Human Services. (1994). *Public health in America.* Washington, DC: Author.

U.S. Department of Health and Human Services. (2000, November). *Healthy people 2010: Introduction.* Retrieved November 24, 2003, from http://www.healthypeople.gov/document/html/uih/uih_1.htm

U.S. Department of Health and Human Services. (2001). *Public health's infrastructure: A status report.* Washington, DC: Author.

U.S. Department of Health Education and Welfare. (1979). *Healthy people: The surgeon general's report on health promotion and disease prevention* (DHEW [PHS] Publication No. 79-55071). Washington, DC: Author.

Wenger, E., McDermott, R. A., & Snyder, W. (2002). *Cultivating communities of practice: A guide to managing knowledge.* Boston: Harvard Business School Press.

World Health Organization. (2000). How well do health systems work? In *The world health report 2000: Health systems: Improving performance* (pp. 21–46). Geneva: Author.

Yasnoff, W. A., O'Carroll, P., Koo, D., Linkins, D., & Kilbourne, E. M. (2000). Public health informatics: Improving and transforming public health in the information age. *Journal of Public Health Management and Practice, 6*(6), 67–75.

Zerhouni, E. (2003, October 3). The NIH roadmap. *Science, 302,* 63–72.

NAME INDEX

A

Abbott, D. H., 196, 226
Abbott, R., 135, 167
Aber, J. L., 153, 158
Acheson, D, 55, 58, 130, 158, 205, 206, 224, 225, 227, 297, 328
Acosta, C. M., 265, 279
Adams, C. F., 256, 270, 279
Adams, V., 142, 164
Aday, L. A., 1, 2, 6, 10, 25, *28*, 29, 32, 33, 65, 73, 86, 87, 88, 98, 100, 218, 227, 228, 236, 262, 266, 280, 285, 301, 303, 311, 317, *321*, 328, 330, 331
Adelman, H. F., 137, 177
Adlaf, E., 141, 181
Adler, N. E., 45, 58
Ågren, G., 52, 57, 58, 298, 328
Ahern, M., 265, 282
Ala-Mursula, L., 128, 158
Albert, M. S., 138, 158
Albrecht, G., 19, *20*, 32, 320, 328
Aldwin, C. M., 127, 160
Allen, C. A., 283
Allred, C. G., 137, 164

Altomare, M., 93, 94, 95, 96, 97, 100
Alvarez-Dardet, C., 52, 61
Anda, R. F., 164
Anderpeciva, S., 64
Anderson, B. J., 119, 166
Anderson, L. M., 153, 158
Anderson, O. W., 296, 328
Anderson, R. E., 162
Andrews, A. B., 133, 158
Aneshensel, C. S., 47, 58
Annan, K. A., 211, 227
Anthony, J. C., 137, 161
Anton, R. F., 196, 232
Antonelli, V., 33, 283
Antonucci, T. C., 126, 158
Arendt, J. N., 139, 158
Arndt, C., 203, 227
Arnstein, S., 310, 328
Ary, D. V., 141, 158
Auerbach, J. A., 54, 58, 298, 328
Auffrey, C., 138, 166
Auinger, P., 120, 171
Austin, J. T., 51, 61
Avendaño, M., 128, 159
Awofeso, N., 18, 26, 32

B

Backlund, E., 136, 182, 192, 193, 227, 232, 233
Badgley, R., 266, 283
Baicker, K., 54, 58
Baker, D. W., 136, 181
Baker, E. L., Jr., 292, 328
Baker, W. L., 124, 175
Bakker, M. J., 206, *207*, *208*, 231
Balfour, J. L., 172, 197, 229, 230
Balkrishnan, R., 2, *28*, 32, 218, 227, 301, 328
Baltes, M. M., 127, 159
Baltes, P. B., 127, 159
Bandura, A., 112, 123, 137, 159
Baranowski, T., 123, 159
Bardos, A. N., 139, 171
Barer, M. L., 37, 59, 120, 164, 300, 329
Barker, D.J.P., 48, 58, 120, 129, 159, 165
Barro, R. J., 201, 227
Bartlett, S. J., 162
Bartley, M., 107, 108, 161, 172, 173

Basen-Engquist, K., 125, 159
Bashir, S. A., 194, 227
Basolo, V., 59
Bates, J. E., 130, 159
Baum, F. E., 244, 280
Bauman, K. E., 176
Baumler, E., *151*, 171, 172
Bavelier, D., 121, 175
Beaglehole, R., 13, 34, 98, 99
Bearman, P. S., 176
Becker, A. B., 254, 281
Becker, B., 133, 172
Becker, E., 186, 227
Becker, G. S., 108, 159
Bedimo, A., 59
Begley, C. E., 2, *28*, 32, 218, 227,
   285, 301, 328
Bell, C. C., 135, 159
Bell, R. M., 142, 164
Belli, P., 200, 232
Benach, R. J., 206
Ben-Arieh, A., 133, 158
Bennett, D., 142, 179, 216, 217,
   220
Bennett, J., 227
Bennett, N. G., 153, 158
Ben-Shlomo, Y., 49, 61, 107, 108,
   109, 131, 159, 170
Benson, P. L., 133, 134, 159, 171
Benzeval, M., 198, 229
Bercovitch, F. B., 226
Berg, L. R., 68, 101, 102
Bergen, D., 123, 159
Berglund, M. L., 134, 160
Berkman, L. F., 45, 47, 58, 59, 60,
   63, 137, 159, 191, 195, 227
Berkowitz, B., 271, 283, 310, 318,
   328, 331
Berkowitz, W. R., 328
Berry, S., 182
Berthelot, J. M., 177
Best, J. A., 125, 164
Best, K. M., 133, 173
Bettcher, D., 214, 234
Bhandari, M. W., 319, 332
Bhargava, A., 199, 201, 202, 227
Bienias, J. L., 128, 164
Birren, J. E., 126, 159
Black, C., 331
Black, D., 205, 227, 297, 328
Blackwell, A. G., 51, 62, 246, 258,
   273, 280

Blair, S. N., 119, 178
Blair, T., 13, 205
Blakely, T. A., 197, 198, 227
Blakley, T. L., 124, 175
Blane, D., 206, 228, 296, 297, 329
Blazer, D., 45, 59, 63
Bloom, D. E., 186, 187, 199, 201,
   212, 227
Bloom, F. E., 112, 119, 175
Blum, R. W., 135, 176
Blyth, D., 134, 159, 171
Boardman, J., 126, 159
Boeke, A.J.P., 63
Boettke, P. J., 218, 228
Boisjoly, J., 141, 160
Booher, D., 244, 281
Bopp, M., 159
Bornstein, M. H., 121, 170
Borrell, C., 159
Bosma, H., 137, 143, 160, 172
Bossé, R, 127, 160
Bourdieu, P., 14, 32, 322, 328
Bourgeois, J. P., 120, 176
Bourguignon, F., 187, 227
Boutilier, M., 266, 283
Boyer, E. L., *321*, 328
Brand, R. J., 60
Brandtjen, H., 123, 160
Breslow, L., 133, 160
Brindis, C., 318, 331
Bromley, D. W., 218, 227
Bronfenbrenner, U., 112, 160
Brook, J. S., 123, 168
Brooks-Gunn, J., 113, 122, 128,
   130, 132, 133, 141, 153, 160,
   163, 165, 169, 195, 230
Brown, B. V., 118, 160
Brown, C. K., 319, 328
Bruce, T. A., 310, 328
Bruer, J. T., 122, 160
Bruner, J. S., 123, 160
Brunner, E., 49, 59, 137, 160, 172
Bryant, T., 9, 26, 33
Bryk, A. S., 51, 63
Buchanan, C. M., 124, 161, 163
Bulkow, L. R., 46, 59
Burdine, J. N., 243, 282
Burke, G. L., 166
Burkham, D. T., 140, 171
Burnett, R. T., 83, 100
Bush, G. W., 143, 145, 148, 149
Busnel, M. C., 120, 162

Busse, R., 269, 284
Butler, S. M., 273, 280

C

Cafferata, G. L., 127, 179
Cairns, B. D., 141, 160
Cairns, R. B., 141, 160
Caldji, C., 173
Callahan, L. F., 48, 63
Cameron, N., 131, 160
Campbell, C., 261, 280
Campbell, T. L., 123, 160
Canning, D., 186–187, 227
Caplan, M., 133, 181
Cardarelli, K. M., 35, 106, *151*,
   171, 228, 236
Carlson, E., 137, 139, 163, 168
Carrino, G., 33, 283
Carroll, A. B., 74, 90, *91*, 92, 97,
   100
Carta, J., 123, 181
Carvajal, S. C., 181
Case, A. C., 217, 228
Case, R., 128, 160
Cassel, J., 49, 59
Casswell, S., 123, 161
Catalano, R. F., 134, 142, 160, 167
Catlin, A., 296, 328
Caughy, M. O., 254, 256, 280
Cauthen, N. K., 146, 160
Cavelaars, A.E.J.M., 61
Chalmers, I., 206, 230
Chambers, S., 250, 280
Chandola, T., 107, 161, 178
Chandra, A., 54, 58
Chao, S. S., 283
Chavis, D. M., 243, 282
Chechik, G., 122, 161
Chen, J. M., 171, 230
Chen, J. T., 316, 330
Chilcoat, H. D., 137, 161
Chipuer, H. M., 243, 280
Chung, W. S., 142, 161
Cicchettie, D., 133, 172
Cioffi, J. P., 319, 328, 330
Claeson, M., 270, 280
Clark, N. M., 319, 328
Clark-Lempers, D., 141, 171
Claussen, B., 128, 161
Cleland, J. G., 138, 161
Clifford, R. M., 114, 177

Clinton, B., 13, 18, 143
Coatsworth, J. D., 133, 177
Coburn, D., 9, 12, 19, 26, 32, 41, 42, 59, 63
Cohen, D. A., 47, 48, 59, 137, 161
Cohen, H. W., 241, 280
Cohen, M., 331
Cohen, P., 123, 168
Cohen, R. D., 60, 63, 172, 197, 229, 230
Cohen, S., 45, 59
Coleman, J. S., 45, 59, 108, 135, 161
Colletta, N. J., 243, 244, 280
Collins, J. W., 46, 59
Colmenar, R., 246, 258, 273, 280
Colombo, J., 131, 161
Comfort, C., 134, 167
Conger, R. D., 125, 127, 165, 181
Conley, D. C., 153, 158
Connolly, G. M., 123, 124, 161
Connolly, S. D., 161
Constanza, R., 100
Conway, L., 218, 228
Corburn, J., 322, 328
Cornoni-Huntley, J., 136, 164
Corso, L. C., 319, 328
Costa, F. M., 125, 168
Costa, G., 206
Costanza, R., 75, 100
Côté, S., 167
Cowan, C., 296, 328
Cox, C., 120, 171
Cox, C. L., 141, 170
Cox, M. J., 125, 135, 162
Crespo, C. J., 123, 162
Crocker, J. P., 135, 176
Crockett, L. J., 125, 162
Croner, C. M., 316, 331
Cronin, P., *151*, 172
Crouter, A. C., 135, 162
Culica, D., 237
Cullen, M. L., 243, 244, 280
Culyer, A. J., 270, 280
Cummins, S., 195, 230

D

Daft, R. L., 311, 328
Dahlgren, G., *21*, 32, 209, 228
Daily, G. C., 74, 75, 100
Daly, H., 69, 84, 100

D'Angiulli, A., 132, 172
Daniels, N., 43, 59
d'Arge, R., 100
Darling, N., 123, 134, 162
d'Avernas, J. R., 125, 164
Davey, S. G., 128, 161, 171
David, R. J., 59
Davidson, N., 205, 233
Davis, W., 125, 176
Daw, N. W., 121, 162
Dawson, G., 121, 162
Day, J. C., 121, 171
Day, L. E., 164
de Groot, R., 100
de Moor, J. S., 35, 106
Dearing, E., 153, 162
Deaton, A., 113, 135, 162, 193, 195, 199, *200*, 206, 212, 214, 216, 217, 220, 228
DeCasper, A. J., 120, 162
DeCoster, C., 331
Deeg, D.J.H., 63, 127, 162
Demerath, E. W., 131, 160
Denny, K., 32, 59
Denson, S. E., 162
Denzin, N. K., 16, 32, 260, 280
D'Estelle, S., 138, 181
DeWitt, S. J., 120, 162
Dickens, W. T., 139, 162, 238, 244, 247, 281
Dickinson, D. K., 107, 175
Dierker, L., 120, 163
Dietrich, K., 120, 171
Dietz, W. H., Jr., 123, 162
Diez-Roux, R., 38, 63
Dillman, K. N., 247, 280
Diorio, J., 121, 171, 173
Dishion, T. J., 137, 162
Docteur, E., 53, 54, 59
Doherty, G., 107, 163
Donnerstein, E. I., 134, 178
Donovan, J. E., 125, 168
Dora, C., 230
Douglas, M. J., 218, 228
Dowling, J. E., 119, 163
Drager, N., 13, 34
Drake, D. R., 171
Driscoll, A. K., 130, 174
Dryfoos, J. G., 141, 142, 163
Duan, N., 48, 63
Duan, W., 127, 173
Duff, E. M., 141, 181

Duhl, L., 241
Duncan, C., 48, 59, 64
Duncan, G. J., 122, 128, 130, 132, 141, 153, 160, 163, 192, 231
Duncan, M., 33, 283
Duncan, S. C., 137, 141, 158, 163
Duncan, T. E., 137, 141, 158
Dunn, J., 39, 52, 59, 60, 123, 167, 177
Durlak, J. A., 153, 163
Dusek, J. B., 123, 173
Dwyer, D. S., 126, 163
Dwyer, L., 59
Dyer, A. R., 166

E

Eakin, J., 41, 63
Earley, P. C., 137, 163
Earls, F, 46, 63, 244, 283
Eaves, R. C., 139, 163
Ebrahim, S., 128, 171
Eccles, J. S., 124, 163
Eckenrode, J., 137, 163
Edmonds, R., 163
Edmundson, E., 119, 125, 137, 159, 163, 169
Edwards, L. N., 140, 178
Edwards, V., 164
Egeland, B., 137, 139, 140, 163, 168, 178
Ehrenberg, H. M., 163
Einstein, A., 15
Eisenberg, L., 130, 163
Ekelund, R. B., Jr., 84, 100
Elder, G. H., Jr., 109, 125, 127, 163, 165, 181
Elder, J., 163
Ellaway, A., 47, 61, 195, 230
Ellen, I. G., 247, 280
Ellickson, P. L., 135, 142, 163, 164
Elliot, M., 182
Elo, I. T., 135, 164
Else, J. G., 196, 233
Ensminger, M. E., 176
Epp, J., 56, 59, 297, 329
Erickson, D. L., 318, 329
Erickson, R. A., 274, 280
Eriksen, H. R., 107, 170
Erikson, E. H., 124, 164
Ernst, D., 45, 64

Escobar-Chaves, S. L., 123, 125, 134, 164
Etienne, W., *321*, 329
Etzi, S., 256, 281
Evans, A. E., 176
Evans, D. A., 128, 164
Evans, D. B., 296, 331
Evans, R. G., 9, 19, 26, 32, 37, 39, 40, 41, 42, 59, 66, 100, 108, 109, 120, 135, 141, 142, 143, 164, 192, 206, 216, 220, 228, 230, 295, 297, 300, 329, 330, 331
Evans, T., 123, 167
Everson-Rose, S. A., 128, 164
Exworthy, M., 206, 228, 296, 297, 329

F

Fagan, J., 137, 164
Faggiano, F., 206
Falk, I., 253, 281
Farber, S., 100
Farley, J., 69, 84, 100
Farley, T. A., 59
Fassin, D., 206
Fee, E., 107, 158, 170
Feeney, A., 62, 128, 142, 172
Feldman, H. A., 163
Feldman, J. J., 136, 140, 164
Felitti, V. J., 121, 164
Ferguson, R. F., 238, 244, 247, 281
Field, J., 253, 281
Field, S., 167
Fielding, J. E., 153, 158
Fiese, B. H., 127, 177
Finn, J. D., 137, 164
Fischhoff, B., 125, 164, 176
Fisher, E., 25, 34
Fisher, G., 136, 175
Flanagan, C., 163
Flay, B. R., 125, 137, 164
Flint, B. M., 123, 165
Floud, R., 191, 228
Flynn, J. R., 139, 162
Foege, W. H., 125, 173, 300, 331
Fogel, R. W., 152, 165, 202, 228
Fogelman, K., 141, 167
Folger, R., 137, 177
Forrest, C. B., 176
Forrest, R., *245*, 281
Fortmann, S. P., 136, 182

Fox, J., 131, 176
Fozard, J. L., 127, 162
Francis, D., 121, 130, 165, 171, 173
Frank, E., 136, 182
Frankel, K. A., 130, 159
Franzini, L., 183, 197, 228
Fredman, L., 45, 63
Freeman, S., 19, *20*, 32, 320, 328
Freidman, S. W., 274, 280
Freire, P., 16, 32, 248, 249, 254, 255, 259, 261, 281
Frenk, J., 296, 331
Friedman, M., 93, 100
Friedman, S. W., 280
Frierson, T., 134, 178
Frohlich, N., 331
Fuchs, V. R., 139, 140, 165
Fullerton, C. S., 125, 134, 165
Fullilove, M. T., 153, 158
Fuqua, J., 112, 166
Furubotn, E. G., 72, 93, 94, 100

G

Gabrijelcic-Blenkus, M., 230
Gaebler, T., 18, 33
Gallup, J. L., 203, 228
Gannon-Rowley, T., 244, 283
Ganzel, B., 112, 165
Garbarino, J., 112, 165
Garmezy, N., 133, 165, 173
Garson, G. D., 269, 281
Gates, C. T., 246, 250, 283
Gazzaniga, M. S., 119, 165
Ge, X., 125, 165
Gebbie, E. N., 319, 329
Gebbie, K. M., 318, 319, 329
Gehlert, S, 50, 60
Gentile, D. A., 123, 165
Gentleman, J. F., 192, 233
Gershman, J., 186, 228
Gershoff, E., 114, *115*, 115, 122, 146, 149, 153, 154, 165
Geurts, J. J., 61, 128, 170
Giampaoli, S., 128, 181
Giddens, A., 13, 14, 32
Gilliland, J., 182
Gingiss, P. M., 181
Ginsburg, H. P., 124, 165
Glass, R., 46, 60, 135, 169, 197, 229
Glass, T., 45, 58, 195, 227

Glei, D. A., 130, 174
Glouberman, S., 9, 19, 26, 32, 266, 281
Glynn, R., 63
Godfrey, K. M., 120, 165
Godin, I., 178
Goldman-Rakic, P. S., 120, 176
Goodwin, J. S., 50, 60
Gore, S., 137, 165
Gorman, D., 218, 228
Gortmaker, S. L., 123, 162
Gostin, L. O., 318, 329
Gould, M. S., 123, 165
Graber, J. A., 132, 165
Graham, H., 22, 32, 113, 165, 322, 323, 329
Grandjean, H., 206
Grandjean, P., 69, 100
Granier-Deferre, C., 120, 162
Grantham-McGregor, S. M., 141, 181
Grasso, M., 100
Gravelle, H., 197, 228
Gray, B., 33, 263, 283
Gray, J. N., 119, 178
Green, B. F., 176
Greenlund, K. J., 137, 166
Greenough, W. T., 108, 119, 166
Greenwood, C., 123, 181
Griffin, C. C., 280
Griffin, S., 128, 160
Griffin, S. F., 176
Grimson, R., 256, 281
Groenhof, F., 61
Grootaert, C., 244, 281
Grosse, R. N., 138, 166
Grossman, M., 135, 140, 151, 166, 178
Grove, B., 126, 159
Grubel, H. G., 150, 166
Gruber, J., 193, 228
Grunbaum, J. A., 118, 125, 141, 166, 181, 182
Grunfeld, N., 120, 166
Gruskin, S., 230
Grzywacz, J. G., 112, 166
Guerra, N. G., 134, 179
Guo, Z., 127, 173
Gupta, M., 319, 329
Guralnik, J., 45, 63
Gusmano, M., 33, 283
Guthrie, J. W., 144, 178

Gutmann, A., 248, 250, 251, 252, 259, 281

H

Habermas, J., 14, 15, 16, 32, 248, 249, 250, 251, 252, 254, 258, 259, 281
Hacker, C. S., 65
Hadden, W., 136, 175
Hains, S. M., 169
Halfon, N., 108, 109, *110*, 113, 132, 141, 166, 318, 331
Hall, A. J., 111, 166
Hall, E. M., 194, 229
Hall, L., 317, 331
Hallet, J. D., 75, *76*, 100
Hallqvist, J., 49, 61, 107, 170
Halverson, P. K., 292, 305, 318, 319, 328, 330, 331
Handler, A., 29, 32, 59, 292, 317, 329
Hanlon, P., 218, 228
Hannon, B., 100
Hardt, M., 12, 32, 322, 329
Hardy, R., 128, *129*, 170
Harkness, S., 126, 166
Harper, S., 230
Harris, B., 191, 228
Harris, K. M., 135, 141, 160, 176
Harris, L. J., 176
Harris, R. C., 123, 182
Harrison, D., 52, 60
Harrison, L. H., 46, 59
Hart, B., 107, 123, 166, 181
Hart, G., 138, 181
Harter, K.S.M., 125, 162
Hartman, K. A., 141, 171
Hartup, W. W., 134, 166
Harvey, B., 75, *76*, 100
Harwood, R. L., 133, 181
Hassmiller, S., 299, 329
Hatcher, M. T., 317, 331
Hauser, P. M., 192, 229
Hauser, R. M., 141, 153, 166
Haveman, R., 141, 166
Havighurst, R. J., 124, 125, 166
Hawkins, J. D., 134, 135, 141, 142, 160, 166, 167
Hawkins, L., 166
Hayes, M. V., 39, 52, 59, 60
Hays, R. D., 142, 164
Head, J., 62, 172, 231

Healy, T., 108, 167
Heck, K. E., 172, 230
Hedeker, D., 164
Helliwell, J. E., 167
Hemingway, H., 137, 160, 172
Hendryx, M., 265, 282
Hertzman, C., 49, 60, 107, 108, 109, 111, 120, 122, 123, 127, 128, 129, 130, 131, 132, 133, 141, 153, 167, 168, 169, 172
Heyne, P., 218, 228
Hibbett, A., 141, 167
Hicks, L. E., 139, 167
Higginbotham, N., 19, *20*, 32, 320, 328
Hill, E. J., 142, 182
Hill, K. G., 135, 167
Hillemeier, M., 230
Himes, J. H., 141, 181
Hippocrates, 36
Hobdell, M. H., 199, 228
Hochstein, M., 109, *110*, 113, 132, 141, 166
Hockfield, S., 121, 167
Hohenadel, J. M., 230, 330
Holberg, C. J., 46, 60
Hollis, J. F., 45, 64
Honoré, P. A., 318, 331
Hops, H., 137, 141, 158, 163
Horton, R., 206, 230
House, J., 45, 60, 61, 137, 167, 171, 192, 197, 230, 231
Hu, F. B., 164
Huang, H., 169
Hughes, D. C., 318, 331
Huisman, M., 159
Hurford, J. R., 121, 169
Hurley, J. E., 230
Hurley, L. P., 141, 167
Huston, A. C., 153, 167
Hutchinson, T. C., 71, 101
Huttenlocher, P. R., 120, 167
Huynh, P., 52, 60, *151*, 172, 204, 229
Hwang, I., 319, 329
Hyman, J. B., 244, 281
Hymel, S., 134, 167

I

Ingersoll, G. M., 124, 168
Innes, J., 244, 281
Inui, T., 25, 34

Ireson, C., 317, 331
Irwin, A., 186, 228
Irwin, C., 112, 168
Ison, E., 319, 331
Israel, B. A., 23, *24*, 33, 254, 255, 256, 261, 281
Issel, M., 29, 32, 292, 329

J

Jack, W., 200, 229
Jackson, B., 128, 168
James, W.P.T., 194, 229
Jamison, D. T., 187, 199, 227, 229
Jan, S., 266, 281
Janus, M., 116, *117*, 168
Jatulis, D. E., 136, 182
Jefferis, B. J., 130, 168
Jenkins, P., 141, 177
Jessiman, B., 83, 100
Jessor, R., 125, 142, 168
Jessor, S. L., 142, 168
Jimerson, S., 139, 140, 168
Joffe, M., 319, 331
Johnson, C. C., 163
Johnson, J. G., 123, 168
Johnson, J. V., 45, 62, 194, 229
Johnson, L. B., 13, 143
Johnson, N. J., 192, 227
Johnson, T. G., 229, 236
Johnston, T. A., 280
Jolly, A., 123, 160
Jones, J., 176
Jones, K., 48, 59, 64
Jordan, W. J., 153, 168
Jovchelovitch, S., 261, 280
Judge, K., 198, 229

K

Kaestner, R., 135, 166
Kagan, J., 121, 168
Kagan, S. L., 114, 145, 168
Kahn, A. J., 116, 168
Kamerman, S. B., 113, 116, 147, 168, 169
Kaminski, M., 206
Kandel, D. B., 137, 169
Kang, M., 176
Kann, L., 166
Kaplan, B. H., 63
Kaplan, D., 60

Kaplan, G., 44, 45, 51, 60, 61, 63, 135, 136, 169, 172, 177, 182, 197, 198, 209, 226, 229, 230, 233
Kaprio, J., 139, 169
Karasek, R., 126, 142, 169
Kardaun, J.W.P.F., 127, 162
Karron, R. A., 46, 59
Kasen, S., 123, 168
Kawachi, I., 45, 46, 47, 60, 135, 152, 169, 182, 191, 196, 197, 198, 200, 201, 227, 229, 232
Kearns, A., *245*, 281
Keating, D. P., 107, 108, 111, 112, 120, 122, 128, 129, 130, 131, 153, 169
Keefe, K., 134, 169
Keefer, C. H., 166
Keefer, K., 126
Kegler, M. C., 243, 282
Keil, J. E., 169
Kelder, S. H., 119, 169, 181
Keller, J. B., 192, 232
Keller, L. O., 313, 330
Kelly, A. V., 319, 332
Kelly, W. M., 128, 160
Kendall, P. C., 134, 179
Kennedy, B. P., 46, 60, 135, 169, 197, 198, 200, 201, 227, 229, 232
Kennedy, S., 138, 139, 169
Kersell, M. W., 125, 164
Kesler, J. T., 241, 281
Keverne, E. B., 226
Kickbusch, I., 9, 18, 26, 33, 322, 330
Kiefe, C. L., 166
Kilbourne, E. M., 316, 332
Kilgour, M., 123, 165
Kilpatrick, S., 253, 281
Kimbrell, J. D., 317, 330
Kinchen, S. A., 166
Kindig, D., 4, 33, 302, 330
Kirby, S., 121, 169
Kisilevsky, B. S., 120, 169
Kitagawa, E. M., 192, 229
Kivimaki, M., 128, 143, 158, 181
Klein, D., 142, 178
Kleinbaum, D. G., 45, 63
Kleiner, A., *321*, 332
Kleinman, J. C., 136, 164
Knapp, A., 239, 284

Knight, E. A., 319, 332
Knudsen, L., 45, 63
Kochtcheeva, L., *80*, *81*, *82*, 83, 100
Kohen, D., 123, 130, 132, 133, 167, 169, 172
Kohout, F., 63
Koivusilta, L. K., 140, 170
Kolar, V., 126, 170
Kolbe, L. J., 118, 134, 170
Koné, A., 283
Koo, D., 316, 332
Koplan, J. P., 292, 328
Korpi, B. M., 146, 147, 170
Koskela, K., 137, 173
Kosterman, R., 135, 167
Krasnik, A., 209, 216, 229, 266, 281
Krause, N, 47, 61
Kretzmann, J. P., 261, 282
Krewski, D., 83, 100
Kriebel, D., 230, 319
Krieger, J., 283
Krieger, N., 22, 33, 36, 37, 41, 46, 49, 61, 107, 109, 158, 170, 191, 193, 195, 196, 218, 220, 230, 316, 319, 330
Kriegsman, D.M.W., 63
Krimgold, B. K., 54, 58, 210, 232, 298, 328
Kristenson, M., 107, 142, 170
Kristjansson, B., 22, 33, 43, 62, 320, 331
Kubzansky, L. D., 128, 168
Kuh, D., 49, 61, 107, 108, 109, 111, 128, *129*, 131, 133, 143, 159, 170, 178
Kuhl, P. K., 121, 170
Kuhn, T., 15, 33
Kulbok, P. A., 141, 170
Kumpfer, K. L., 134, 170
Kunst, A. E., 61, 128, 136, 140, 159, 170
Kuper, H., 107, 161

L

La Parra, D., 52, 61
Laber-Laird, K., 196, 232
Labonte, R., 189, 190, 230
LaBree, L., 137, 161
Lacroix, A., 63

Ladd, G. W., 122, 170
Lafronze, V., 271, 283
Lahelma, E., 108, 172
Lai, C.K.W., 46, 64
Lairson, D. R., 2, *28*, 32, 218, 227, 301, 328
Lalonde, M., 33, 36, 56, 61, 204, 230, 297, 330
Lamb, M. E., 121, 170
Lambson, T., 175
Landis, K. R., 137, 167
Landry, S. H., 121, 141, 162, 170
Lane, D. S., 256, 281
Lang, T., 206
Langenberg, C., 128, *129*, 170
Langer, J. A., 137, 171
Langham, R. A., 139, 167
Lankau, M. J., 143, 177
Lanphear, B. P., 120, 171
Lantz, P. M., 137, 171, 193, 194, 230
LaPlante, P., 173
Lara, J., 153, 168
Larsson, B., 64
Lassiter, K. S., 139, 171
Lau, L. J., 199, 227
Lau, R. R., 141, 171
Lavin, C., 139, 171
Lavis, J. N., 204, 205, 230, 297, 330
Lawlor, D. A., 128, 171
Lawrance, E. C., 139, 171
Leather, S., 194, 229
Leatherman, S., 25, 34
Lebowitz, M. D., 60
Lecanuet, J. P., 120, 162
Leclerc, A., 206
LeDoux, J. E., 119, 165
Lee, K., 169
Lee, P., 18, 33
Lee, V. H., 140, 171
Leffert, N., 134, 159, 171, 177
Lefkowitz, B., 54, 58, 210, 232, 298, 328
Legowski, B., 52, 61
LeGrand, J., 194, 231
Leidy, L. E., 109, 171
Leigh, J. P., 45, 61
Lempers, J. D., 141, 171
Lempert, L. B., 23, *24*, 33
Lepkowski, J. M., 171, 230
Lerner, R. M., 133, 171
Levenson, M. R., 127, 160

Leventhal, T., 195, 230
Lewis, J. D., 203, 227
Li, J. L., 153, 158
Li, L., 130, 176
Lia-Hoagberg, B., 313, 330
Liang, J., 45, 64
Lichtveld, M. Y., 319, 328, 330
Lincoln, Y. S., 16, 32, 260, 280
Linder, L. H., 25, 33, 311, 330
Lindsey, E., 238, 282
Link, B. G., 2, 22, 33, 39, 49, 61, 246, 282
Linkins, D., 316, 332
Lipson, D., 13, 34
Lituchy, T. R., 137, 163
Liu, D., 121, 171
Liu, K., 166
Liu, X., 45, 64
Lleras-Muney, A., 138, 171
Lochner, K., 46, 60, 197, 227
Lock, K., 218, 230
Loe, H. D., Jr., 285
Lombroso, P. J., 121, 167
Lonczak, H. S., 134, 160
Longest, B. B., Jr., 100
Love, R., 32, 59
Low, B. J., 35, 106, 123, 137, 141, *151*, 164, 171, 172
Low, M. D., 35, 106, *151*, 171, 172
Lowry, R., 166
Lu, H.-H., 146, 160
Lurie, N., 25, 34, 50, 61, 209, 210, 223, 230, 300, 330
Lustbader, L. L., 141, 167
Luster, T., 126, 172
Luthar, S. S., 132, 133, 172
Lynch, J., 49, 61, 136, 170, 182, 198, 233
Lynch, J. W., 44, 45, 61, 107, 136, 172, 177, 185, 194, 196, 197, 198, 217, 226, 229, 230
Lytle, L. A., 119, 169

M

Macaskill, P., 142, 179
MacCallum, R. C., 51, 61
MacDermid, S. M., 135, 162
Macera, C. A., 162
Macintyre, S., 47, 61, 107, 128, 172, 195, 206, 230

Mackenbach, J. P., 45, 61, 206, 207, *208*, 209, 231
Maggi, S., 132, 172
Magruder, C., 319, 332
Makuc, D. M., 136, 164
Mann, L., 139, 163
Manor, O., 108, 130, 131, 167, 176
Marceau, L. D., 38, 53, 58, 62
Margalit, M., 126, 172
Markham, C., 123, 164
Markman, E. M., 121, 182
Marmor, T. R., 37, 59, 120, 164, 300, 329
Marmot, M., 37, 44, 52, 55, 61, 62, 107, 108, 113, 128, 129, 136, 137, 142, 143, 160, 161, 172, 178, 185, 192, 193, 194, 195, 196, 206, 228, 231, 232, 296, 297, 329
Marshall, P. C., 132, 178
Martikainen, P., 108, 111, 172
Martin, N., 139, 173
Martinez, F. D., 60
Martuzzi, M., 230
Maslin, C. A., 130, 159
Mason, K., 59
Masten, A. S., 124, 133, 172, 173, 174, 177
Mathers, C., 42, 62
Matheson, M. P., 47, 64
Mathur, S. K., 6, 33, 65, 73, 86, 87, 88, 98, 100
Mattessich, P., 242, 247, 282
Matthews, S., 108, 130, 167, 176
Mattson, M. P., 127, 173
Maugeais, R., 120, 162
Mays, G. P., 292, 305, 330
McAlister, A., 137, 173
McBrier, D. B., 142, 177
McBroom, J. R., 134, 173
McCain, M. N., 128, 141, 156, 173
McCarthy, M., 266, 282
McCartney, K., 153, 162
McClenaghan, P., 246, 282
McCulloch, A., 256, 282
McDaniel, K. L., 125, 182
McDermott, R. A., 310, *321*, 329, 332
McDonough, P., 32, 59, 192, 231
McDougall, P., 134, 167
McDowell, I., 22, 33, 43, 62, 320, 331

McEwen, B. S., 49, 62
McGee, D. L., 138, 181
McGinnis, J. M., 125, 173, 300, 331
McGroder, S. M., 144, 173
McGuffog, I. D., 52, 62
McGuigan, K. A., 135, 142, 163, 164
McGuinness, L., 238, 282
McHale, S. M., 135, 162
McIntyre, J. G., 123, 173
McKane, S. U., 310, 328
McKay, L., 52, 61
McKenzie, F. D., 123, 173
McKinlay, J. B., 38, 53, 58, 62
McKnight, J., 119, 173, 242, 261, 265, 282
McLachlan, M., 280
McLean, S. A., 123, 167
McLeod, C. B., 230, 330
McLeroy, K. R., 243, 282
McLoyd, V. C., 153, 173
McMahon, R. J., 137, 162
McMichael, A., 83, 98, 99, 100
McMillan, D. W., 243, 282
McNeely, J., 238, 247, 255, 282
McPartland, J. M., 153, 168
Meaney, M. J., 111, 120, 121, 130, 165, 171, 173
Mechanic, D., 276, 282
Medoza, S. P., 226
Meilijson, I., 122, 161
Meisels, S. J., 114, 173
Mendes de Leon, C. F., 128, 164
Mercer, B. M., 120, 163
Mercier, J. R., 218, 231
Mero, R. P., 171, 230
Merrill, J., 319, 329
Metzner, H. L., 45, 60
Meyer, K. K., 123, 182
Micklewright, J., 114, 116, 173
Midgley, C., 163
Mijanovich, T., 247, 280
Millar, J., 9, 19, 26, 32, 266, 281
Miller, B. C., 142, 182
Miller, F. K., 111, 112, 169
Miller, J. Y., 142, 167
Miller, P., 139, 173
Miller-Loncar, C. L., 121, 141, 170
Milluzzi, C., 120, 163
Mindell, J., 319, 331
Miner, K., 319, 328

Minkler, M., 51, 62, 248, 255, 256, 282
Miringoff, M., 320, 331
Miringoff, M.-L., 320, 331
Mirowsky, J., 45, 48, 62, 63, 136, 137, 177
Mitchell, O. S., 126, 163
Mitchell, S. M., 265, 282
Mizuno, M., 138, 182
Molinari, C., 265, 282
Monsey, B., 242, 247, 282
Montgomery, S. M., 107, 173
Moon, G., 48, 59
Moore, K. A., 130, 174
Moore, S. G., 134, 166
Morenoff, J. D., 244, 282, 283
Morgan, L. M., 260, 261, 266, 282
Morgenstern, H., 43, 62
Morison, P., 124, 174
Morris, J. A., 139, 174
Morrisson, C., 187, 227
Mortimore, P., 153, 174
Moser, C.O.N., 261, 282
Moulton, A. D., 318, 331
Mroczek, D. K., 127, 160
Mueller, P., 105
Muir, D., 121, 174
Mulhall, S., 10, 33
Mulligan, J. A., 198, 229
Mullooly, J. P., 45, 64
Mulvey, C., 139, 173
Muntaner, C., 254, 280
Murakami, Y., 183
Murray, C.J.L., 42, 62, 199, 227, 296, 331
Mustard, J. F., 128, 174
Mustard, J. M., 128, 141, 156, 173
Muthen, B. O., 51, 62
Muurinen, J. M., 194, 231
Mykhalovskiy, E., 32, 59

N

Nabeshima, T., 138, 182
Nader, P. R., 123, 159
Narayan, D., 135, 182
Nattrass, B. F., 93, 94, 95, 96, 97, 100
Navarro, V., 10, 33, 206, 214, 231
Neckerman, H. J., 141, 160
Negri, A., 12, 32, 322, 329

Neiss, M., 139, 175
Nelson, C. A., 112, 119, 121, 175, 179
Nelson, M., 194, 229
Neuman, M., 113, 169
Neuman, S. B., 107, 175
Neville, H. J., 121, 175
Newacheck, P. W., 318, 331
Newman, K., 45, 58
Nicholson, A. C., 160
Nicola, R. M., 271, 283, 310, 317, 328, 331
Nicolopoulou, A., 175
Niedhammer, I., 107, 142, 175, 178
Nijhuis, H.G.J, 52, 53, 62
Noble, P., 218, 228
Nordenberg, D., 164
Nordgren, P., 209, 228
Nordhaus, W. D., 186, 187, 188, 189, 220, 231, 232
Norris, T., 241, 283
North, D. C., 72, 93, 100
North, F., 62, 128, 172, 231
Northridge, M., 230, 241, 280, 322, 331
Norton, B. L., 243, 282
Norton, M. C., 142, 182
Novick, L. F., 316, 331
Nurss, J. R., 136, 181
Nutbeam, D., 142, 179

O

O'Campo, P. J., 254, 280
O'Carroll, P., 316, 332
O'Carroll, P. W., 142, 177
O'Conner, D., 246, 250, 283
Offord, D., 116, *117*, 168
O'Hara, N. M., 119, 178
Okagaki, L., 126, 172
Oldenburg, B., 52, 55, 62
Olson, L., 156, 175
Omenn, G. S., 98, 101
Opper, S., 124, 165
Ordway, N., 137, 164
Orth-Gomer, K., 45, 62
Osborne, D., 18, 33
Osler, M., 107, 175
Osmond, C., 48, 58, 129, 159
Otorepec, P., 230
Owens, D. E., 144, 178

P

Paavola, J., 218, 227
Paikoff, R. L., 124, 161
Pamuk, E. R., 172, 197, 229, 230
Panter-Brick, C., *110*
Pappas, G., 136, 140, 175
Parcel, G. S., 119, 125, 159, 163, 178
Pardeck, J. T., 142, 161
Parker, E. A., 254, 281
Parker, R. M., 136, 138, 176, 181
Parkerbohannon, A., 139, 163
Parra-Medina, D., 176
Paskett, E. D., 50, 62
Pate, R. R., 119, 178
Patel, C., 172, 231
Patz, J. A., 83, 101
Paxman, D., 18, 33
Paxton, C., 135, 162
Penninx, B.W.J.H., 45, 63
Pentti, J., 143, 158, 181
Perkins, R., 126, 159
Perry, B. D., 124, 175
Perry, C. L., 163
Perry-Jenkins, M., 135, 162
Petersen, A. C., 125, 162
Petraitis, J., 164
Pfannensteil, J. C., 154, 175
Phelan, J., 2, 22, 33, 39, 49, 61, 246, 282
Philipson, T., 150, 175
Piaget, J., 124, 175
Pickles, A., 132, 175
Pierre-Louis, M., 283
Pincus, T., 48, 63
Pittman, M., 241, 283
Pogson, P., 126, 179
Poland, B., 41, 42, 63, 266, 283
Pollard, R. A., 124, 175
Poole, D. L., 141, 176
Pope, C. R., 45, 64
Porter, R., 191, 231
Potapchuk, W. R., 135, 176
Powell, K. E., 142, 177
Power, C., 49, 61, 107, 108, 128, 130, 131, 167, 168, 170, 176
Prescott, E., 107, 175
Preston, S. H., 135, 164, 231
Pretty, G.M.H., 243, 280
Price, J. M., 122, 170
Prothrow-Stith, D., 46, 60, 197, 229

Prychitko, D. L., 218, 228
Pulkkinen, L., 139, 169
Puska, P., 60, 137, 173
Putnam, R., 45, 63, 135, 176, 244, 283

Q

Quadrel, M. J., 125, 141, 171, 176
Queen, S., 136, 175
Quill, B. E., 25, 33, 237, 285, 311, *321*, 330, 331
Quinn, M., 230

R

Raghunathan, T., 230
Rahi, K., 255
Rakic, P., 120, 176
Ralph, A., 194, 229
Rao, M. J., 190, 232
Raphael, B., 127, 176
Raphael, D., 9, 26, 33
Rapport, D. J., 71, 74, 77, 79, 98, 99, 101
Rasmussen, N. K., 209, 216, 229, 266, 281
Rasu, R. S., 183
Ratzan, S. C., 138, 176
Raudenbush, S. W., 46, 51, 63, 244, 282, 283
Raven, P. H., 68, 101, 102
Ray, C. G., 60
Reagan, R., 12, 269
Rebbeck, T., 50, 63
Redd, Z., 130, 174
Regier, H. A., 71, 101
Rehkopf, D. H., 316, 330
Rehme, G., 146, 157, 176
Reininger, B., 134, 176
Reise, S. P., 48, 63
Reklis, D. M., 140, 165
Repetti, R. L., 49, 64, 130, 176
Resnick, M. D., 125, 135, 141, 176
Reuman, D., 163
Ribble, J., 197, 228
Richards, M., 128, *129*, 170
Richards, T. B., 316, 331
Richardson, J., 137, 161
Richmond, J., 36, 123, 173
Riley, A. W., 117, 128, 141, 176, 179
Rimpela, A. H., 140, 170

Rimpela, M. K., 140, 170
Risley, T. R., 107, 166
Robbins, C., 45, 60
Robèrt, K.-H., 78, 101
Roberts, C., *321*, 332
Robertson, A., 32, 41, 59, 63
Robertson, J., 128, 179
Roccella, M., 120, 176
Rock, D. A., 137, 164
Rodgers, G. B., 197, 232
Rogers, E. M., 46, 63
Rohrer, J. E., 260, 262, 283
Roisman, G. L., 133, 177
Roos, N. P., 313, 331
Roosevelt, F.D., 12, 13
Rose, G., 37, 37–38, 55, 62, 63, 98, 101, 194, 196, 231, 232
Rose, R. J., 139, 169
Roseland, M., 73, 86, 101
Rosenau, R. V., 260, 283
Rosenberg, M. L., 142, 177
Rosenfield, D., 137, 177
Ross, C. E., 45, 48, 62, 63, 107, 135, 136, 137, 140, 177
Ross, J. G., 166
Ross, N., 136, 177, 182, 198, 230, 232, 233
Ross, R., *321*, 332
Ross, S. E., 230, 330
Rowe, D. C., 139, 175
Rowe, G., 192, 233
Rowentree, B. S., 191, 232
Ruppin, E., 122, 161
Rutter, M., 109, 125, 126, 132, 133, 175, 177
Ryan, J.A.M, 134, 160
Ryan, K. B., 125, 164

S

Sachs, J., 187, 203, 228, 229
Saegert, S., 246, 283
St. Peter, R. F., 54, 64
Salomon, J. A., 42, 62
Salonen, J. T., 60, 137, 173
Saltzman, W., 226
Saluja, G., 114, 177
Sameroff, A. J., 127, 177
Sampson, R. J., 46, 63, 244, 254, 282, 283
Samuelson, P. A., 186, 188, 189, 220, 232

Sangl, J., 127, 179
Sapolsky, R. M., 49, 63, 196, 232, 233
Scales, P. C., 134, 159, 171, 177
Scandura, T. A., 143, 177
Schaffer, M. A., 313, 330
Schaie, K. W., 126, 159
Schechter, W. H., 135, 176
Schieman, S., 142, 177
Schlesinger, M., 25, 33, 263, 283
Schoenbach, V. J., 45, 63
Schonert-Reichl, K., 134, 167
Schulz, A. J., 23, *24*, 33, 254, 281
Schunk, D. H., 137, 177
Schwartz, S., 38, 63
Sclar, E., 322, 331
Scott-Little, C., 114, 177
Scribner, R., 59
Scrimshaw, S. C., 153, 158
Scutchfield, F. D., 292, 305, 317, 319, 330, 331, 332
Seccombe, K., 153, 177
Seeman, T., 45, 49, 63, 64, 130, 176
Selye, H, 49, 64
Sen, A., 152, 177, 186, 187, 224, 232, 276, 283
Senge, P. M., 17, 33, 320, *321*, 332
Sensenig, A., 296, 328
Seydlitz, R., 141, 177
Shaffer, D., 123, 165
Shakotko, R., 140, 178
Shakow, A., 186, 228
Sharma, A. R., 171
Shaw, M., 230
Shea, S., 98, 101
Shepherd, G., 126, 159
Shi, L. Y., 10, 33
Shipley, M., 55, 62, 128, 172, 196, 231
Shively, C. A., 196, 226, 232
Shonkoff, J. P., 132, 143, 178
Shore, R., 120, 178
Shortell, S. M., 265, 282
Showstack, J., 25, 34
Shy, C. M., 37, 64
Siddiqui, O., 164
Siegel, D. J., 111, 121, 178
Siegel, J. M., 124, 182
Siegrist, J., 107, 142, 143, 172, 175, 178
Silva, P. A., 123, 161

Silver, R. C., 127, 182
Simeonsson, N. W., 119, 178
Simeonsson, R. J., 127, 141, 178
Simmonds, S. J., 129, 159
Simons-Morton, B. G., 119, 178
Sims, P. G., 144, 178
Singer, M. I., 134, 178
Singh, A., *80, 81, 82,* 83, 100
Singh-Manoux, A., 107, 161
Singleton, R. J., 46, 59
Slater, A., 121, 174
Slovak, K., 134, 178
Sluiter, J. K., 107, 170
Smailes, E. M., 123, 168
Smit, E., 162
Smith, B., *321,* 332
Smith, C., 296, 328
Smith, G. D., 44, 61, 128, 133, 143, 170, 172, 178, 181, 197, 230, 231
Smith, J. P., 193, 201, 232
Smith, K., 121, 141, 162, 170
Smith, R., 206, 230
Smith, R. S., 123, 133, 181
Smith, S. L., 134, 178
Smrekar, C., 144, 145, 156, 178
Smylie, C. S., 119, 165
Snyder, W., 17, 34, 310, *321,* 329, 332
Soares, R. R., 150, 175
Sorlie, P. D., 192, 227, 232
Soucat, A.L.B., 280
Soule, E., 69, 101
Sparks, J. W., 162
Spasoff, R. A., 22, 33, 43, 62, 320, 331
Spears, W., 197, 228, 237
Spiro, A., III, 127, 160
Spitz, A. M., 164
Sprague, T., 127, 176
Sroufe, L. A., 137, 139, 140, 163, 168, 178
Stajduhar, K., 238, 282
Stansfeld, S., 47, 64, 137, 160, 172, 231
Starfield, B., 128, 176, 179
Starke, D., 107, 170, 175, 178
Steinberg, L., 123, 134, 162
Sterner, J. M., *151,* 171
Stewart, K., 114, 116, 173
Stieb, D., 83, 100
Stiglitz, J. E., 189, 199, 213, 214, 232

Stoddart, G. L., 4, 9, 19, 26, 32, 33, 39, 40, 41, 42, 59, 66, 100, 108, 109, 141, 164, 230, 302, 330
Stone, R., 127, 179
Strohschein, S., 313, 330
Stuart, M., 206, 228, 296, 297, 329
Subramanian, S. V., 48, 64, 197, 198, 200, 201, 202, 232, 316, 330
Sucoff, C. A., 47, 58
Suen, J., 319, 332
Sugisawa, H., 45, 64
Suleman, M. A., 196, 233
Sullivan, M., 243, 283
Sumaya, C. V., 243, 282
Suomi, S. J., 130, 133, 179
Super, C. M., 126, 166
Suppanz, H., 53, 59
Svardsudd, K., 64
Swank, P. R., 121, 141, 162, 170
Swift, A., 33
Swint, J. M, 183
Sylva, K., 123, 160
Syme, S. L., 45, 59, 60, 62, 128, 137, 159, 172, 210, 224, 225, 232
Symons, R., 59
Szreter, S., 18, 34, 302, 332

T

Takenaka, J., 139, 167
Tamir, H., 51, 62
Tarara, R., 196, 233
Tarlov, A. R., 22, 34, 54, 64, 265, 283
Taussig, L. M., 60
Taylor, B. A., 153, 162
Taylor, S. E., 49, 64, 130, 176
Tek, M. L., 107, 175
Tellegen, A., 133, 177
Tennant, M., 126, 179
Tesh, S. N., 18, 34
Testa, D., 120, 176
Teti, D. M., 121, 170
Teven, J. J., 137, 179
Thatcher, M., 12, 205
Thelle, D., 128, 161
Theodore, K., 203, 232
Theorell, T., 126, 142, 169, 172
Thielen, L., 319, 328
Thomas, S. L., 111, 166

Thompson, D. F., 248, 250, 251, 252, 259, 281
Thompson, J. P., 246, 283
Thompson, M., 51, 62
Thompson, R. A., 108, 111, 119, 121, 179
Thrall, T. H., 248, 256, 283
Tibblin, B., 64
Tickner, J., 319, 330
Tobin, S., 266, 283
Tolan, P. H., 134, 179
Tollison, R. D., 84, 100
Tomiak, M., 192, 233
Tortolero, S., 123, 164, 181, 182
Townsend, P., 205, 233
Tremblay, R. E., 131, 179
Tresidder, J., 142, 179
Troiano, R. P., 162
Tucker, K., 50, 64
Tuomilehto, J., 137, 173
Turner, C. W., 134, 170
Turnock, B., 29, 32, 292, 329
Turrell, G., 52, 62

U

Umberson, D., 137, 167
Uno, H., 196, 233
Ursano, R. J., 125, 134, 165
Ursin, H., 107, 170
Usher, D., 187, 233

V

Vahtera, J., 128, 143, 158, 181
Valois, R. F., 176
van Bastelaer, T., 244, 281
van den Berg, B. J., 128, 170
van der Maesen, L. J., 52, 53, 62
Van Doorslaer, E., 270, 284
van Eijk, J.T.M., 63
van Ginneken, J. K., 138, 161
Van Gundy, K., 142, 177
van Lenthe, F., 159
van Tilburg, T., 63
Van Willigen, M., 45, 63, 107, 135, 177
Vance, R. H., 139, 163
Vasilescu, I. P., 319, 332
Veenstra, G., 254, 284
Verny, T., 123, 160
Vescio, M. F., 128, 181

Vidal, A. C., 273, 284
Vigilante, D., 124, 175
Villermé, L., 36
Vincen, M. L., 176
Vingilis, E., 141, 181
Vogt, T. M., 45, 64
Voigt, K. H., 142, 178
Vojvodic, R. W., 237
Volpe, B. T., 119, 165
Vondracek, F. W., 124, 181

W

Wade, T. J., 141, 181
Wadsworth, M. E., 108, 128, 129, 170, 172
Wagstaff, A., 270, 280, 284
Waldfogel, J., 113, 169
Walker, D., 123, 181
Walker, S. P., 141, 181
Wall, S. N., 59
Wallace, L., 187, 224, 233
Wallace, L. E., 127, 181
Wallace, P., 230
Wallerstein, N., 248, 255, 282
Walsh, D. A., 123, 165
Wan, R., 127, 173
Wang, J., 187, 229
Warren, M. R., 246, 283
Warrick, C., 237
Waterman, P. D., 316, 330
Weinberg, A. S., 73, 86, 101
Weiss, B. D., 138, 181
Weiss, S. T., 128, 168
Weissberg, R. P., 133, 181
Weist, E., 319, 328
Welin, L., 45, 64
Weller, N. F., 142, 181
Wenger, E., 17, 34, 310, 311, 320, 321, 332
Werner, E. E., 123, 133, 181
Whitehead, M., 21, 32, 209, 228

Whiteis, D. G., 13, 34, 233, 235, 262, 284
Wickrama, K. A., 127, 137, 181
Widdowson, J., 173
Wield, G. A., 129, 159
Wiens, M., 49, 60, 111, 131, 133, 167
Wiesner, P. J., 319, 328
Wigfield, A., 163
Wilcox, R., 239, 284
Wilkinson, D. L., 137, 164
Wilkinson, R. G., 37, 44, 46, 62, 64, 107, 173, 181, 185, 191, 195, 196, 197, 233
Williams, B., 166
Williams, D., 23, 24, 33, 171, 192, 230, 231
Williams, M. V., 136, 181
Williams, S., 141, 181
Williamson, D. F., 164
Willis, H. D., 153, 181
Willms, J. D., 122, 128, 132, 181, 182
Wills, T. A., 59
Wilson, D. H., 119, 165
Wilson, M. E., 83, 101
Wilson, R. S., 128, 164
Wilson, W. J., 46, 64
Windham, J., 156, 182
Windle, M., 118, 182
Windsor, D., 92, 101
Winick, M., 123, 182
Winkleby, M. A., 136, 143, 182
Wise, D. A., 193, 228
Wismar, M., 269, 284
Withers, G. S., 119, 166
Witt, W. P., 128, 179
Wolfe, B., 141, 166
Wolff, T., 310, 328
Wolfson, M., 136, 177, 182, 192, 198, 232, 233
Wong, G.W.K., 46, 64
Woo, J., 53, 59
Woodward, A., 152, 182

Woodward, A. L., 121, 182
Woodward, C. A., 230
Woodward, D., 13, 34
Woolcock, M., 135, 182, 302, 332
Worthman, C. M., 109, 110, 182
Wortman, C. B., 127, 182
Wright, A. L., 60
Wright, R. J., 128, 168
Wu, C. L., 45, 63, 107, 136, 137, 140, 177
Wu, P., 137, 169

X

Xie, X., 169

Y

Yach, D., 214, 234
Yamada, K., 138, 182
Yancey, A. K., 124, 182
Yarnell, V., 175
Yasnoff, W. A., 316, 332
Yazbeck, A. S., 280
Ye, H. H., 169
Yee, L. J., 111, 166
York, P., 134, 178
Yoshikawa, H., 132, 182
Young, I. M., 248, 249, 250, 251, 252, 254, 259, 284
Young, M. H., 142, 182
Young, T. K., 133, 182
Yunis, C., 166

Z

Zaslow, M. J., 130, 174
Zerhouni, E., 292, 332
Zhang, J. F., 123, 161
Ziersch, A. M., 244, 280
Zigler, E., 132, 172
Zollner, H., 209, 234

SUBJECT INDEX

A

Absolute deprivation, 195
Absolute income, 196
Absolute poverty, defining, 199
Academia, role of, 306
Academic achievement, 114, 115, 122, 123, 141–142, 145–146, 153. *See also* Education
Academic Achievement for All Act, 143
Academy for Health Services Research, 298
Access to Care task force, 274
Access to health care: and child development, 122; community development policy aimed at, 274–275; focusing on inequalities in, 296; increasing, 225, 240, 242; in the U.S., 36, 53, 54, 194–195
Access to Health Care Commission, 274
Access to medicine, policies to increase, 211
Access to resources: differential, 44–45, 194; equity of, 152

Accountability, 218, 248, 251, 252, 258, 259, 317, 319
Accountability systems, creating, 264
Acheson report, 55, 205, 206, 224, 225
Achievement experience, 137
Achievement gap, 154
Achievement indicators, 149
Action guidelines, creating, 249, 257
Activist view, 261
Ad Hoc Committee on Health Literacy for the Council on Scientific Affairs, 113
Adaptation, and stages of life-course development, 119–120
Adaptative process, health development as an, 109
Adaptive ability, 131, 132
Adaptive behaviors, importance of, 107
Adaptive capacities, 124
Adaptive efficiency, 72, 93, 94
Additive effects, chain of risk involving, 111
Additive protective effects, 134–135

Adolescence: and academic achievement, 153, 193; community development policy aimed at reducing violence during, 273; development during, 124–125; and education, 141–142; expression of risk exposure from, 130; health during, shifting traditional paradigm of, 112; and health-risk behavior, 125, 142, 153; leading causes of mortality and morbidity during, 125, 142; link between physical environment and health outcomes during, 47; supporting and strengthening development during, 133–134; transition from, to young adulthood, 125–126; vocational training during, 226
Adolescent, defined, 124
Adolescent Health Attitude and Behavior Survey, 134
Adult literacy, 150
Adult mortality: in developing countries, 199; and socio-economic position, 128, 129

Adulthood: development during different stages of, 126–127; expression of risk exposure from, 128, 130; transition from adolescence to, 125–126

Adult-onset diabetes (Type 2), 129, 193

Adults. *See specific age group*

Africa, 203

African Americans: breast cancer survival rates of, tracking, 55; complex factors influencing mortality of, 193; discrimination of, 46, 193; and infant mortality rates, 240; mortality and poverty rates for, 192; segregation of, 46; and social capital, 246. *See also* Racial and ethnic health disparities; Racial segregation

Afrol News, 203, 227

After-school programs, 146

Agency and action, inclusion of, in the conceptual model, issue of, 41

Agency for Healthcare Research and Quality, 54, 58, 255, 280

Agents of change, communities as, 243

Aggregate measures, 43, 276, 320

Aging, rapid, 196

Agriculture and food policy, 218

AIDS. *See* HIV/AIDS

Alaska RSV Study Group, 46, 59

Alcohol and drug use, during adolescence, 125, 142

Allocative efficiency, 29, 138, 218, 219, 220, 221, 222, 289

Allostatic load, 49

Alma Alta Declaration, 26

Altruism, 93

Ameliorative interventions, focus on, 22

America 2000: An Education Strategy (USDE), 119

American Academy of Pediatrics, 123, 158

American Journal of Public Health, 226

American Medical Association (AMA), 113, 138, 158

Analytic framework: conclusion on, 30–31; fields of study in the, 4,

5; fundamental determinants in the, 4, 5; issues and aspects framing the, 2–3; key aspects in the, 1–2; and major public health trends, 17–27; for moving toward a healthy (re)public, 4–9; policy criteria in the, 27–30; policy domains in the, 4, 5, 6–9; policy models and examples in the, 5, 9–17; summary of, 5; units of analysis in the, 4, 5. *See also specific policy domains, fields of study, and policy models*

Analytic techniques, choice of, importance of, for future research, 51

Anemia, 202

Anheuser-Busch, 97

Annie E. Casey Foundation, 117, 125, 153, 158

Anti-globalization movement, 16

Appalachian region, impact of globalization on, 236

Aquatic changes, examples of, and potential health impacts, *81*

Area-based measure, 42–43

Arkansas standardized test scores, 150

Asia, 152, 199

Asian Development Bank, 214, 227

Assessment: assets, 261; community, 271–272; environmental impact, 217; health impact, 217–218, 224; needs, 260, 261; risk, 83

Assessment function, 239, 291, 313, *314*, 316

Assessment Protocol for Excellence in Public Health (APEX/PH), 317

Asset development, local, 241

Asset model, 261

Assets and resources. *See* Resources

Association for Community Health Improvement, 257, 258, 280

Associational activity, local polices to support, *245*

Associations, collective, 242–243

Assurance function, 239, 291, *315*, 318

Asymmetrical partnerships, 312

Asymmetrical power, 313

Atmosphere, defining, 75

Atmospheric changes, examples of, and potential health impacts, *80*

At-risk children, 122, 127–128, 130–131, 133–134

Auspices, blueprint of, *308*

Australia, 2, 52, 55, 150, 266

Australian Institute of Family Studies, 116, 159

Authoritarian communist regimes, 10, 12, 14

Avian flu, 216

B

Bangladesh, 214, 221–222

Bangladesh Central Bank, 214

Barriers to health care, types of, 241

Basic material needs, meeting, in developed countries, 194

Behavioral model, 78

Behavioral risk factors, research focusing on, 50. *See also* Health-risk behaviors

Belgium, 150

Belonging, sense of, 243, *245*

Bias, example of, 47

Biodiversity, preservation of, 77, 78

Biologic embedding, 49

Biologic mechanisms, 49–50

Biological risk factors, research focusing on, 50

Biological/genetic endowments, 39, 138–139

Biomedical approach, prevailing, 40, 50

Biomedicine, business of, impact of, 53

Biophysical realities, recognizing, 69

Biosphere, defining, 75

Birth, learning starting at, 120

Black Americans. *See* African Americans

Black report, 205

Blair administration, 13, 205

Bonding. *See* Social bonds

Boston Community Policing (Ten Point Coalition), *267, 268*, 272–273, 275

Brain damage, 202

Brain development, aspects of, 119, 120, 121, 122

Brain drain, 216, 226

Brazil, 215

Breast cancer survival rates, tracking, 55

Bretton Woods exchange system, 189

Bright From the Start program, 155

Britain. *See* United Kingdom/Great Britain

British Columbia, 205, 220

British military school, 191

Bureau of Justice Statistics, 141, 180

Bush administration, 143, 145, 148, 149

Business decision making. *See* Corporate decision making

Business law, partnership models rooted in, 311

Business models, 94

Business objectives, reconciling, with public health objectives, 85, 86

Business responsibilities, 74. *See also* Corporate social responsibility (CSR)

Business sector, 305, 312

Business-related policies, 188

C

California Smoke-Free, *267*, *268*, 270–271

Canada: balance sought in, 9; and community development, 266, 269; controversy within, 26; economic policies in, 204–205; economic policies of, 220–221; educational approach in, 152; and HDI ranking, 150; health policy agenda of, 2, 52; human development policies in, 146; income inequality and mortality in, 198; intersectoral collaboration in, 224; and the Lalonde report, 17–18, 36; monitoring child development in, 116–117; population health policies in, 56–57, 297; school readiness in, 140–141; vulnerable children in, 122

Canadian Centre for Studies of Children at Risk, 155

Canadian Federal, Provincial and Territorial Early Childhood Development Agreement, 116

Canadian Institute for Advanced Research (CIAR), 3, 9, 19, 26, 32, 37, 52, 56, 204

Canadian Institute for Health Information, 205, 227

Cancer, 125

Capacity concept, 289. *See also specific capacities*

Capital-intensive development, 190

Capitalism, 10

Cardiovascular disease, 125, 136, 142, 143, 193

Caregiver roles, 126, 127

Caregiving, impact of, on early childhood development, 122–123, 130, 140

Caribbean, 203

Carnegie Corporation of New York, 120, 153, 160

Causal modeling, need for, 302

Causal models, 51, 111

Causation, multiple, tenet of, field guided by, 37

Center for Healthier Children, Families and Communities, 113

Center for Law and Social Policy, 154, 160

Center for the Study of Social Policy, 155, 161

Centers for Disease Control and Prevention (CDC), 118, 123, 125, 161, 180, 223, 277, 291, 292, 317, 331

Centers for Population Health and Health Disparities, 50

Centre for Educational Research and Innovation, 167

Centrist political strategy, 13

Chain of risk, 111

Change: community, view of, 26; thinking and acting globally and locally for, 322. *See also* Ecosystem change

Change agents, communities as, 243

Change process, beginning, foundation for, 250

Charitable responsibilities, 90, 91

Child abuse and neglect, 114

Child care: access to, 122; formal, linking, to K-12 education, 155, 158; recommendations on, 154–158. *See also* Early childhood care

Child development: inequalities in, contributing factors in, 122; influence of physical environment on, 48; supporting and strengthening, 133–134; unsatisfactory, 114. *See also* Early childhood development

Child Development Centre, 116

Child development measures, 114–119

Child health index, 117

Child Health Initiative, 318

Child health measures, 114–119

Child literacy, 150

Child mortality, in developing countries, 199

Child poverty: and access to preschool, 154; cumulative effects of, 130; and developmental outcomes, 116, 123, 133; economic policies to address, 146; and literacy, 150; policies to reduce, 206; and school readiness, 114–115; and standardized test scores, 115, *151*; in the U.S., 114, 130, 150

Child rearing, stage of, 126

Child tax credits, 225

Child well-being index, 118

Childhood: adult mortality related to socioeconomic position during, 128, *129*; health during, shifting traditional paradigm of, 112; latent effects from, 129–130; transitional period of, development during, 123–124, 129. *See also* Early childhood development

Childhood diseases, international policies addressing, 211, 212

Children. *See specific age group*

Children at risk. *See* At-risk children

Children Families and Learning Network, 146, 147, 161

Children's Defense Fund, 125, 153, 161

Children's Fund International, 116

Children's Health Insurance Program (CHIP), state-level, 53

China, 10, 203, 215

Chronic disease, 38, 109, 125, 130, 203

Chronic stress, 49, 120, 194, 195–196, 197

Church membership, 246

Citizen participation. *See* Civic participation

City infrastructure, deterioration of, 235

Civic engagement: as a measure of social capital, 254, 255; policies lacking in details of, 275

Civic participation: developing minimum standards for, 263; diverse, 241; highest rate of, 246; ladder of, 310; levels of, 270, 271, 272, 273, 274, 275; local polices to support, *245*; in young adulthood, 126. *See also* Community building

Civil rights movement, 10

Civil society, 14, 15, 16, 23, 244

Clean water, 194, 212

Climate change, 83

Clinical medicine, 23, 42

Clinton administration, 13, 18, 143

Clinton Health Care Plan, 18

Closed economic system model, 84–85, 88

Closing the Health Care Gap Act, 54

Clusters of risk, accumulation of, relative to time, 111

Coalition for Healthier Cities and Communities, 256, 270

Coalitions, political, 16, 310

Codification: levels of, of CSR components, 90, 91; of public health concerns, 98

Cognitive capacity, 120, 121–122, 124

Cognitive decline, protection against, 138

Collaboration: example of, 265; increased, generating, 263; legitimacy of, 307. *See also* Partnerships

Collaborative decision making models, 307, 309, 310–313

Collaborative relationships, importance of, 292–293, 317. *See also* Public-private partnerships

Collective action, manifestation of, 68

Collective assets, 135

Collective associations, 242–243

Collective efficacy, 243, 244, 248, 252, 254, 261, 290

Collective governmental responsibility, maintaining, 307, 309

Collectivist view, 52, 53, 55, 57

Columbia University, 155

Command-and-control processes, use of, 84

Commission on Macroeconomics and Health, Working Group 1, 9, 19, 34, 190, 199, 201, 202, 203, 211, 214, 215, 216, 225, 233

Committee on Understanding and Eliminating Racial and Ethnic Disparities in Health Care, 54

Committee for the Study of the Future of Public Health, 4, 19, 32, 68, 100, 238, 281, 290, 330

Committee on Assuring the Health of the Public in the 21st Century, 4, 9, 19, 20, *21*, 25, 32, 224, 229, 242, 261, 262, 263, 264, 293, 306, *321*, 330

Committee on Educating Public Health Professionals for the 21st Century, 4, 9, 19, 25, 33, 293, 319, *321*, 330

Committee on Integrating the Science of Early Childhood Development, 111, 174

Committee on Prevention and Control of Sexually Transmitted Diseases, 125, 168

Committee on Prevention of Mental Disorders, 142, 168

Committee on Public Education, 123, 158

Committee on Summary Measures of Population Health, 42, 43, 60, 296, 330

Committee on Understanding and Eliminating Racial and Ethnic Disparities in Health Care, 46, 60

Committee on Using Performance Monitoring to Improve Community Health, 263, 281

Communication: improving, across sectors, 263–264; role of, exploring, 16–17

Communicative action theory, 16, 249

Communism, 10, 12, 14

Communitarian philosophy, 10, 15

Communities of practice, 17, 311

Community: broad definition of, use of, 241; as a critical tool, 265; defining, 242–243; reinventing, 14; sense of, 243

Community and market models: of collaborative decision making, *310*; political and economic philosophies behind, *11*, 13–14; selected, summary of, *287*. *See also specific examples*

Community assessment, 271–272

Community benefit, 290. *See also* Collective efficacy

Community building, 238, 246–248, 252, 256, 265

Community buy-in, lack of, 279

Community capacity, 242–243, 256

Community decision making, 241, 270, 271

Community development: concepts and perspectives presented by, 8, 9; consideration of, lack of, 2–3; and current policies addressing fundamental determinants, 259–264; defining, 6, 238; and evidence regarding research on determinants, 252–259; and fields of study, 242–248; focus on, in determining sustainable development, 73; ideals integral to concept of, 241; importance of, 23; international initiatives informing understanding of, 266, 269; introduction to, 238–252; key aspects involving, 237–238; and key policies,

summary of, 287; and major evaluation issues, 290; and measurement of assets associated with child development, 119; overview of, 238–242; and policy domains, 248–252; recommendations for, 276–279, 326–327; role of public health in, 239; and strengths and limitations of current policies, 264–276; successful, prospects of, enhancing, 9; and typology of selected policies, *267*
Community development model, 252, *253*
Community empowerment, 16, 241, *245*, 248, 256, 260, 261, 316–317
Community Food and Nutrition Program, 269
Community health partnerships (CHPs), 265
Community health planning, 260
Community infrastructure: creating, 241; and racial segregation, 23, *24*
Community interests, respecting, 279
Community models: of collaborative decision making, *310*; of community development policies, 243, 260–261, 264, *267*, *268*, 271–273; political and economic philosophies behind, 10, *11*; selected, summary of, *287. See also specific examples*
Community organizing, 238, 265
Community Services Block Grant (CSBG), *267*, *268*, 269–270
Community stability, as requisite, 247
Community support, and academic achievement, 141
Community sustainability: defining, 73; foundation for, 244, 260–261
Community underdevelopment, 262
Community values, 137, 238, 241, 255, 261, *267*, 279
Community-based interventions, categories of, 153

Community-based participatory research (CBPR), 51, 248, 252, 255–259, 260, 261, 277
Community-building activities, examples of, 247
Community-centered advocates, view of, 261
Community-level assets, 135
Company (firm), defined, 85–86
Competence, 112, 128, 133, 153, 154
Competing policy contexts, 8
Complex interrelationships, consideration of, importance of, for future research, 51
Complex open systems, 74, 265
Complex reality, failure to address, issue of, 41
Complex Systems, 15, 32
Complexity, previously unexamined, new lenses for revealing, 320
Complexity theory, 15
Compliance with physical laws, 90, *91*, 92
Conceptual model, 39–42
Conflict, 243–244, 255
Conflict management, 244
Connective mechanisms, direct and strong, absence of, 83
Connectivity, rate of, 16–17
Consensus, 249, 250, 257
Conservation, law of, 71
Conservativism, rise of, 26
Consultative Group on Early Childhood Care and Development, 155, 161
Consumer Product Safety Commission, 98
Context: as changing, 109; defining, 131; viewing as a barrier, 261
Continuous quality improvement, implementation of, 17
Control, sense of, 48, 143
Controlled experiments, need for, 302
Controversy, over population health, 26
Conventional corporate policy, 85–86, 88, *89*, 99
Cooperative behavior, 243
Copenhagen Declaration on Reducing Social Inequalities in Health, 209

Copernican understanding of the universe, 15
Coping skills, acquisition of, 112
Coronary heart disease, increased risk for, 129
Corporate decision making, 68, 69, 71, 86, 88, 92
Corporate ecological responsiveness. *See* Ecologically responsive corporate policy
Corporate industry impacts, 263
Corporate investment, 263
Corporate morality, 92
Corporate policies, 74
Corporate policy: domain of, 73–74; evaluating, 88, 93; exploring, 66; relevance of, 68. *See also* Conventional corporate policy; Ecologically responsive corporate policy
Corporate profit motive. *See* Profit maximization (motive)
Corporate responsibility, 72, 86
Corporate social performance, example of, 94–95
Corporate social responsibility (CSR): case study demonstrating, 94, 96; and community development, 263; defining, 74; evaluating, 289; and IKEA, 94; modifying the framework of, 92–93; pyramid of, 90–91
Corporate taxes, 188
Corporate wealth, maximizing. *See* Profit maximization (motive)
Corrective action, 87, 88
Cost shifting, 261–262
Cost-effectiveness: defining, 69; supporting more research on, 224
Costs and benefits, 71–72, 86
Costs of health care. *See* Health care costs
Criminal activity, and education, 141
Critical periods, defining, 131
Critical theory, 16
Critical thinking, achieving, 261
Cuba, 10
Cultural capital: as a determinant, 4; importance of, 238. *See also* Community development

Cultural diversity, growing, challenges from, 15
Cultural ideology, 55
Culture, viewing as a barrier, 261
Cumulative effects, 128, 130, 131, 132
Cumulative exposure, health consequences of, evidence highlighting, 113
Cumulative risk, product of, 111
Current generation, focusing on, versus future generation, issue of, 187
Customs and traditions, use of, 84

D

Data and information systems, 291–292, 313, 316
Data collection and analysis model, 275
"Deadly Poisoned Bookshelves" controversy, case study involving, 93–98
Deadweight loss, 217
Death rates. *See* Mortality
Debt relief program, 213–214, 222–223
Decentralization, 66, 72, 87, 93
Decision-making domains: in the analytic framework, 10; summary of, *11. See also specific domains*
Decision-making environments, 72, 87, 93
Decisions, interdependence and impact of, acknowledging, 7
Deficiency model, 261
Deforestation, *80, 82,* 83
Deliberation, process of, 250
Deliberative democracy: calls for, 14–15, 23; community characteristics allowing for, 254; community development policy grounded in, 248, 278; in community models, 261; principles of, 248, 249–252, 253, 255; ways of achieving, examples of, 258, 259
Deliberative justice, 30, 220, 221, 222, 223, 266, 290, 313, 317

Demand and supply, 72, 83–85, 189
Demand-stimulation strategy, 13
Democracy: and community development, 248; essential component of, 224; and inequalities, 254; support and actualization of, policies providing, 275. *See also* Deliberative democracy
Department of Defense (DoD) schools, 145–146, 155, 156
Department of Defense Education Activity, 145, 162
Department of Health, 56, 59, 205, 228, 240, 280
Dependency, decreased, 125
Depopulation of rural areas, 236
Deregulation, 13
Developed countries: characterization of, 191; economic policies of, 204–210; evaluation of economic policies in, 220–221; and evidence regarding research on economic determinants, 191–198; and trade polices, 188–189
Developing countries: characterization of, 191; economic policies of international organizations affecting, 210–216; evaluation of economic policies in, 221–223; and evidence regarding research on economic determinants, 199–203; and globalization, 189–190; industry moving to, 235; lending bank to, 189; policy recommendations for, 225, 226
Development: balancing, with sustainability, 7; focusing on, reason for, 6; further defining, 187; goal of, 7; issue over objective of, 187. *See also* Community development; Economic development; Human development; Sustainable development
Developmental assets, 132–135, 152

Developmental Assets Framework, 134
Developmental outcomes, 116, 123
Developmental perspective of health, 108–109, *110. See also* Life-course perspective
Developmental trajectories, 111–112, 118
Devolution of government, 10, 12, 25
Diabetes (Type 2), 129, 193
Diagnosing and investigating, practices for, 316
Dialogical theory, 249
Dialogue guide, 257, 258
Dialogue, manner of, 249–250, 253, 256, 258, 261
Differences versus levels, 322, 323
Direct causal pathways, 28, 29, 135–136, 137–138
Disability-adjusted life expectancy (DALE), 296
Disabled population, health insurance for, 53
Disciplinary research paradigm, 19, *20*
Discourse principle, 248, 249–250. *See also* Participatory discourse; Rational discourse
Discrimination: impact of, 46, 193; role of, in population health research, 50; and social networks, 246. *See also* Racial segregation
Disease: depiction of, in the conceptual model, 39, 40; as health care system defines, 41; international policies aimed at addressing, 211; philosophical orientation toward, 52–53; treatment of, policies to encourage, 211. *See also* Morbidity
Disease prevention: addressing education in, 141; continued focus on, new strategy extending beyond, recommending, 99; corporate investment in, 263; extension of research on, 99; and managed care, 25; national goals for, 119, 239; research into, policies to

encourage, 211; strategy
toward, shift in, call for, 38;
transferring responsibility for, to
managed care system, 263; in
the workplace, 263
Disease surveillance systems, 291,
316
Diseases. *See specific type*
Distal factors, defining, 22
Distributive justice, 30, 43, 221,
222, 223, 266, 289, 312
Distributive measures, 43, 276
District of Columbia, State Center
for Health Statistics Admin-
istration, 240, 280
Downstream category, 53, 302
Dropouts. *See* School failure
(dropouts)
Drug and alcohol use, during
adolescence, 125, 142
Drug pricing, 211
Dynamic efficiency, 29, 290. *See also*
Social capital

E

Early Child Care Research
Network, 118, 123, 174
Early childhood: development
during, 122–123; importance of,
120, 153; risk exposure from,
expression of, 128, 129, 130
Early Childhood and Family
Education Section, 147, 179
Early childhood care: as a
contributing factor, 108;
focusing policies on, importance
of, 113; funding of, issue of, in
the U.S., 148, 149, 156–157. *See
also* Child care
Early childhood development: and
education, 140–141; focusing
policies on, importance of, 154;
initiative addressing, in the U.S.,
149; recommendations on, 154–
158; and resilience to risk, 133
Early childhood education: focusing
policies on, importance of,
112–113; recommendations for,
154–158. *See also* Preschool
programs

Early childhood intervention
programs, 144–148, 157, 289
Early Childhood Longitudinal
Study, 114
Early Development Instrument
(EDI), 116
Early Head Start, 144, 155, 156
Early risk, human ecology of, 112
Earned Income Tax Credit, 146
Ecological determinants: current
policies addressing, 85–90;
drawing out, 69; evidence
regarding, 66, 70, 71, 78–83,
98; and potential health
impacts, 79, *80*, *81*, *82*
Ecological dysfunction, treating
symptoms of, versus addressing
fundamental causes, 67
Ecological effectiveness, 73, 74, 88,
89, 90, 92, 93, 288
Ecological epidemiology, 67
Ecological imbalance, 71, 83
Ecological model, 4, 70, 77, 112, 141
Ecological paradigm, community
models grounded in, 260–261
Ecological responsibility, 92, 94, 96
Ecologically responsive corporate
policy, 69, 73, 74, 88, *89*; case
study involving, 93–98; defining,
92, 93. *See also* Corporate social
responsibility (CSR)
Ecology: defined, 68; drawing on
contributions from, 66, 68
Econometric model, 138
Economic activity: by-product of,
71–72; and corporate social
responsibility, 92; distribution of
environmental risks resulting
from, focus on, 67; driving
aquatic system changes, *81*;
driving atmospheric changes,
80; driving terrestrial ecosystem
changes, *82*; ecosystem change
due to, 66, 69, 71, 78, 79–83;
examples of, 71; exposure to
stress from, 77; inconsistencies
between, and economic function, 79, 83; issue with addressing, 69; overview of, 67
Economic allocations, and health
equity, 152

Economic conditions, education
influencing, 136
Economic cycles: in a closed system,
84–85; in opposition with
natural cycles, 69–70, 78
Economic determinants: current
policies grounded in, 204–216;
of ecosystem change, evidence
on, 67, 70, 71, 83–85; evidence
regarding, 191–203; focus on,
22; recognition of, enhancing,
218, 223. *See also* Economic
development
Economic development: as a
broader concept, 186; and
community development, 262,
270, 273; concepts and perspectives presented by, 8, 9; consideration of, lack of, 2–3; and
current policies addressing
fundamental determinants,
204–216; defining, 6, 184;
degree of, importance of, 190; in
developing countries, impact of,
on health, 199–201; and evidence regarding research on
determinants, 191–203; and
fields of study, 185–187; focus
on, in determining sustainable
development, 73; impact of
health on, in developing countries, 201–203; introduction to,
184–190; key aspects involving,
183–185; and key policies, summary of, 287; and major evaluation issues, *288*, 289; measures
of, 186–187; overview of,
184–185; and policy domains,
187–190; recommendations for,
223–226, 326; and strengths and
limitations of current polices,
216–223. *See also* Income
Economic efficiency, 73, 74, 87, 88,
89, 90, *91*, 92, 94, 186, 188, 289
Economic ends, competing, issue of,
69–70
Economic environment, focus on,
55, 56
Economic factors: importance of,
20, *21*; role of, pointing out, 8.
See also specific factors

Economic growth: defined, 186; emphasis on, 262; measures of, 184; promoting, 157, 225. *See also* Gross domestic product (GDP)

Economic inequalities: and racial segregation, 23, *24. See also* Income inequality

Economic models, standard, 84, 85

Economic Opportunity Act, 269

Economic policies: to address child poverty, 146; barriers to, 216–217; defined, 187–188; of developed countries, 204–210; evaluation approach for, 218–220; evaluation of, 220–223; fundamental goal of, 187; as health policies, argument for, 209, 226; of international organizations affecting developing countries, 210–216; potential of, in affecting poverty, 185; relationship between, and population health, 190; supporting more research on, 224

Economic power, 17, 313

Economic resources, as requisite, for community building, 247

Economic responsibilities, 74, 90, 91, 94, 96

Economic sector, 306, 312

Economic systems: defined, 68; operations of, approach to, 69; reliance of, on ecosystems, 72

Economic theory, 72, 87

Economic vitality, community development policy aimed at, 273–274

Economics: defined, 68, 186; drawing on contributions from, 66, 68

Ecosocial paradigm, 20, *21,* 49, 109, 316, 320. *See also* Life-course perspective

Ecosystem behavior, 77–78, 88

Ecosystem change: aquatic, examples of, *81;* atmospheric, examples of, *80;* case study involving, 102–105; consequences of, 69; as a constant, 77; and corporate policies, 90; due to economic activity, 66, 69,

71, 78, 79–83; evidence on economic determinants of, 67, 70, 71, 83–85; examples of, 70–71; impacting ecosystem services, 77; overview of, 67; terrestrial, examples of, *82*

Ecosystem degradation, 67, 77, 83

Ecosystem function: case study involving, 102–105; defining principles of, 77–78, 88; general model of, *76;* inconsistencies between economic activity and, 79, 83; normal, evidence on, 70, 74–78

Ecosystem integrity, 98

Ecosystem modification. *See* Ecosystem change

Ecosystem services, 75–77

Ecosystems: assessing well-being of, approaches used in, 77; defined, 68, 74; focus on, 66; persistence and stability of, dependency of, 71; reliance of economic systems on, 72; resilience and biodiversity of, preservation of, 77, 78; stressed, looking beyond sick people to, 98–99; as a unit of analysis, 7

Education: affecting income, 193; alternative approach to, 152; alternative explanations for effects of, 138–140; and cardiovascular disease, 136, 143; and community development, 270; as a contributing factor, 108; corporate investment in, 263; in developing countries, improving, calls for, 212; direct and indirect causal pathways of, 135–137; direct effects of, on health, 137–138; focusing policies on, importance of, 154; and the human development index, 149; impact of, evidence for, 140–142; as an indicator of socioeconomic position, 44, 45, 48; and influence of fertility, 202; optimizing, focusing policies on, importance of, 140; parent, level of, 122; of parents with students in DoD schools, 145; pursuing, in young adult-

hood, 126; and racial segregation, 23, *24;* relationship between health and, evidence for, 135, 193; role of, pointing out, 8; spending on, 188, 197. *See also* Early childhood education; Human development

Education Excellence for All Children Act, 143

Education policies: economists favoring, 217; in other countries, 146–148; recommendations for, 226; right, benefits of, recognizing, 157–158; in the United States, 144–146

Education sector, 305

Educational attainment, 107, 113, 134, 140, 150, 157, 184, 186

Educational Excellence for All Children Act, 163

Educational Excellence for All Learners Act, 144, 163

Educational goals, national, 119

Edudata Canada, 117, 163

Effectiveness: in child care and education, issue of, 149; of collaborative decision making models, 313; of community development policies, 266, *268,* 270, 271, 272, 274, 275; critical element of, 307; defining, 2, 29; of early childhood development programs, 153; of economic policies, 219, 220, 221; and globalization, 215; of human development policies, 149, 150, 151; and measuring population health, 43; models operationalizing, importance of, 265; objective of, defining, 301; of partnerships, 312; research needed on, 303, *304;* and resource allocation to priority health issues, 292; standards of, precedence of, in questions of policy, 152; supporting more research on, 224; use of, for evaluating policies, *28,* 29, *288. See also* Ecological effectiveness

Efficiency: of collaborative decision making models, 313; of community development policies, 266, *268*, 270, 272, 274, 275; defining, 2, 29; of economic policies, 219; and globalization, 215; of human development policies, 149, 151, 152; and measuring population health, 43; models operationalizing, importance of, 265; objective of, defining, 301; of partnerships, 312; research needed on, 303, *304*; and resource allocation to priority health issues, 292; supporting more research on, 224; and sustainable development, 7; use of, for evaluating policies, *28*, 29–30, *288*. *See also* Allocative efficiency; Dynamic efficiency; Economic efficiency; Technical (production) efficiency

Effort-reward imbalance, 142

Elderly population, 47, 53, 236

Emergency Preparedness Centers, 292

Emotional attachment and commitment, 134

Employees. *See* Working population

Employer-based insurance, 53, 262

Employment: community, policy aimed at, 273–274; as an indicator of socioeconomic position, 45; pursuing, in young adulthood, 126; and racial segregation, 23, *24*. *See also* Economic development

Employment protection, 209, 225

Empowerment. *See* Community empowerment

Empowerment evaluation, 248

Enforcing laws and regulations, 318

England: and community development, 266; early childhood education in, 146, 147. *See also* United Kingdom/Great Britain

Enterprise Zone, *267*, *268*, 273–274

Entitlement programs, spending on, 188

Environmental change, 71

Environmental criteria, 7

Environmental equity, 73–74, 88, *89*

Environmental factors, importance of, 20, *21*. *See also specific factors*

Environmental hazards, incidence and distribution of, 67

Environmental impact assessment, 217

Environmental impacts: consideration of, 69; of corporate industry, 263; ecological events representing, 79, *80*, *81*, *82*, 92; minimizing, 92

Environmental justice, 73–74, 90, 248

Environmental justice movement, 10, 16, 47

Environmental measures, 43

Environmental pollution, shifting focus to, in prevention strategies, call for, 38

Environmental protection, 90, 99

Environmental Protection Agency (EPA), 98, 263

Environmental regulation, 270–271

Environmental resources and risks, focusing on, 67. *See also* Sustainable development

Environmental stressors, individual response to, 39, 49

Epidemiologic transition, 203

Epidemiological change, 99

Epidemiology: early studies in the field of, 36; ecological, 67; life-course, 109, 128; modern, critique of, 37, 98

Epidemiology of the marketplace, 67, 70–72, 78

Equal opportunity for participation. *See* Political equity

Equity: in child care and education, issue of, 149; of collaborative decision making models, 312–313; of community development policies, 266, *268*, 270, 272, 274, 275; defining, 2, 29; of economic policies, 219, 220, 221, 222, 289; and globalization, 215; health, reach of, 152; of human development policies, 149, 153; and measuring population health, 43; models operationalizing, importance of, 265; objective of, defining, 301;

of partnerships, 312; of planning models, 317; political, 248; research needed on, 303, *304*; serving dimensions of, 73, 90; standards of, precedence of, in questions of policy, 152; and sustainable development, 7, 73–74, 289; use of, for evaluating policies, *28*, 30, *288*. *See also* Deliberative justice; Distributive justice; Environmental equity; Intergenerational justice; Social justice

Erikson's stages of development, 124

Ethical implications, of measuring population health, 43

Ethical leadership, *321*

Ethical responsibilities, 90, 91, 97

European countries: and community development, 266; economic policies in, 206–209; educational streaming practices in, 152; funding of education and child care in, 157; intersectoral collaboration in, 224; participatory approach in, 224; political and economic philosophy of, 12. *See also specific countries*

European Network on Interventions and Policies to Reduce Inequalities in Health, 206, *207*, *208*, 231

European Union, 69, 196

Evaluating policies. *See* Policy evaluation

Evaluating services, 319

Evidence-based approach, 52, 264, 303

Evolutionary processes, 75

Exchange-rate system, 189

Exclusion, vulnerable to, 251, 262

Existing models, evaluation of, recommending, 277

Experience-dependent brain plasticity, 119–120

Experience-driven brain development, 120, 121

Explicit policies, supporting, designed to improve population health, 8

External investment, as requisite, for community building, 247

Externality, defining, 71–72. *See also*
  Market externalities
Exurbia, growth of, 235

F

Family dysfunction, 133
Family support, 114, 123, 141, 142.
  See also Social capital
Federal Interagency Forum on
  Child and Family Statistics,
  117–118, 124, 164
Federal oversight, as a starting
  point, for child care, 157
Federal, Provincial and Territorial
  Advisory Committee on Popu-
  lation Health, 56, 59, 329
Federal spending: areas dominating,
  188; on community develop-
  ment, 269
Feedback loop, health care and
  disease depicted in context of,
  40
Fertility, influence of, in developing
  countries, 202
Fields of study: in the analytic
  framework, 4; summary of, *5.
  See also specific fields of study*
Fight-or-flight mechanism, 195–196
Finance, international, 189, 212–214
Financial barriers, 241
Financial (earning) incentives, 205,
  210
Financial flows, shift in, from
  developed to developing
  countries, 13
Financial resources sector, 312
Finland, 207
Firearm-related deaths, 240
Firm (company), defined, 85–86
Fiscal policy, defined, 188
Fixed exchange rate, 189
Floating exchange rate, 189
Food and Drug Administration, 98
Food chain balance, 78
Food Quality Protection Act, 69
Foreign aid, composition of,
  changing, 211
For-profit managed care industry,
  growing dominance of, effect
  of, 18

Foster Grandparents, 269
Foundation for Child Development
  Index of Child Well-Being
  Project, 118, 165
Founder's Network, 117, 165
Fourth-grade literacy levels, 150
Fourth-grade standardized math
  scores, *151*
France: concurrent policy devel-
  opment in, 206; labor market
  policies in, 225; universal child
  care in, 146, 147–148
Fraser Institute, 149
Free markets, issue with, 213
Free or reduced-cost lunch pro-
  gram, percent of children
  eligible for, *151*
Free trade, income inequality asso-
  ciated with increase in, 190
From Vision to Reality (Department of
  Health), 205, 228
Full income, 186–187
Functions and programs, blueprint
  for designing, *309*
Fundamental causes: versus
  intervening mechanisms, 22, 26;
  and racial segregation, 23, *24*;
  treating symptoms of ecological
  dysfunction versus, 67
Fundamental determinants: in the
  analytic framework, 4; summary
  of, *5. See also specific determinants*
Fundamental determinants of population health: calls for reform
  grounded in, 19; conceptual
  model of, 39–42; current policies
  attempting to address, 52, 53–
  58; evidence regarding research
  on, 74–85; focus on, 22; impact
  of development on, understanding, importance of, 6; importance
  of examining, 3, 36–37;
  influences on, 2; key aspects
  involving, 35–36; list of, 2, 4;
  measuring and modeling, issue
  of, 20, 22; and measuring
  population health, 42–44; overview of, 36–39; racial segregation
  as, framework for examining, 23,
  24; reform grounded in, 293;
  research on, key findings in,

  44–51; sustainable development
  policies addressing, 85–90
Funding: of early child care and
  development programs, 148,
  149, 156–157; of interventions
  in developing countries, 211;
  matched, 277; mixed, allowing
  for, 300; of research on
  population health, 204
Funding streams, 318
Future generations, focusing on,
  versus current generation, issue
  of, 187
Future of Public Health, The (Institute
  of Medicine), 290, *308*
*Future of the Public's Health in the 21st
  Century* (Institute of Medicine),
  19, 262
Future research, 50–51
Future-oriented time horizon,
  grounding the, 8

G

Galileian understanding of the
  universe, 15
General Agreement on Tariffs and
  Trade (GATT), 13, 189
General knowledge, 115
Generalizing programs and
  products, 260
Genetic/biological endowments,
  39, 138–139
Geographic information systems, 316
Geographic jurisdiction: blueprint
  of, *308*; system focus based on,
  306
Georgia Department of Early Care
  and Learning, 155, 165
Georgia, integrated policymaking
  in, example of, 155, 156
Germany, 266
Gestation period, development
  during, 120, 193
Gini coefficient, 196
Global and local thinking and
  action, 322
Global climate change, *80*, 83
Global continuum, 75
Global economy, governing
  financial transactions in, 189

Global health agenda, broad, calling for, 322

Global Health Council, 202

Global measures, 43, 320

Global trading partners, increased strength of, 212

Globalization: description of, 189; and developing countries, 189–190, 214, 215–216; forces of, consequences of, 322; and local urban and rural economies in the U.S., 235–236; political and economic philosophies behind, 10, 12, 13; protests against, 16; recommendations on, 226

Goal 1 Technical Planning Group, 114, 174

Goals 2000: Educate America Act, 119, 165

Goals, balancing, 302

Goal-setting experience, 137

Goods and services, flow of, 84, *89*

Government: devolution of, 10, 12, 125; reinventing, call for, 18

Government and community models: of collaborative decision making, *310*; political and economic philosophies behind, *11*, 14; selected, summary of, *287*. *See also specific examples*

Government decision making, 188, 190

Government models: of collaborative decision making, *310*; of community development policies, 243, 260, 264, *267*, *268*, 269–271, 279; dominance of, 277; political and economic philosophies behind, 10, *11*, 12; selected, summary of, *287*. *See also specific examples*

Government sector, 305, 312

Government values, *267*

Governmental public health: critiques of, 23, 290; investment in, level of, 25; leadership role of, in an intersectoral public health system, 306; moving beyond, 9, 68, 292; period of reassessment and redesign of, 18; role of, 264

Governmental responsibility, collective, maintaining, 307, 309

Government-centered proponents, view of, 261

Gradient effect, 130

Grameen Bank, 214, 221–222

Grameen Communications, 214, 228

Great Britain. *See* United Kingdom/Great Britain

Great Society Initiatives, 13

Greece, 206

Gross domestic product (GDP): and the human development index, 149; increase in, 184, 186; and life expectancy, 199, *200*, 201, 203; percentage of, devoted to health care, 2, 53

Ground rules, establishing, for dialogue, 258

H

Habitat dimension, looking beyond, 98

Hazard dimension, broadening perspective from, 98

Hazards, environmental, incidence and distribution of, 67

Head Start, 144–145, 147, 154, 155, 269, 270

Health: broad definition of, use of, 241; as a consequence of multiple determinants, 109; differentiating between definitions of, 41; distribution of, and health equity, 152; functional definition of, change in, 203; overall improvement in, 157; philosophical orientation toward, 52–53; strong association between income and, 184, 185, 191–192, 193, 201

Health and education policy, 135

Health Canada, 301, 302, *321*, 323, *324*, 330

Health care: approaches for addressing, *208*; depiction of, in the conceptual model, 40, 42; distribution of, and health equity, 152; quality, providing, 225. *See also* Access to health care

Health Care Access initiative, *267*, *268*, 274–275

Health care costs: and education level, 136; focusing on rising, 296; issue of, 2, 53–54; rising, 261; society reducing, and promoting population health, 67; very high national (U.S.), 113

Health care policies, recommendations for, 226

Health care quality, 54, 225

Health care reform: agendas of, proposed shift in, 300; debate over, 295–296; promise of and failure of, 18

Health care sector, role of, 306

Health care spending: findings on, and quality of care and health status, 54; in the U.S., 209

Health departments and laboratories, improving, 291, 292

Health development, dynamics shaping, 131–132

Health development framework, 109, *110*

Health disparities: arising from the work environment, 143; criteria for evaluating, 322–325; differing perspectives on population health and, 22, 276, 323; focus on, *294*, 295; as an outcome; overview of, 2; recognition of, 242; reducing, focus on, 20; requirement for reducing, 3; root of, 241; significant, across the population, 113; socioeconomic, 2; unfair and unjust, 152. *See also* Racial and ethnic health disparities

Health equity, reach of, 152

Health for All initiative, 26

Health gap, 22, 322, 323

Health gradient, 22, 322, 323

Health impact assessment (HIA), 217–218, 224

Health imperialism, 217

Health indicators, leading, 118, 191

Health inequities, defined, 152

Health insurance, 53, 146, 262. *See also* Medicaid; Medicare

Health insurance companies, 261

Health literacy, definition of, 138

Health outcomes: during adolescence, 47, 125; criteria for evaluating, 322–325; focus on, *294*, 295; impact on, documenting, 8; and the life-course health development framework, 109, *110*; and racial segregation, 23, *24*, 46; and socioeconomic position, 128. *See also specific outcomes*

Health policies: attempting to address fundamental determinants, 53–58; broadening scope of, 2, 295–300; different orientations forming, 52–53; economic policies as, argument for, 209, 226; focusing on, 206, 207. *See also* Population health–centered policies; Public health policies

Health process measures, 43

Health promotion: addressing education in, 141; corporate investment in, 263; efforts at, 242; extension of, 99; focus on, 53; and managed care, 25; national goals for, 119, 239; public health revolution involving, 17–18, 36–37; in the workplace, 263

Health Promotion program, 9, 23, 26, 56

Health Resources and Services Administration, 118, 121, 180, 292

Health services: focus on, 57, 98; and the human poverty index, 186

Health trajectories, 111–112

HealthAlert, 291

HealthCare Equality and Accountability Act, 54

Health-compromising behavior, early initiation of, 125

Health-income gradient, 191–193, 205, 206

Health-promoting behaviors, 45, 48, 136, 137

Health-related behaviors: adoption of, in child development, 123, 125; approaches for addressing, *208*; influences shaping, 134; and racial segregation, 23, *24*

Health-risk behaviors: and academic achievement, 142, 153; and child development, 123, 125, 134; and education, 136, 141; examples of, 127; and income, 194; presence of, 23; research focusing on, 50; surveillance of, 134; youth avoiding, greater likelihood of, 134

Healthy behaviors, promoting, 242

Healthy Cities and Healthy Communities initiatives, 26, 295

Healthy Communities agenda, 241–242, 252, 256–258, 263, 270, 272, 317

Healthy Community Agenda Dialogue Guide, 257

Healthy community, defining, 239

Healthy development: supporting and strengthening, focusing on, 133–134; timing and context of, 131–132

Healthy environments, creating, 242

Healthy lifestyles: and education, 136; and income, 195; maintaining, 126, 127

Healthy Passages project, 118

Healthy People 2000, 119, 239

Healthy People 2010, 54, 118, 119, 138, 223, 239–240, 242, 252, 256, 265, 291, 295, 296

Healthy People in Healthy Communities, 239, *240*, 241–242

Healthy People: The Surgeon General's Report on Health Promotion and Disease Prevention, 296

Healthy Pregnancy task force, 274

Healthy public: contribution of, 3; dimensions and criteria of, *294*, 295

Healthy Public Policy Network, 52, 63

Healthy republic: defining, 3, *294*; dimensions and criteria of, *294*, 295

Healthy (re)public, moving toward: analytic framework for, 4–9;

community development model for, 252, *253*; and comparison of political and economic philosophies, *11*; context for, present realities forming, 290–294; dimensions and criteria for, 294–325; key aspects involving, 285–286; overview of, 295; policy issues and examples for, 286–294; recommendations for, 325–327

Healthy Start program, 256, 258–259

Heart disease, 125, 129, 136, 142, 193

Heavily Indebted Poor Countries Initiative (HIPC), 213–214, 222–223, 225

Hierarchical bureaucracies, challenging, 17

High blood pressure, increased risk for, 129

High school dropouts. *See* School failure (dropouts)

Higher-risk pregnancies, 202

Hispanic Americans, 192

HIV/AIDS: during adolescence, 125; and globalization, 216; influence of, in developing countries, 202, 203; international policies addressing, 211, 212

Holistic approach: of community building, 246, 256; countries taking a more, 36, 55; defining, 53

Home environment, as a contributing factor, 108

Homicide, during adolescence, 125, 273

Hospitals, spending on, 188

Housing, access to, and income, 194

Human capacities, enhancing, throughout the life course, goal of, 8

Human capital: contribution to, focusing on, 108; creating, 246, 255; defined, 108; as a determinant, 4; development of, impact of, on health, 135–143; production of, alternative approaches to, range of, 152;

strengthening stock of, 157; underinvestment in, 197. *See also* Human development

Human development: and community development, 270, 271, 273, 275; concepts and perspectives presented by, 7–8; consideration of, lack of, 2–3; and current policies addressing fundamental determinants, 143–148; defining, 6, 108; and evidence regarding research on determinants, 113–143; and fields of study, 108–112; focus on, in determining sustainable development, 73; healthy, timing and context of, 131–132; introduction to, 107–113; key aspects involving, 106–107; and key policies, summary of, 287; and major evaluation issues, *288*, 289; measuring, 149; overview of, 108; and policy domains, 112–113; recommendations for, 154–158, 326; and strengths and limitations of current policies, 148–153. *See also* Education

Human development index (HDI), 149–150, 186

Human health impacts of ecosystem change, 71, 79, *80*, *81*, *82*, 83. *See also* Disease; Morbidity; Mortality

Human poverty index, 186

Human resources sector, 312

Hydrosphere, defining, 75

Hypertension, increased risk for, 129

I

Identity formation, 124, 125

IKEA Corporation, case study of, 93–98

IKEA Systems, 94, 100

Incentive systems, creating, for collaboration, 263

Inclusion, 248, 250, 251, 252, 258, 259, 270. *See also* Community-based participatory research (CBPR)

Income: creating, policies directed toward, issue with, 66; delay in

earning, to stay in school, 139; distribution of, 185, 191, 197, 199–201, 217, 220; and education, 136, 141; effect of globalization on, 12; family, and child development, 122; full, 186–187; and the human development index, 186; increase in, 190, 199; as an indicator of socioeconomic position, 44–45; levels of, measuring, 191; and life expectancy, 136; measures of, and the human development index, 149–150; strong association between health and, 184, 185, 191–192, 193, 201; types of policies affecting, 184. *See also* Economic development

Income disparities: associated with poor health, 113; increased, 13

Income flows, 84, *89*

Income inequality: defining, 185, 196; determining importance of, to health, 196–198; in developing countries, 190, 199–200; economists questioning, 217; measures of, 196

Income policies, 188, 205, 220

Income redistribution, 157, 188, 200–201, 217

Income transfer programs, 205

Income-based gradient, 191–193

Independent Inquiry into Inequalities in Health (Acheson), 55

Independent risk, accumulation of, relative to time, 111

India, 203, 215

Indirect causal pathways, 27–28, 29, 136–137

Individual biology: depiction of, in the conceptual model, 39; focus on, 57; research on, key findings on, 48, 49–50

Individual health: depiction of, in the conceptual model, 39; effects on, in dynamic pathways, 40; focus on, 23, 37; shifting focus from, 37–38

Individual health behaviors: and causal pathways, 38; depiction of, in the conceptual model, 39; effects on, in dynamic pathways,

40; focus on, 56; research on, key findings on, 48

Individual responses, 39, 48–50, 132

Individualistic view, 52, 53, 54

Industry sector, 312

Infancy: development during, 111, 112, 121–122; latent effects from, 129–130

Infant mortality: in developing countries, 199, 201; and income inequality, 197; national plan to reduce, 56; in the U.S., 54, 240, 258

Infant mortality gradient, 191

Infectious diseases, 125, 202–203, *321*. *See also specific disease*

Information age, 16–17

Information revolution, 319–320

Information systems: geographic, 316; improving, 291–292; population health, 313, 316

Informational uncertainty, firms operating under, 93

Informing, educating, and empowering, practices for, 316–317

Injections, 84, 85

Injuries, unintentional and intentional, during adolescence, 125

Inner cities. *See Urban entries*

Innovative approaches, engaging unconventional allies for, 7

Input flows, 84, *89*, 219

Institute for Defense Analyses, 156, 168

Institute of Medicine, 4, 9, 19, 20, *21*, 25, 32, 33, 42, 43, 46, 54, 60, 68, 100, 125, 142, 168, 224, 229, 238, 242, 248, 261, 262, 263, 264, 281, 290, 293, 296, 306, *308*, 319, *321*, 330

Institutions, influence of, 2

Integrated child-care and education/development programs: funding of, creating new models for, 156–157; models of, 155; quality standards for, developing and applying, 155–156; recognizing benefits of, 158

Integrated policy domains:
  embracing, 56; lack of, 2–3, 4
Integrated policymaking models,
  155
Integration, social, 23, *24*
Intelligence quotient (IQ), 139
Interdisciplinary research, 19, *20*,
  306
Intergenerational justice, 30, 73, 90,
  220, 221, 222, 223, 266, 289,
  312, 317
Intergovernmental Panel on
  Climate Change, 98
International Bank for
  Reconstruction and
  Development (IBRD), 213. *See
  also* World Bank
International Conference on
  Reducing Social Inequalities in
  Health, 229
International development
  assistance, 218
International Development
  Association (IDA), 213. *See also*
  World Bank
International finance, 189, 212–214
International Monetary Fund
  (IMF), 13, 16, 189, 212–213,
  222–223, 225
International organizations,
  economic policies of, 210–216.
  See also specific organizations
International sector, 312
International trade policies, 189,
  209, 214–216, 235
Interpersonal relationships: forming
  and maintaining, 125; quality
  of, influence of, 112
Intersectoral capital, 312
Intersectoral collaboration,
  generating, 263, 300
Intersectoral design, 293
Intersectoral local public health
  agency, blueprint for, 307,
  308–309
Intersectoral policies, need for, 217
Intersectoral public health system:
  accountability challenges in,
  319; building, 322; changes
  compelling design of, 26, 27;
  and comparison of political and

economic philosophies, *11*;
  consideration of, 23; designing,
  304–310; elements in
  developing, *11*; identifying roles
  in, 316–317; importance of
  partnering to create an, 25;
  important rationale for, 307;
  move toward, 9; need for, 224;
  paradigm guiding development
  of, 19, 20; raising questions of
  professional training and
  development, 319; requisites of,
  323
Intersectoral responsibility,
  enhancing, 218
Intervening mechanisms,
  fundamental causes versus, 22,
  26
Investments, balancing, 302
Iowa prairie ecosystem case study,
  102–105
Iowa standardized test scores, 150
Italy, 146, 206

J

Job creation policies, 146
Johnson administration, 13, 143
Justice: defining, 250; dimensions
  of, 30. *See also* Deliberative
  justice; Distributive justice;
  Intergenerational justice; Social
  justice

K

Kaiser Family Foundation, 123,
  125, 168
Kansas community development
  policy, 274
Kansas Health Foundation, 54
Kauai Longitudinal Study, 133
Kaunas University of Medicine,
  206–207
Kindergarteners, 114–115, 117,
  122, 140, 151
K-12 education: and adoption of
  standardized curricula, 151;
  focusing on, 107; linking formal
  child care and, 155, 158;
  strengths and limitations of,
  148–149, 157; traditional, 140

L

Labor absorption, policies to
  encourage, 211
Labor market: and appropriate
  policies, 190, 225–226;
  improving entry into the, 206,
  225, 270; promoting
  participation in the, 8, 209, 225;
  regulation of the, 188; and
  working conditions, approaches
  addressing, *208*
Labor-intensive development, 190
Ladder of citizen participation, 310
Lag times, 217
Lalonde report, 17, 36, 56, 204
Larger good, the, serving, 249, 250
Late adulthood, development
  during, 126–127. *See also* Elderly
  population
Latent conflict, 243–244
Latent effects, 128, 129–130, 131
Latin America, 199
Law of conservation, 71
Laws: physical, compliance with,
  90, *91*, 92; public health, 17,
  264, 318
Laws of demand and supply, 72,
  83–85
Leadership: assuming, 327; ethical
  and principled, *321*; providing,
  223; requiring, from multiple
  sectors, 305, 309; as requisite,
  286
Leadership training and
  development, 292, 320
Leakages, 84–85
Learned capacities, 137
Learning: continued capacity for,
  126, 157; of new material, in
  older adults, effects of, 138; start
  of, 120. *See also* Education
Learning communities, 17, 311,
  320
Learning organizations, 17, 320
Leave No Child Behind Act, 144,
  171
"Lee Closes Meeting with White
  House Plan to Reinvent Public
  Health," 15, 33
Legal responsibilities, 90–91, 92,
  94, 96

Legal Services, 269
Legitimacy, 90, 307
Levels versus differences, 322, 323
Liberal democracies, 10, 12, 13
Libertarian philosophy, 10, 12
Life expectancy: and education, 135, 138, 141; and full income, 187; and gross domestic product (GDP) per capita in developing countries, 199, *200*, 201, 203; and the human development index, 149, 150, 186; and income, 136; and income‘ distribution, 199–200; and income inequality, 197; and income redistribution, 200–201; influence of, in developing countries, 201; as a measure, 184, 296; national plan to reduce, 56; U.S. ranking in, 54, 150
Life exposures to risk: expression of, overview of, 127–128; moderators of trajectories of, 131–135; trajectories of, 128–131
Life-course development: dynamics of, 127–135; stages of, 119–127
Life-course effects model, 108
Life-course epidemiology, 109, 128, 289
Life-course health development framework, 109, *110*, 111
Life-course perspective, 49, 52, 108, 109, *110*, 111, 193
Life-exposure trajectory, reflection of, 128
Life-span development, 109
Lifetime learning, centered on, *321*
Lifeworld concept, 249, 279
Linking people to services, 318
Literacy rates, 150
Lithosphere, defining, 75
Lithuania, 206
Local and global thinking and action, 322
Local assets and resources, development of, 241
Localized materials, 77
Loka Institute, 255
Long-term perspective, 7
Low birth weight, impact of, 121

Low-income population. *See* Poor population; Poverty
Luxembourg Income Study, 114, 172, 198

M

Macrocontextual factors, 109
Macroeconomics: defined, 186; government decision making grounded in, 188, 190
Macrosocial factors, 22, 23, *24*
Maine standardized test scores, 150
Making Cancer Health Disparities History (National Cancer Institute), 54
Malaria, 203, 211, 212
Malnutrition, and the human poverty index, 186
Managed care consolidation, 18
Managed care industry: challenges of, 25; transferring responsibility for disease prevention to, 263
Managerial resources, defined, 68
Managerial strategies, 85–86, 88
Manpower Demonstration Research Corporation, 210, 221, 231
MAP-IT approach, 256–257, 258, 278, 279
Mapping, 316
Marine Society, 191
Market environments, 93
Market externalities: accounting for, in corporate decision making, 86; aspects of, 72; identifying, 78; as stimulants of ecological determinants, 79
Market models: of collaborative decision making, *310*; of community development policies, *260*, 261–264, *267*, *268*, 273–275; political and economic philosophies behind, 10, *11*, 12–13, 14, 16; selected, summary of, *287*. *See also specific examples*
Market outcomes: intended versus unintended, difference between, acknowledging, 67; unintended, 79, 83
Market rate, 189

Market sector, 312
Market values, *267*
Marketplace, questions resolved in the, 66, 68, 83–84
Marriage, probability of, 193
Mass media, 14, 123, 125, 134, 306
Matched funding, 277
Material capital, as a determinant, 4. *See also* Economic development
Material conditions, 22, 194–195
Material deprivation, 195
Material incentives, use of, 84
Material privilege, 254
Material resources, access to, and income, 194
Maternal and Child Health Bureau, 118, 180
Maternal conditions, international policies addressing, 212
Mathematica Policy Research, 144, 173
Mathematics achievement, 115, 140, 150, *151*
MATISS Research Group, 128, 181
McMaster University, 155
Measures: of child health and development, 114–119; of a healthy public, 295; of income inequality, 196; of population health, 42–44, 133, 320; of social capital, 244, 254
Mechanism component, 109, *110*, 111
Mechanistic orientation, 52–53
Media. *See* Mass media
Medicaid, 10, 18, 53, 98, 188
Medical care perspective, shift toward, from a population health perspective, 203
Medical technology: access to, 195; rapid diffusion of, and health care costs, 53
Medicare, 10, 53, 54, 98, 188
Mental retardation, 202
Mexico, 201
MHIP Social Conditions and Health Action Team, 54
Microcontextual factors, 109
Microcredit initiatives, 214, 221–222, 225

Microeconomics: corporate decision making grounded in, 68, 186; defined, 186
Microfinance initiatives, 214, 221–222
Microsocial factors, 22
Middle adulthood, development during, 126
Midlife stage, 126
Milbank Memorial Fund, 300, 331
Millennium Development Goals, 211, 213
Minimum wage, 146, 206, 225
Minister of Public Works and Government Services, Canada, 116, 173
Ministry of Health and Social Affairs, Sweden, 207
Ministry of Social Affairs and Health, Finland, 207
Minnesota Department of Health, 210, 299
Minnesota Family Investment Program (MFIP), 210, 221
Minnesota Health Improvement Partnership (MHIP), 54, 299
Minnesota Health Improvement Partnership Social Conditions and Health Action Team, 62, 210, 231, 299, 331
Minnesota standardized test scores, 150
Minority adolescents, 141
Minority Health and Health Disparities Research Act, 54
Minority populations: and infant mortality rates, 240; in inner cities, impact of globalization on, 235. *See also* African Americans; Hispanic Americans
Minority students, 145, 153
Mission-driven responsibility and externally mandated accountability, balancing, 319
Mississippi standardized test scores, 150
Mixed funding, allowing for, 300
Mobility rates, 145
Mobilize, assess, plan, implement, and track (MAP-IT) approach, 256–257, 258, 278, 279

Mobilizing community partnerships, practices for, 317
Mobilizing for Action through Planning and Partnerships (MAPP), 317
Modeling, 123, 137
Modern epidemiology, critique of, 37
Modern society, critics of, arguments of, 14–15, 16
Monetary policy, defined, 188
Monitoring, practices for, 313, 316
Monologue versus two-way dialogue, 250
Moral management, 92
Morbidity: adolescent, 125, 142; in the child health index, 117; and higher-risk pregnancies, 202; from infectious disease, in developing countries, 202, 203; influence of physical environment on, 46; influence of social environment on, 44, 45; as a measure of population health, 42, 43, 133; racial and ethnic disparities in, in the U.S., 241; and workplace hierarchy, 55. *See also* Human health impacts of ecosystem change
Mortality: adolescent, 125, 142; in the child health index, 117; in developing countries, 199, 200; early studies involving, 36; and education, 136, 137; and higher-risk pregnancies, 202; and the human poverty index, 186; and income inequality, 197, 198; and income-based gradient, 192; from infectious disease, in developing countries, 202, 203; influence of physical environment on, 46, 48; influence of social environment on, 44, 45; as a measure of population health, 42, 43, 133; national health targets to reduce, 239; overall, national plan to reduce, 56; percent related to unhealthy lifestyle choices, 125; premature, and health literacy, 138; and psychosocial mechanisms, 196;

racial and ethnic disparities in, in the U.S., 192, 241; related to ecological imbalance, 83; related to socioeconomic position during childhood, 128, *129*; shift in focus from reducing, to improving quality of life, 203; and the work environment, 143; and workplace hierarchy, 55, 128, *129*, 136, 143, 192. *See also* Human health impacts of ecosystem change
Motor development, delayed, 202
Motor vehicle accidents, during adolescence, 125
Multiculturalism, growing, challenges from, 15
Multidisciplinary research paradigm, 19, *20*
Multilevel analysis, benefit of, 48, 275
Multilevel modeling, 51, 302, 316
Multiple causation, tenet of, field guided by, 37
Multiple determinants, changing, 109
Multiple systems, acknowledgement of, 260–261
Multisectoral focus: calls for, 26; of intersectoral public health systems, *305*, 306, 307
Mutual dependency, 72
Mutual support, 243

N

National Agency for Education, 147
National Assessment of Academic Progress, 146
National Association for State Community Services Programs, 269, 282
National Association of County and City Health Officials, 271, 272, 274, 282, 292, 317, 331
National Board of Health, 206
National Cancer Institute, 54, 62
National Center for Children and Families, 155
National Center for Children in Poverty, 114, 154

National Center for Chronic Disease Prevention and Health Promotion, 123, 125, 161, 180

National Center for Education Statistics (NCES), 113, 150, 153, 180

National Center for Health Statistics, 33, 174, 180, 231, 331

National Center for Health Statistics (NCHS), 25, 119, 121, 125, 141, 142, 153, 192, 296

National defense spending, 188

National Education Association, 153, 174

National Education Goals Panel, 114, 174

National Healthcare Disparities Report (Agency for Healthcare Research and Quality), 54

National health care system. *See* Universal health care

National Health Service, 205, 206, 297

National Institute of Health Working Group on Health Disparities, 174

National Institutes of Child Health and Development (NICHD), 118, 123, 174

National Institutes of Health (NIH), 50, 113, 174, 180, 292

National Library of Medicine, 113, 180

National Longitudinal Mortality Study, 192

National Policy Association, 54, 298

National Public Health Performance Standards, 292

National Research Council, 111, 143, 149, 174

National Strategy for Neighborhood Renewal, 56

National Youth Sports, 269

Nation-state political philosophies, 10, *11*

Natural capital, as a determinant, 4. *See also* Sustainable development

Natural cycles: economic cycles in opposition with, 69–70, 78; as a general model of ecosystem function, 75, *76*; policies

addressing, 88; principles involving, 77, 78

Natural environment, focus on, 66

Nature's life supports: disruption in, 75; maintaining, aspects of, 73; potential damage to, awareness of, 99

Needs assessment, 260, 261

Negative externality, 72

Neighborhood associations, 244

Neighborhood conditions, 46–48, 122

Neighborhood institutions and resources, 247

Neighborhood revitalization, 273–274

Neighborhood-based networks and norms, 248

Neighborhood-level risk factors, research focusing on, 50

Neoliberalism, 12–13, 14, 18

Neonatal period, 120

Nested factors, 109, 131

Netherlands, 207, 209

New Brunswick, 205, 220

New Community Schools Initiative, 147

New Deal, the, 12, 13

New models, promising, 262–264

New Perspective on the Health of Canadians, A (Lalonde), 36

Newtonian understanding of the universe, 15

No Child Left Behind Act, 143, 149, 175

Nongovernmental organizations, funding by, 211

Nongovernmental sector, 305

Nonmedical determinants, greater recognition of, 218, 223–224. *See also* Economic determinants; Social determinants

Nonparticipation, 310

Normative economics, defined, 186

North American Free Trade Agreement (NAFTA), 13

North Carolina standardized test scores, 150–151

North Dakota standardized test scores, 150

Norway, 10, 150

"Nurturing Economic Growth Through Nutrition," 202, 231

Nurturing experience, 130

Nutrient cycles: case study involving, 102–105; defined, 102

Nutrition, 194, 202, 212

O

Observational studies, research relying on, 50, 51

Occupation: dangerous, likelihood of working in a, 194; and education, 136; as an indicator of socioeconomic position, 44, 45. *See also* Economic development

Occupational Health and Safety Agency, 98

Occupational success, predictor of, 140

Office of the Assistant Secretary for Planning and Evaluation, 115, 145, 180

Office on Smoking and Health, 123, 180

Offord Centre for Child Studies, 155, 175

Oklahoma, community development policy in, 272

On Airs, Waters and Places (Hippocrates), 36

One-size-fits-all approaches, 152, 260

Open economic system model, 88

Organisation for Economic Co-operation and Development (OECD), 53, 54, 55, 62, 108, 150, 157, 167, 197, 210, 215, 296

Organization theory, 17

Organized labor, weakening of, 12

Ottawa Charter, 9, 23, 26, 56

Outcomes criteria, 322–325

Out-of-pocket medical costs, 193

Output flows, 84, *89*, 219

P

Parental education programs, availability of, expanding, 154

Parental influence, 123, 125, 134, 137, 142, 146

Parental transfers, 145

Parenthood stage, 126

Parenting style, 122, 123

Participation. *See* Civic participation; Social participation

Participatory action research, role of, 51

Participatory and inclusive approach, 19, 293. *See also* Deliberative democracy

Participatory discourse: recommending, 224, 226; role of, exploring, 16

Partnership formulation and function, symmetry of, addressing questions of, 311

Partnerships: benefit of, 265; building, 292–293; challenges of, 25–26; evaluating, 312; forging, 9, 311; importance of, 25; successful, central element of, 312. *See also* Public-private partnerships

Patent protection, 215, 226

Pathway effects, 128, 130–131, 132

Payroll tax burden, 146

Peer influence, 124, 134, 137, 141

People's Republic of China. *See* China

Performance, corporate social, of IKEA, 94–95

Performance indicators, designing, 263

Performance measurement, 260, 275, 292, 327

Performance standards, shift in, 317

Performance-based standards, 319

Perinatal period, importance of, 120

Personal barriers, 241

Personal Responsibility and Work Opportunity Reconciliation Act, 269, 283

Personal taxes, 188

Pharmaceutical industry, 211, 215, 226

Pharmaceuticals, expensive, 53–54

Philanthropic responsibilities, 90, 91

Philanthropic sector, 312

Physical environment: and child development, 121; effect of, 39, 40; focus on, 55, 56; impact of corporate industry on, 263; link between social environment and, 46–47, 51; and racial segregation, *24*; reducing stressors in, 247; research on, key findings on, 46–48

Place, defined, and significance, 107

Planned Approach to Community Health (PATCH), 317

Planners and planning models, misplaced perception about, 87

Planning models, 317

Plasticity, 119–120, 132

Polarization, conflict arising from, 243–244

Policy advancement, further, framework for, 275

Policy development cycle, stages of, 301

Policy development function, 9, 239, 291, *314*, 316

Policy domains: in the analytic framework, 4, 6–9; summary of, *5. See also specific domains*

Policy evaluation, 27–30, *288. See also* Effectiveness; Efficiency; Equity

Policy implications, of measuring population health, 43–44

Policy interventions, differing focus of, 22

Policy models: in the analytic framework, political and philosophical underpinnings of, 9–17; summary of, *5. See also specific models*

Policy perspectives, contrasting, 52–57

Policy questions, 152, 303, *304*

Policy sectors, collaborations across, 265, 305, 306

PolicyLink, 258, 259, 283

Policy-steering mechanisms, 207, *208*

Polio, 211

Political action, 26, 278–279

Political agendas, issues dominating, 187

Political and economic philosophies, changing, implications of, 9–15, 26

Political coalitions, 16, 310

Political command-and-control processes, use of, 84

Political continuum, 10, *11*

Political economy perspective, acknowledging, 41

Political environment: focus on, 56; inclusion of, in the conceptual model, 41

Political equity, 248, 250, 251, 252, 258, 259

Political left, 10, *11*, 12, 14

Political power, 17, 254, 313

Political right, 10, *11*, 14

Political will, lack of, 217

Pollution, *80, 81, 82,* 83

Poor population: concentration of, in rural areas, 236; in developing countries, 189–190, 200; health insurance for, 53; and health-risk behavior and risk factors among, 194; in inner cities, impact of globalization on, 235; and material conditions facing, 194–195. *See also* Poverty; Socioeconomic position (SEP)

Poorer health: and education, 136, 140; relatively, across the population, 113; and work environment, 143

Population health: addressing and improving, specific remedy for, 8; aspects directly and indirectly affecting, 39, 40; controversy over, 26; and corporate social responsibility, 92–93; defining, 39; differing perspectives on health disparities and, 22, 276, 323; as a field of study, 4, 6, 36, 37; focus on, 23; increase in research funding for, 204; measuring, 42–44, 133, 320; origination of the term, 56; promoting, and society reducing health care costs, 67; reconciling profit maximization with, 85, 86. *See also* Fundamental determinants of population health

Population health–centered policies: basis for designing, 31; broader, examples of, 296–299; calls for, 19, 293; designing and evaluating, framework for, 322–325; developing, practice of, 317; end point of, 8; focus on, issue of, 2, 3; formulating, steps for, 295–304; framework for designing and evaluating, 323, *324*, 325; lack of emergent, 2, 36, 53, 54, 143, 209–210, 296, 299; and major issues related to evaluation of, 288–290; multisectoral focus in, calls for, 26; national-level development of, various stages of, examples of, 52, 53–57; requisites of, 323; selected examples of, by policy domain, 286–287; ultimate goal of, 8; and universal health care financing, 18

Population health–centered public health practice, engaging in, shift to, 313–320, *321*

Population health model, 39–42, 108, 109

Population health objectives and criteria, defining, 300–302

Population health perspective, 37–38, 52, 66, 203, 225

Population health–relevant resources, 198

Population health research: agenda of, 50–51; intention of, issue with, 22; key findings of, 44–50; leader in, 55; need for, highlighting, 302–304

Population Health Research Program, 9, 23, 37, 204

Population Reference Bureau, 153, 158

Population Strategic Policy Directorate of the Population and Public Health Branch, 301, *321*, *324*, 330

Positive economics, defined, 186

Positive youth-development interventions, 134

Positivist science, 15–16

Post-modern society, critics of, arguments of, 14–15

Postmodernism, 16

Potential impacts of ecosystem change, 71, 79, *80*, *81*, *82*, 83

Poverty: defining, in relative versus absolute terms, 196; in developing countries, 199; and DoD school students, 145; early studies examining, 36; and globalization, 190; historical records on negative effect of, on health, 191; infectious disease associated with, 202, 203; material deprivation of living in, mediating negative effects of, 107; perpetuation of, 46; potential of economic policies in affecting, 185; and social participation, 195; transition out of, effect of, on perspective, 203. *See also* Child poverty; Poor population; Socioeconomic position (SEP)

Poverty cycle, 187, 222

Poverty rates, 150, 192, 270

Poverty reduction: calls for, 211, 213; community development policy aimed at, 269–270; growth leading to, 13; recommending targeted programs for, 225; supporting, 8. *See also* Economic development

Power balance, maintaining, 25–26

Power differentials, 254–255

Power levels, increased, 310

Power shift, 248, 279

Pragmatic view, 260

Precautionary principle, 69, 83, 319

Predictive models, developing, challenge of, 83

Pregnancy: during adolescence, 125, 134; healthy, community development policy aimed at, 274–275; tobacco use during, 193; unintended or unwanted, in developing countries, 202

Prenatal nutrition, 193

Preschool period, development during, 122–123, 129. *See also* Early childhood development

Preschool programs, 144–145, 146, 147, 148, 154, 156

Prevention Research Centers, 292

Preventive health care: access to, 195; use of, and education level, 136. *See also* Disease prevention

Principled leadership, *321*

Pristine ecosystems, 77, 78

Private health–relevant resources, 198

Private policymakers, 265

Private sector, 265

Private-public collaboration. *See* Public-private partnerships

Privatization, 12, 13, 18, 25

Proaction, defining, 69

Problem analysis, 303, *304*

Process component, 109, *110*

Process criteria, 310–320

Productive capacity: development of, 125, 126; enhancing, throughout the life course, goal of, 8

Productive efficiency. *See* Technical (production) efficiency

Profit, defined, 86

Profit maximization (motive), 72, 73, 74, 85, 86, 87, 88, *91*, 92–93, 263, 289

Profit-stimulation approach, 13

Progressive distributional policies, 205

Progressive taxes, 188

Pronatalism, 147

Proportionate good, 251

Protective factors, 111, 123, 127, 130, 132, 133. *See also* Developmental assets

Proximate causes, defining, 22

Psychological distress, vulnerability associated with, 125

Psychological risk factors, research focusing on, 50

Psychosocial mechanisms, 195–196, 197

Psychosocial stages of development, 124

Psychosocial theory, defined, 49

Psychosocial-behavioral factors, 22, 45, 107–108

Public decision making, in a healthy republic, 1, 3, 294

Public, defining, 3, 294

Public education, shared commitment to, 148

Public expenditures, levels of, 188

Public health: business of biomedicine subsuming, 53; and comparison of political and economic philosophies, *11*; defining, 4, 68; delimited, 23, 24; focus of, since inception, 23; in general, focus of, 37; ideals integral to concept of, 241; and implications of changing political and economic philosophies, 9–15; major trends in, 17–27; opportunity to reinvent, health care reform proposal as, 18; past history and future potential of, understanding, *321*; as a policy domain, 4, *5*, 6; recommendations for, 325–326; strengthening the role of, in community development, 277–278; vision for reinventing, 3, 18–19

Public Health Agency of Canada, 52, 56, 58, 63

Public health community, expanding, beyond traditional participants, 277

Public health finance, 318

Public Health Foundation, 257, 258, 283

Public health functions: core, 238–239, 290, 291, 313, *314–315*, 316, 318; serving all, *315*, 319–320, 319–320

Public Health in America, 290

Public health informatics, 316

Public Health Information Network, 291

Public health infrastructure: community resources partnering with, 252, 253; defining, 292; fundamental components of, 291; quality and capacity of, service delivery contingent upon, 290; strengthening, 263, 264, 271

Public health insurance. *See* Medicaid; Medicare

Public health interventions: addressing, 23; recommended strategies for, 262–264

Public health laws and regulations, 17, 264, 318

Public Health Leadership Institutes, 292

Public Health Leadership Society, *321*, 331

Public health objectives: breadth of, 57; reconciling, with business objectives, 85, 86

Public health–planning models, 317

Public health policies: blueprint for designing, *308*; context of, 290–294; focus of, on outcomes, 317; influence of, 2; integration of other policy domains into, lack of, 2–3, 4. *See also* Population health–centered policies

Public health policy agendas: broader, 2, 6, 18, 23, 153, 286, 293–294; different aspects informing and motivating, 20–22; embracing population health in, 56; new directions suggested for, 293; proposed shift in, 300

Public health practice: context of, 290–294; current, 291–292, *314–315*; population health–centered, shift to, 313–320, *321*

Public health practitioners: testing and credentialing of, 319; training of, to facilitate change, 9

Public health principles, guided by, *321*

Public health–relevant resources, 198

Public health revolutions, 17–18, 36

Public health schools, recommendation for, 278

Public health services, 239, 291, 313, *314–315*, 316, 317, 318, 319

Public health surveillance systems, expanding, 277–278

Public health systems: context of, 290–294, 290–294; defining, 305. *See also* Intersectoral public health system

Public Health Training, 292

Public health university model, 320, *321*

Public health workforce: competency of, assuring, 319; development and training of, 278, 291, 292, 306, 318–319

Public institutions, shutting down of, 236

Public policymakers, 265

Public schools, excellent, providing access to, 225

Public sector, 265

Public support, diminishment of, 235

Public, the, philosophical orientation toward, 52

Public transportation, 226

Public-private partnerships: benefits of, 265; building, 292–293; challenges of, 25–26; emergence of, 14; forging, aspects of, for a healthy (re)public, 311–313; growth of, 25; promoting, 277; role of, in an intersectoral public health system, 306–307

Q

Quality health care, providing access to, 225, 240, 242. *See also* Access to health care

Quality of life: measures reflecting, 43, 184, 186; pursuit of, 241; shift toward improving, versus mortality reduction, 203

Quality standards, for integrated programs, 155–156

Quantitative and qualitative methods, evolution of, 316

Quantum physics, 15

Quebec, 146

Quotas, 188, 189, 215

R

Racial and ethnic health disparities, 2, 23, *24*, 50, 54–55, 192

Racial segregation: examining, framework for, 23, *24*, 48, 320; in inner cities, 235; social isolation resulting from, impact of, 46; and social networks, 246

Randomized control trial feasibility, 216

Rapid epidemiological appraisal, 248
Rational discourse, 250, 258, 259
Raw materials sector, 312
Reading achievement, 115, 150
Reagan administration, 12
Real income, increase in, 184, 186
Reasonableness, 248, 250–251, 258, 259
Recapitalization, 13
Reciprocal determinism, 112
Reciprocity, 243, 244, *245*, 248, 251, 252, 258, 259, 279
Regressive distributional policies, 205
Regressive taxes, 188
Regulatory system, existing, inadequacy of, 98
Reinforcement, 137
Relative deprivation, 195, 197
Relative income, 196
Relativity theory, 15
Religious right, the, 10
Reporting bias, 47
Representation, participation through, 220
Republic, defining, 3, 294
Research agenda, 50, 302–304
Research design: choice of, importance of, 51; paradigm guiding, 19, 20. *See also* Community-based participatory research (CBPR)
Research emphasis, 303, *304*
Research focus, 50
Research funding, 204
Research involvement, 248
Research paradigms, 19, *20*
Research, population health. *See* Population health research
Research practice, 319–320
Residential segregation, race-based. *See* Racial segregation
Resilience to risk, 132–135, 153
Resource allocation, 84
Resource development, local, 241
Resource distribution, issue of, 198. *See also* Distributive justice
Resource reallocation, 99
Resource usage, measurement of, complication of, 217
Resources: access to, 44–45, 152, 153, 246; assessment of, 261;

communities as, 243; defined, 68; essential, 2, 4; galvanizing, 248; investment in and distribution of, requisites for, 325; partnering of, 252, 253. *See also specific resources*
Respect, 254, 255, 279
Response patterns, adopting new, 132. *See also* Individual responses
Responsibility: collective governmental, maintaining, 307, 309; corporate, 72, 86; intersectoral, 218; mission-driven, 319; for sustainable development, 87; transferring, for disease prevention, 263. *See also* Corporate social responsibility (CSR)
Retirement, 193
Return flows, 84
Reverse causation, 47, 140, 193
Right education policy, benefits of, recognizing, 157–158
Rio Declaration, 69
Risk: defined, 127; early, human ecology of, 112; inequity in distribution of, 67; pathways leading from, 111; resilience to, 132–135, 153. *See also specific risks*
Risk assessment, 83
Risk exposure: during childhood, 127; forces at play in, acknowledgement of, 18. *See also* At-risk children; Life exposures to risk
Risk factors: distribution of, 198; focus on, different approaches to, 37–38; and income, 194; research focusing on, 50
Risk pools, 262
Risk reduction, public health revolution involving, 17
Risky behavior. *See* Health-risk behaviors
Robert Wood Johnson foundation, 271, 299, 318
Roosevelt administration, 12, 13
Roundtable on Environmental Health Sciences Research and Medicine, 248, 281

Royal Military Academy, 191
Rural development, 190, 214
Rural economies, impact of globalization on, in the U.S., 235–236
Russia/Soviet Union, 10, 12, 199

S

Safe Drinking Water Act Amendment, 69
Safety, 122, *245*, 248
Sales taxes, 188
Sanitation services, 186, 194, 212
SARS disease, 216
Scholarship, excellence in, *321*
School Act, 147
School failure (dropouts), 133, 140, 141, 142, 151, 153
School personnel, influence of, 134, 137, 141, 146
School readiness, 114, 116–117, 119, 123, 130, 140–141, 151, 154
School resources, access to, 153
School vouchers, 148
School-age years, expression of risk exposure from, 128. *See also* Adolescence; Childhood
Scientific certainty, issue of, 69, 83
Scientific Commission for the Study of Health Inequalities in Spain, 206
Scientific Council for Government Policy, 207
Scientific paradigms, revolutionary changes in, 15–17
Scotland: early childhood education in, 146, 147; and the health impact assessment tool, 218. *See also* United Kingdom/Great Britain
Scottish Council Foundation, 52, 63, 147
Secondary benefits, sustaining, 275
Selection. *See* Reverse causation
Self-efficacy, 136
Self-regulation, 112
Self-reliance, 125
Self-Sufficiency Projects (SSP), 205, 220–221
Self-worth, establishment of, 124

Sensitive periods, defining, 131
Service delivery, effective, requirement for, 290
Settings, communities as, 243
Sexual activity, in adolescence, 134–135, 142
Sexually transmitted diseases (STDs), 125. *See also* HIV/AIDS
Shared values, local polices to support, *245*
Shared vision, 241, 249, 319
Short-term perspective, 7
Simple altruism, 93
Single-parent families, students from, percentage of, 145
Slavery, 50
Slovenia, 218
Smallpox, 211
Social and psychological resources, pathway between education and health mediated by, 136–137
Social bonds, 137, 238, 243, 244
Social capacity, 246, 247, 248. *See also* Community building
Social capital: aspects of, 244–246; assets linked to, at the community level, 135, 252; building, 278; creating, 246; defining, 135, 244; as a determinant, 4; domains of, and supporting policies, *245*; importance of, 238; level of measuring, 45; lowering, 197; measures of, 256–257; producing, 248; promoting development of, 135; as requisite, for community building, 247; research on, key findings of, 45–46; as a resource for community development, 253–255, 261; studying, use of multilevel models for, 252–253. *See also* Community development; Family support
Social choice theory, 186
Social cohesion, 41, 45, 146, 197, 243–244, 254, 256
Social conditions. *See* Social environment
Social Conditions and Health Action Team, 54
Social democracies, 10, 12

Social determinants: current policies grounded in, 143–148; evidence regarding, 113–143; field of, perspectives provided by, 23; frameworks for understanding, 22; proposed agenda for addressing, 298–299; recognition of, enhancing, 218. *See also* Human development
Social disparities, 46, 55, 57
Social dysfunction, adolescent, 125
Social environment: and child development, 121; effect of, 39, 40, 49; embodiment of, mechanisms for, 195; enhancing, 248; focus on, 55, 56; inclusion of political environment in, 41; link between physical environment and, 46–47, 51; quality of, influence of, 112, 246; and racial segregation, 23, *24*, 46; reducing stressors in, 247; research on, key findings in, 44–46
Social equity, 16, 73
Social exclusion, 116
Social Exclusion Unit, 116, 178
Social factors, importance of, 20, 21. *See also specific factors*
Social good, 244
Social hierarchy, 195
Social identity, 261
Social institutions, improving, through community-based interventions, 153
Social integration, 23, *24*
Social isolation, impact of, 45, 46, 195
Social justice, 152, 266, 289, 313, 317; borrowing elements of, 263; building, means of, 250; defining, 30; and economic development, 217, 220, 221, 222, 223; promoting, 147
Social learning theory, 16, 261
Social medicine, involvement in, tradition of, 224
Social movements: change resulting from, inclusion of, in the conceptual model, 41; major,

discourse arising in, 16; supporting, 278
Social networks, 45, 135, *245*, 246, 254, 255–256
Social order, collapse of, 14
Social organizations, 135
Social participation, 195
Social philosophy, 52, 55
Social production of disease-political economy of health, 49, 50
Social progress, measures of, 186
Social relationships, improving, through community-based interventions, 153
Social Research and Demonstration Corporation, 205, 220, 232
Social resources, relying on, to deal with stress, 133
Social roles and behavior, many factors influencing, 126
Social sector, role of, 306
Social Security, 10
Social security programs, 188, 209
Social spending, reduced, 197
Social stratification. *See* Socioeconomic position (SEP)
Social support, 23, *24*, 45, 133, 136, 137, 195
Social ties. *See* Social bonds
Social welfare spending, cutbacks in, 12, 13, 18
Social welfare states, 10, 12
Socially responsible business practice: constraint in, 288–289; foundation for, 73. *See also* Corporate social responsibility (CSR)
Socially responsive corporate governance, 311
Social-structural factors, 22
Sociocultural sector, 312
Socioeconomic health disparities, persistence of, 2
Socioeconomic inequalities, 207, *208*, 262
Socioeconomic position (SEP): and academic achievement, 153; adult mortality related to, 128, *129*, 192; and child development, 114–116, 117, 123, 191;

commonly used indicator of, 48; discoveries illuminating influence of, 37; early studies involving, 36; gradient of, 127, 130, 196; importance of, 107; and life exposure to risk, 127–128; marker for, 195; and marriage, 193; and physical environment, 47; potential influence of, 39; research on, key findings in, 44–45; shifting focus to, in prevention strategies, call for, 38. *See also* Poverty

Sociology, early studies in the field of, 36

Solution analysis, 303, *304*

South Africa, 203, 215

Soviet Union/Russia, 10, 12, 199

Spain, 206

Spanish Black report, 206

Spiritual resources, 137, 152

Standardized test scores, 115, 145, 150–151

Standards of quality, for integrated programs, 155–156

State and local spending, areas dominating, 188

State Children's Health Insurance Program (SCHIP), 53

State of Public Health: Local and State Government Issues in Texas: Report Resulting from House Concurrent Resolution 44 of the 75th Legislature, 307, 332

Stop TB Partnership Secretariat, 202, 234

Strategic altruism, 93

Strategic approach, corporate, 69, 73, 74

Streaming practices, 152

Stress: issue of, 107; from life transitions, 126, 132; women facing additional, 143; and the work environment, 143. *See also* Chronic stress

Stressed ecosystems, looking beyond sick people to, 98–99

Stressors: and economic activity, 77; and racial segregation, 23, *24*; reducing, 247–248; response to, 39, 49, 111

Structural barriers, 241

Structural design, *309*

Structural equation modeling, value of, 51

Structure criteria, 295–310

Structure of Scientific Revolutions, The (Kuhn), 15

Study of Early Child Care, 118

Sub-Saharan Africa: infectious disease in, 202, 203; policies aimed at, 212; poverty in, 199

Subsidies, 209, 215, 226

Substance use, during adolescence, 125, 134, 142

Successful Societies Program, 3

Suicide, during adolescence, 125, 142

Supply and demand, 72, 83–85, 189

Support networks. *See* Social networks

Sure Start, 56

Surroundings, improving, through community-based intervention, 153

Surveillance systems, 291, 316

Sustainability: balancing development with, 7; of collaborative decision making models, 313; community, 244, 260–261; defining types of, 73; goal of, 7

Sustainability practice: corporate strategy for, 95–97; defining, 88; distinguishing, from other practices for public health, 97–98; elements in, *89*; moving toward, 95. *See also* Corporate social responsibility (CSR)

Sustainable business policy, defining, 86. *See also* Ecologically responsive corporate policy

Sustainable community development. *See* Community building

Sustainable development: case study involving, 102–105; commonly understood expectation of, 87–88; concepts and perspectives presented by, 7; consideration of, lack of, 2–3;

and current policies addressing fundamental determinants, 85–90; defining, 6, 73; and evidence regarding research on determinants, 74–85; and fields of study, 68–70; introduction to, 66–74; key aspects involving, 65–66; and key policies, summary of, 287; and major evaluation issues, 288–289; overview of, 67–68; and policy domains, 73–74; recommendations for, 98, 326; responsibility for, 87; and strengths and limitations of current policies, 90–98

Sustainable development policy, 73, 86–87

Sweden: and community development, 266; concurrent policy development in, 207, 209; early childhood education in, 146, 147; focusing on, 209; and HDI ranking, 150; health policy agenda of, 2, 52; labor market policies in, 225; political and economic philosophy of, 10; population health policies in, 57, 298

Switzerland, 2

Symmetry of partnerships, 311–312

Synaptic pruning, 122

Syphilis, 240

Systems approach, 239–240, 327

Systems, as a critical tool, 265

Systems change, 241

T

Target populations, system focused on specific, 306

Targets, communities as, 243

Tariffs, 188, 189, 211, 215, 226

Task Force on Community Preventive Services, 153

Tax base, local, diminishment of, 236

Tax credits, 206, 225

Tax cuts, 12, 13

Tax policy, in Canada, 205

Taxation: and deadweight loss, 217; inclusion of, in policy recommendations, 209; lowering, in developing countries, to compete for capital, 216; types and rates of, 188

Technical (production) efficiency, 29, 138, 218, 219, 220, 221, 222, 289

Technocratic (expert-dominated) approach, 260

Technology, medical: access to, 195; rapid diffusion of, and health care costs, 53

Technology sector, 312

Teenage pregnancies, 125, 134. *See also* Adolescence

Ten Point Coalition (Boston Community Policing), *267, 268,* 272–273, 275

Terrestrial ecosystem changes, examples of, and potential human health impacts, *82*

Territorial approaches, *208*

Texas: income inequality in, and mortality, 197; standardized test scores in, 150–151

Texas County Turning Point project, 272

Texas Model Public Health Practice Subcommittee, 307

Thatcher administration, 12, 205

Theoretical democracy, 254

Third Way, the, 13–14, 25

Third-factor hypothesis, 138–139

Time, effect of, recognition of, in the conceptual model, 42

Time frames, community development versus political, 279

Time preference, 138, 139

Time spent, 279

Timing: and context, 109, 131–132; and sequence, 111

Tobacco use: during adolescence, 125, 142; during pregnancy, 193; regulating, 270–272; and stress, 194, 195

Tobacco-related illness, international policies addressing, 212

Tokensim, 310

Trade agreements, 189

Trade barriers, 199, 209, 214, 215, 226

Trade benefits, balance of, improving, 8

Trade policies, 188–189, 199, 209, 226, 235

Trade protection, 215

Trading partners, global, increased strength of, 212

Trajectory, defined, 128

Transdisciplinary development, recommendations to assist, 276–279

Transdisciplinary research, 19, *20,* 293, 306, 320, 323

Transition periods, defining, 132

Transparency, enhancing, 218

Transportation policy, 218, 226

Trigger effects, chain of risk involving, 111

Trust: within and across partnerships, 312; associations built on, 242; building, 256; establishing, 249, 254, 255, 279; gaining, 259; local polices to support, *245;* as a measure of social capital, 254; producing, 248; and social bonds, 244; social capital subsuming, 135

Tuberculosis (TB), 202, 211, 212

Turning Point, *267, 268,* 271–272, 299, 309–310, 318, 332

Turnover, defined, 95

Two-way dialogue, benefit of, 250

Type 2 diabetes, 129, 193

U

UCLA Center for Healthier Children, Families and Communities, 179

Unemployment, 193

Unemployment benefits, 225

Unhealthy lifestyles: mortality related to, 125; transmission of, 127

Uninsured population, 53, 262

Uninsured women, policy aimed at health care for, 274–275

Unintended market outcomes, 67, 79, 83. *See also* Ecological determinants

United Kingdom/Great Britain: broader population health–centered policies in, 297, *298;* concurrent policy development in, 207; and cumulative effects, 130; current population health policies in, 55–56; economic policies in, 205–206, 209; health policy agenda of, 2, 52; income per capita growth in, historical increase in, 202; influence of physical environment in, 48; innovative research in, 37; labor market policies in, 225; and latent effects, 129–130; mortality across job classifications in, study of, 128, *129,* 136, 143, 192; political and economic philosophy of, 12–13, 13–14. *See also* England; Scotland

United Nations, 116

United Nations Children's Fund International Child Development Centre, 179

United Nations Conference on Environment and Development, 69

United Nations Development Programme (UNDP), 149, 179, 186, 233

United Nations Educational, Scientific, and Cultural Organization, 147, 179

United States: access to care in, 36, 53, 54; adult mortality in, 125; approach gaining attention in, 38; charting new directions in the, 9; child poverty in, 114, 130, 150; community development policies in, 269–271; community-based participatory research in, 256–259; compulsory education in, 122, 138; desirable child care model for, 147; dominant strategy for disease prevention in, 38; economic policies in, 209–210; education policies in, 144–146; educational approach in, 152; funding of education and child care in, issue of, 148, 149, 156–157, 235–236; general recommendations for, 223, 224; government expenditures in, levels of, 188; HDI ranking of, 150; health care costs in, 53–54, 261; health care spending by, 209; and the health impact assessment tool, 218; health orientation in, 52–53; health policies in, 53–55; health policy agenda of, 2, 295, 296, 303; improving education in, 140; income inequality and mortality in, 197, 198; infant mortality ranking of, 54, 258; innovative research in, 37; intersectoral collaboration in, lack of, 224; lack of emergent population health policy in, 2, 36, 53, 54, 143, 209–210, 296, 299; leading health indicators in, 118; life expectancy in, 54, 150; literacy rates in, 150; low birth weight in, 121; market-dominated health care system of, 261–262; measures of child health and development in, 117–118; medical care delivery system in, 25; and medical technology, 300; national child health and education goals in, 119; new health goals in, establishment of, following the Lalonde report, 36–37; persistence of racial and ethnic disparities in, 2, 192; philosophical orientation toward health and disease in, 52–53; policy potential of, due to vast resources, 113; political and economic philosophy of, 10, 12–13, 13–14, 18; population health research agenda in, 50–51; poverty rate in, 150; precautionary principle adopted in, 69; premature mortality in, and health literacy, 138; promotion of academic success in, 141; public health system in, 290–294; race-based segregation in, 23; regulatory agencies in, 98; school readiness in, 140; state and local population health policies in, 54–55,

298–299; steps to advance a population–health centered agenda in, 300; trade polices of, 215; unique history of, 50; vulnerable children in, 122
U.S. Census Bureau, 53, 64, 150, 153, 179, 192, 233
U.S. Department of Defense (DoD), 145–146
U.S. Department of Education (USDE), 113, 119, 150, 153, 179, 180
U.S. Department of Health and Human Services (USDHHS), 18, 113, 115, 117, 118, 121, 123, 138, 141, 144, 145, 156, 180, 239, 240, 241, 242, 256, 283, 284, 290, 291, 295, 296, 332
U.S. Department of Health Education and Welfare, 296, 332
U.S. Department of Justice, 141, 180
U.S. Environmental Protection Agency, 47, 64, 69
U.S. Health care system, restructure of the, attempt at, 18
U.S. Institute of Medicine. *See* Institute of Medicine
U.S. Surgeon General, 36–37, 223
Units of analysis, 5
Universal access to education, 156
Universal child care, 146, 156
Universal health care: lack of, 53, 193, 194–195; recommending, 226
Universal health care financing, prospect of, 18
Universal health care system, maintaining, 55
Universal primary school, 226
University of California at Los Angeles (UCLA), 113, 179
Upstream category, 53, 301
Urban areas, impact of market models on, 262
Urban development, 190
Urban economies, impact of globalization on, in the U.S., 235
Urban environments, and social capital, 246
Utility, defined, 218
Utility function, 219

V

Veterans Administration, 223
Violence, 142, 254, 272–273
Vision: new and expanded, 327; for reinventing public health, 3, 31; shared, 241, 249, 319
Vision and mission: blueprint of, *308*; example of, 309–310; population health–centered, focused on, *321*; for public health, 290
Vocational development, role for, 124
Vocational training, 226
Vulnerability: general, 196; periods of, 132

W

W. K. Kellogg foundation, 271, 299
Washington, DC, infant mortality rate, 240
Water, clean, 194, 212
Wealth, 4, 36, 66–67. *See also* Income
Web-of-causation interpretation, 37
Welfare economics framework, 218, 219, 289
Welfare programs: participation in, and education, 141; spending on, 188
Welfare reform, 154, 210
Welfare Reform Act, 269
Welfare spending, 12, 13, 18, 188
White Americans, mortality and poverty rates for, 192
Whitehall studies, 55, 136, 143, 192
Women: additional stress facing, 143; providing microcredit to, in developing nations, 214, 222
Work ability, 193
Work environment: approaches for addressing, *208*; as a contributing factor, 108; education influencing, 136, 142; evidence for the impact of the, on health, 142–143; policies aimed at the, 209, 225
Workforce, leaving the, 126

Working conditions. *See* Work environment
Working Group on Health Disparities, 113
Working population: health insurance for, 53, 146, 262; health promotion and disease prevention for, 263
Workplace hierarchy, and mortality, 128, *129*, 136, 143, 192. *See also* Occupation; Socioeconomic position (SEP)
World Bank, 16, 189, 213–214, 222–223, 225
World Bank Group, 199, 213, 214, 222, 233

World Commission on Environment and Development, 87–88, 100
World Health Organization (WHO), 9, 19, 26, 34, 42, 64, 113, 182, 190, 199, 201, 202, 203, 206, 214, 215, 216, 225, 233, 234, 295, 300, 322, 332; broader population health policies of, 296–297; and economic development, 209, 210–212
World poverty, increase in, 199
World Trade Organization (WTO), 16, 189, 214–216

World War II, period following, 189, 235
Wyandotte County Community Health Partners, 274

Y

Young adulthood: development during, 126; transition from adolescence to, 125–126
Youth Risk Behavior Surveillance Survey, 118, 134
Youth-development interventions, 134
Youths. *See* Adolescence; Childhood